THE BODY HEALS

William B. Ferril, M.D.

The Bridge Medical Publishers
Whitefish, Montana

DedicatedTo

Conner, Hayes, and Billy

The Body Heals

Copyright © 2003 by William Ferril

Published by The Bridge Medical Publishing
200½ Wisconsin Ave. Whitefish, MT 59937

Manufactured in the United States of America

Book design by William B. Ferril 1956-

ISBN   0-9725825-0-9

Contents

Author's Note
Acknowledgements
Introduction

IV – The Body Heals

ACKNOWLEDGEMENTS

Mary Stranahan, D.O., who from the beginning of my practicing career challenged me to think about healing and set an example for the importance of seeing each individuals beauty and their personal story.

My wife, Brenda Ferril D.C., who exposed me to the inconsistencies of my educational paradigm and took time to illustrate this book.

Steven Gordon, N.D. for his gentle insights into industrial shortcomings in the treatment of diabetes. I am also thankful for his ability to listen and help me organize 'raw' insights as I labored through the basic medical texts.

Don Beans, Acupuncturist and Homeopath, for his educational expertise that heals disease through a totally different viewpoint.

Stephen Smallsalmon for taking the time to teach me to pray for myself. I am also thankful for his instruction in regard to the futility of indulging in the seductive negative emotions.

Patrick Montgomery, D.C., who read the earlier versions of this text.

Rick Nagle, Esq. who patiently evaluated the text.

Ginny Wilcox,, who possesses the unique ability to be a perfectionist and a workhorse all the time.

Mariko Crumley, who is the mirror of my youth.
Patty Perigo, who is a computer genius, a real miracle worker.

Jim Manley, Esq. for his belief in me to undertake the challenge of writing a book about how one heals.

Leslie Walker, PhD for providing me with a living example of how to live fully through the years.

Barbara deVeer, RN who read and evaluated the earlier versions of this text.

Jaunita Smallsalmon, who I am grateful for her efforts in exposing me to alternative healing ideas and people that understood them.

Karen Ebel, my mother-in-law who read this material.

My parents, for their encouragement.

Disclaimer

This book is intended as an educational tool to acquaint the reader with alternative methods of preventing and treating chronic degenerative disease. Bridge Medical Publishers hopes this book will enable you to improve your wellbeing and to better understand, assess, and choose the appropriate course of treatment. Because some of the methods described in this book are alternative in nature, by definition, some of them have not been investigated and/or approved by any government or regulatory agency.

The seven principles of longevity, contained in *The Body Heals*, are not intended as a substitute for the advice and/or medical care of the reader's physician. Nor are the contents within this book meant to discourage or dissuade the reader from the advice of his or her physicians. The contents within this book are for informational purposes only and are not intended to diagnose or treat illness. The diagnosis and treatment of illness requires a specific exam, tests, history, and an appreciation for each individual's uniqueness of presentation. For these, the reader is advised to seek the counsel of a nutritionally competent and holistic physician.

It is also imperative to understand that individuals who desire weight loss, improved health or healing from chronic disease need close follow up and supervision from their personal physician.

If the reader has any questions concerning the information presented in this book, or its application to his/her particular medical profile, or if the reader has unusual medical or nutritional needs or constraints that conflict with the advice in this book, he or she should consult his or her physician before embarking on the advice contained in this book. If the reader is pregnant or nursing she should consult her physician before embarking on the nutrition and other lifestyle programs contained in the book. The reader should not stop prescription medications without the advice and guidance of his or her personal physician.

The gray areas throughout the book are the personal opinion of the author. They are highlighted so as to not confuse or cause misunderstandings. The rest of this publication contains the medical opinion and ideas of the author supported by scientific evidence.

Dear Reader,

Several memorable events were the inspiration for writing this book. First, many patients had documented benefit from adhering to contrary 'fringe' advice. These cases led to a growing curiosity about exploring the growing list of inconsistencies. These inconsistencies should not happen if one adheres to the official view of the medical universe. Back then it was beyond my education level to explain why a diet high in cholesterol and fat, but low in carbohydrate leads to a drop in harmful cholesterol parameters. Years later I have come to understand how the different hormones, that these diets promote, leads to improved cholesterol profile. The science is all there, but it largely is presented in a convoluted and fragmented manner. The reorganization of these scientific facts is presented throughout the manual.

An additional inconsistency occurred regarding obesity. I could never figure out why no one was organizing the hormones causing obesity as they relate to one another. The science was present, but like cholesterol knowledge it was fragmented and disorganized in its presentation in the medical texts. The obesity chapter provides what science knows about gaining and losing fat.

Another learning opportunity started about ten years ago and occurred shortly after I married a pretty chiropractor named Brenda. Humility describes the feeling about my MD degree as my knowledge base was forced into the captive position. I watched with humility what a competent chiropractor accomplished with two hands following a multitude of musculoskeletal complaints. My world was rocked on its medical underpinnings. Thinking outside the box was the next logical step.

Later, I had the opportunity to work alongside naturopaths, other chiropractors, acupuncturists, and homeopaths. Each of their various educational perspectives provided me with additional inconsistencies for the toxic symptom control paradigm that I had been groomed into believing.

Over the last several years I have had time to think about what is actually known about the aging process. Early on I could only come with five reasons for cellular deterioration. In the second year, it became clear that there was evidence for a total of seven mechanisms for how the body ages.

The Seven Paths to an Old Body
1. Poor informational substance content
2. Rusting processes
3. Hardening processes
4. Low voltage cell syndrome
5. Deficient and/or excessive molecular building parts
6. Failure to take out the cellular trash water
7. A preponderance of energies that maim compared to the energies that heal

VIII– The Body Heals

This manual is about helping the reader understand ways to combat these processes. There is a lot of bad information circulating around. Sometimes bad information continues to circulate because the good information negates the need for help from the medical industrial complex.

Without good information, owners will always be vulnerable to the clever advertising schemes of the medical industrial complex. These informational sound bites are dispersed through various media outlets and are usually the most profitable ways of treating an owner's disease. Many of these popular approaches are based in a symptom control paradigm. Symptom control has little to do with how one heals and always has side effects. Many conventionally trained physicians haven't a clue (neither did I) that their complex funded educations left out many unifying and holistic scientific principles. Owners need to acquire a basic understanding of what is really known about the less profitable ways of treating the common diseases that begin around middle age. Accurate information about how one heals will lower gullibility. This is secondary to living in a profit driven health care system.

I have found that most owners will make life style changes if they understand that it leads to healing. Learning is somewhat painful and depleting. This book is not for the weak minded and lazy types. This manual was written for those owners who possess enough motivation to stay focused on the goal of becoming less gullible regarding their health care choices. The reward for such commitment comes in the form of personal empowerment that is evidenced by acquiring the basics on how to prevent the seven processes from manifesting in our lives.

As the reader endeavors to learn each chapter, awareness will come that the profit driven approaches of mainstream medicine are about symptom control with a price. The price paid to the owner's body is evidenced by side effects and toxicities. Common examples of diseases treated today in the symptom control paradigm instead of the healing paradigm include heart disease, high blood pressure, diabetes, arthritis, asthma, obesity, and menopausal related disease.

Symptom control medicine has nothing to do with healing. True healing can only begin to occur when cause and effect are included in the decision making process. The seven processes are usually involved in this understanding. Science exists to understand and impact these seven processes. Often there is little incentive to publish or advertise this knowledge only because it is less profitable.

Combating these seven processes is fundamental to achieving lasting health. This manual facilitates the reader on ways to begin accessing and applying seven correcting principles that the holism of science revealed long ago.

It is also important to not get overly frustrated when a concept is not clear. Chances are it will be explained later in a way the reader can understand.

At the end of this manual there is a chapter for putting the entire proceeding chapters into practice beginning with a more complete inquiry as to where an owner stands regarding the seven processes in the context of the physical exam. By the time the reader makes it to this section of the manual these principle will make more sense.

William B. Ferril, M.D.
October 2002
Whitefish, Montana

INTRODUCTION

The Seven Operating Aging Principles in a Workable Perspective

1. **Each cell in the body contains a computer program, power plants, and it's own specialized factories**

It helps to view the many different body cells in this way to avoid getting lost in the many complex details involved in living systems. Keeping this mental picture in mind facilitates the understanding that the cell computer program is the DNA. Just like in a computer program, there needs to be instructions given as to which programs is activated and which programs to leave alone. The body's informational substances are the hormones and neurotransmitters. The quality of these reaching a cell determines how wisely the cell is directed in using its available energy. The health of a cell can be thought of as occurring on the continuum of wise all the way down to foolish use of energy.

Which DNA programs are activated determines how functional the power plants are and how much a cell factory produces in the manufacture of their preferred products. This is true for all body cell types whether they are heart cells, brain cells, muscle cells or others. Their computer program (DNA) activation depends on the directions that a cell receives. Healthy owners predictably have high quality informational substances directing their cells in the wise use of available cellular energy. Conversely, unhealthy owners predictably have poor quality informational directions reaching their cells with a resultant diminished wisdom on expenditure of energy.

Many disease processes begin because of this decrease in the quality of the informational substances reaching a cell. This begins to make mechanistic sense when one realizes that their cells are dependent on quality instructions directing the numerous computer programs (DNA) or health consequences follow.

The other side of the story of what science has revealed helps owners to improve the quality of the information directing their cellular activity. In other words, implementation of this knowledge moves owner's cells in the direction of the wise use of available energy. Examples of diseases that often have origins in poor quality hormones are heart disease, high blood pressure, diabetes, arthritis, asthma, obesity, and menopause.

After the completion of section 2 the reader will understand how the typical conventional medicine physical exam and laboratory inquiry are deficient in this regard. In addition, there will be methods explained for recreating real hormones that are more reflective of the youthful state.

Including the best scientific assessment of an owner's hormone report card is important for starting on a path toward healing. In many cases these straightforward ways create better hormonal information directing cells. Better information leads to rejuvenation and optimal performance in the challenges of having an earthling experience.

Rusting and Hardening Processes

The blood vessel chapter explains the importance of preventing the pipes (blood vessels) of the body from starting or continuing the rusting and hardening processes. Blood vessel 'rust' is commonly called oxidation. Oxidation diminishes the ability of the pipes to deliver nutrients and remove waste. Hardening processes lead to other wear and tear in the living pipes. Stiffened living pipes tend to rupture and these events result in the leakage of body fluids into the surrounding space. One cannot have cells that function optimally without pipes that deliver and remove the molecules at the optimal level. The first section concerns preventing the rusting and hardening processes from gaining a hold in the body.

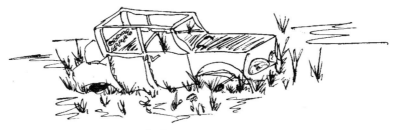

Cellular Force Field

Each cell needs to generate a surrounding force field to protect it from outside unwanted molecules. In the case of a faltering force field, the outside hostile ions will damage the delicate cellular structures and work areas.

This cellular force field is used to perform cellular work much like a car battery allows for the workings of electrical options in a car. Every cell must constantly be recharging the cellular force field. The power plants (mitochondria) in the cell constantly burn up combustible fuel to provide for energy for the force field maintenance.

Similar to brand new car batteries, cells with maximally performing force fields are able to perform optimal amounts of work. There are many owners who suffer from a low cell voltage problem. The fifth section explains the problem and how to heal.

XII – The Body Heals

Molecular Building Parts

One of the cornerstones to health is ensuring that there is a continuous and adequate supply of quality molecular building supplies reaching the different cells. These molecular building parts wear out and become damaged at varying rates. It is important to understand that an owner can't manufacture the correct informational substances if the molecular parts are not available. The nutrition of a cell is only as good as the weakest link in the supply lines because all manufacture stops there. This is much like the assembly line at an auto manufacturing plant where one missing part stops the building process. Old cellular machinery (enzymes) result when there becomes a deficiency in the delivery system and unavailability of molecular parts. They begin to have worn down power plant structures. Inefficient power plants result in a diminished ability to generate energy. With less energy available for work, the cellular force fields begin to falter and damaging substances penetrate the cells. The cellular factories become weak and consequently have a decreased ability to produce their particular cell product. The digestion and immune system chapters help explain ways to optimize the supply of molecular building parts.

Cellular Trash Water

Living cells generate huge amounts of waste every day. Western medicine often fails to counsel owners effectively on ways to take out the trash water. Accumulating trash water leads the body down another path that hastens the old body manifestation.

Body detoxification systems occur in the colon, immune system, kidneys, liver, skin, and lungs. When the reader completes these sections they will begin to hear their cells screaming to take out the garbage. At this point the owner will be qualified to do it.

Energy that Heals and Energy That Maims

This is probably the hardest aging mechanism for the western owner to comprehend. The owner may be well into the book before the powerful forces of rhythmical energy versus chaotic energy become a tangible concept. Without an attempt to bridge this defect in western thinking energies contribution to health versus disease is diminished.

SECTION I

PREVENT RUST AND MAINTAIN FLEXIBILITY

The Principles

All bodies die. Some bodies are on an accelerated path to premature death. This book describes a medical strategy that includes seven steps for creating longevity. The ideas in this book are scientifically sound and are supported by generally accepted medical literature. These ideas do not receive attention because of the nature of the medical industry that is a profit driven business.

The medical industry exchanges health care services for money. The income from patients must exceed the cost of health care services. These business facts require medical practices and treatments that generate this income. These medical practices are the standard of practice taught in medical schools and are applied by the doctors. Consequently, they become the legal standards of medical practice. Research focuses on effective treatments that will return the research cost and provide profit for the investors. Marketing campaigns create a demand for profitable medical procedures and services. In this way the media and 'science' have mutual interests.

Effective treatments that fail to provide a "reasonable" return on investment are marginalized and not advertised. They are not taught. Effective, but unprofitable medical procedures and treatments are ignored because they do not provide the appropriate inducements in a profit driven system.

This book is written for the owners who will use effective and inexpensive medical practices and procedures.   These owners desire to implement medical practices that do not contain the destructive side effects of mainstream medical practices. Side effects occur because the mainstream is largely founded on a symptom control paradigm. Symptom control always has side effects and has little to do with how one heals.

Some owners are willing to do what is necessary for healing to occur. Healing involves understanding how certain diseases occur. There are seven ways that cells function at the optimum level. Failure to identify which ones are operating inefficiently leads to disease, aging, and the need for symptom control measures.   Symptom control includes prescription medications, medical procedures, and surgery. This text is written to facilitate owners who are willing to engage in their health and healing and renounce the convenience of mainstream medical practice.

GROUND RULES

This book is organized according to seven health and healing strategies referred to as principles. Each principle is discussed, developed, and addressed in a separate section. In the first six sections the organ systems that best facilitate an understanding of a principle are grouped together. In addition, that organ system and its relationship to the other principles are discussed. The body story told in this way facilitates owner empowerment that involves learning about the often-omitted principles. These omissions prevent healing from the common deteriorations operating in the middle age body.

The middle-aged body wants to heal. The first two principles, rust prevention and flexibility preservation within the blood vessels, have a strong relationship and are the subject of the first section. The third principle explains how one satisfies the body requirement for high quality hormones. The fourth is about obtaining high quality molecular replacement parts. The fifth principle concerns the removal of the body's trash water by six different organ systems. The sixth principle explains the importance of the quality of the cellular electrical charge. The seventh principle explains the energies that heal contrasted to the energies that maim the cells of the body.

Chapter One

Health of the Blood Vessels

Each human body contains 180,000 miles of waterways that transport liquids, solids, gases, charged particles, and waste products. The waterways that flow away from the heart (arteries) carry fresh supplies of oxygen, nutrients, and recently recruited immune system cells to the tissues. The waterways that travel towards the heart (veins and lymphatics) carry waste, solids, gases, and spent immune system cells from the tissues toward exits.

The quality and integrity of the inside inner surface of these waterways creates a powerful determinant for youth versus aging. The importance of this inner surface arises from the fact that these waterways provide the interface for exchange between the blood stream and all cell types. Healthy bodies have quality surfaces lining their 180,000 miles of waterways. Many unhealthy owners have a problem with the integrity of their inner waterway surface at the root of their disease.

Nutrients, waste, solids, charged particles, and gases are selectively absorbed and eliminated through the inner-lining layer of the blood vessels. This layer distributes nutrients according to the specific nutritional needs of the tissues. An important determinant of longevity is the quality of this lining.

PRINCIPLES 1 and 2: PREVENTION OF RUST AND HARDENING

The first two principles of health are related to the maintenance of the blood vessels. When these principles are ignored the body will age. Most owners possess a visual idea of how rust corrodes when oxygen or some other molecule reacts with a surface. The inside of the blood vessels surfaces are constantly under threat of assault. Processes that increase this assault accelerate the rust formation cycle and require repair. Corroded blood vessel surfaces have either or both an accelerated corrosion rate or/and deficient repair rate. Cholesterol and fat debris collect where the surfaces have been damaged.

Loss of flexibility usually begins in the muscular layer of the vessel. Arteries have the thickest muscular layer and the highest-pressure forces. Processes that increase the muscle layer thickness increase the stiffness that makes them more vulnerable to damage.

The presence of rust and diminished flexibility in the blood vessels diminishes the function of those vessels. Accumulation of rust is a process that occurs in the blood vessels, accelerates the aging process, and diminishes health. Prevention or reversal of these two processes involves several steps.

Aging does not cause the processes of rust and hardening. Rust and hardening processes cause aging. When the rusting and hardening occur in the blood vessels they clog with debris and they perform inefficiently. Medicine describes these concepts as arteriosclerosis (hardening) and atherosclerosis (rust).

A common example of how rust begins will follow. After this the overall scheme between rust and hardening will be outlined. Next will be a discussion on how certain processes become opportunist and accelerate the rust and hardening damage. At the end of these introductory considerations will be a discussion of each risk factor for the development of both rust and hardening. Finally, the opportunistic mechanism will be explored in more detail.

Cells Lining the Water Ways Before Before Rust Damage

The cells that line the waterways appear as elaborate, shiny, flexible tiles. Each tile is glued together with the body's cement by being intricately woven together on the inside of the tubular waterways. Each cell (tiles) possesses a precise, detailed surface that interfaces with the turbulent bloodstream. On the tissue side of the cell (the side opposite of the bloodstream), the cell structure of the blood vessel structure depends on the body part the blood vessel serves. Each tissue type has a specific cell structure. The purpose of a particular cell dictates structure. The structures of the blood vessel cells must be compatible with the cell structure of the tissue that the vessel serves.

Processes that harm the integrity or health of these waterway-lining cells interferes with the transfer into or out of the bloodstream. Damage to blood vessels results from the initial processes of rusting and hardening. The consequence of diminished transfer of hormones, nutritional substances, gases, etc., results in damage to health.

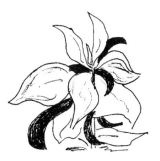

The Basics of Rust

The initial presence of 'rust' in the waterway lining cells creates a 'Velcro' for debris to stick to. Underlying the shinny surface, each tile has an intricate surface made up of numerous types of molecular receiving stations, or receptors. These receptors detect specific molecules moving through the bloodstream. The molecules are designed to initiate the process of transferring the molecular matter from the bloodstream to the tissue cells. The process of rust development tends to damage these precise surfaces. The presence of rust in the vessels diminishes the exchange between the blood stream and the cells. Rust accumulation diminishes the quantity of nutrients transferred to the tissue cells. When the vessels are extremely clogged, tissue cells die.

Rust also damages the blood stream-dependent communication system by damaging the receptors.   Hormones, like insulin, are informational substances that communicate specific messages to the cells. Many hormones can only be detected by a specific receptor in the blood vessel cells. Each cell has a specific type of receptor that depends on the type of tissue cell being served by a blood vessel. Rust clogs these receptors. When the clogging process occurs the tissue cell needing insulin hormone may not be able to receive the message and fail to perform.

Risk Factors for the Development of Rust

The risk factors for the production of rust are; cigarette smoking, male gender, diabetes, high homocysteine level, deficiency of the anti-inflammatory essential fatty acids, obesity, excessive consumption of oxidized fats, nutrition deficiencies, and excessive exposure to oxidizing agents. The presence of abnormal hormone levels is being considered as a factor in developing rust. Increased blood pressure caused by hardening of the vessels increases the rate of rust formation.

The cells lining the blood vessels are under assault from varying amounts of risk factors. Each of these risk factors contributes to the development of rust or increases the probability that rust will occur. Owners must be aware that these factors act on their blood vessels every moment and are affected by choices made during the day.

Anti-oxidants are Rust Retardants

Anti-oxidants can be better understood if one substitutes the word 'oxidation' for 'rust'. Rust is everywhere. Tissue oxidation is rust occurring in the body. When rust forms, a rough, Velcro-like cell surface remains on the waterway lining cells where debris collects. The accumulation of debris begins the clogging process.

Rust is formed by oxidation. Oxygen consumption is necessary to burn fuel aerobically (from processed carbohydrates, fat and protein). Burning fuel creates the energy used for chemical reactions. The combustion of fuel is an oxidation process. Oxygen combustion reactions share many similarities with those of a nuclear power plant. Reactor damage that occurs as a result of the intended reaction has the potential to spill damage outside of the designated confinement area.

Cellular Power Plant Locaations

Oxygen consumption occurs in the mitochondria of the cells, which is equivalent to the cell's nuclear power plant facility. If too much oxygen combustion occurs outside of these 'armored' powerhouses (within the cells) the equivalent of 'nuclear meltdown' occurs.

Oxygen molecules contain two oxygen atoms linked together in a high-energy bond. The paired oxygen formation is the only safe form of pure oxygen outside the mitochondria. Oxygen in this form is found in a clean atmosphere. Air pollution leads to an increase in the unstable, chemically reactive forms of oxygen. All the other forms of oxygen oxidize (rust) body tissues. The mitochondria have the ability to withstand oxygen cleavage explosions (breaking the high-energy bond between the two oxygen atoms). These oxygen combustion reactions allow the breakdown of cellular fuels (food groups) forming energy packets (ATP), heat, water, and the chemically stable gas carbon dioxide.

When the unstable forms of oxygen occur in the cell, these forms need to be minimized to deter oxidation. In healthy states, these oxygen cleavage explosions take place in the 'armor' of the mitochondria. Very small amounts of unstable oxygen leak out of the mitochondria. This property of the mitochondria is like a controlled 'nuclear facility' containment area.

Living in clean air and practicing appropriate nutritional discretion moderates the unstable oxygen that the body is exposed to. A team, comprised of two enzymes, superoxide dismutase and catalase, have the ability to react with the destructive forms of oxygen and render them harmless, stable molecules. There is a limit to their effectiveness. Environmental and dietary sources of unstable oxygen can overwhelm the cell leading to molecular oxidation damage.

Owners who are aware of the destructive effects of unstable oxygen possess a powerful tool against aging by avoiding environmental and nutritional conditions that jeopardize them. It is not difficult for an owner to decrease their exposure to unstable oxygen. Curtail oxygen-free radical exposure by choosing healthy types of nutriceuticals will help. Some nutriceutical companies sell mineral supplements made from salts of oxygen. These salts in general are not very soluble in water so they pass like undigested gravel out of the body. A small portion of these salts dissolves and releases an oxygen atom with a negative charge. This is one of the unstable forms of oxygen. By unpaired oxygen's nature, it can't wait to react with body tissue to create rust. The owner should avoid mineral supplements that contain these reactive oxygen atoms because they defeat the purpose of taking the anti-oxidants. Manufactures denote oxygen salt content with the term, oxide that occurs at the end of the product name. Common examples are calcium oxide, magnesium oxide, and ferrous oxide

Unstable oxygen is just one example of how rust formation begins in the body. With this thought there are other risk factors, which are interrelated in their blood vessel injuring mechanisms and they should be introduced.

Two Mechanisms That Injure Blood Vessels

Two other overall mechanisms injure blood vessels - stiffness and "sticky" (cholesterol). Stiffness is caused by many factors, but high blood pressure is the most conspicuous and highly treatable mechanism. There are also many ways to develop high blood pressure, but the owner controls most of the causes. Stiffness caused by high blood pressure contributes to aging. Prevention of this process is the second principle of longevity.

Sticky (cholesterol), created in the liver, is another mechanism that damages the blood vessels. Sticky accumulates in the blood vessels as an opportunistic mechanism when rust or decreased flexibility is present.

All three blood vessel injury mechanisms can be summarized as follows:

Rust Producing Mechanisms:

> Homocysteine (chapter three)
> Diabetes (liver chapter)
> Nutritional deficiencies (sections three and five)
> Essential fatty acid deficiencies (section three)
> Cigarette smoking
> Oxidant load (section three and six)
> Quality of fat intake (section three)
> Male gender
> Obesity (section two)
> Diminished hormone quality (section two)

Blood Vessel Stiffness Mechanism

High blood pressure states from multiple causes (chapter three)

Opportunist Mechanism Requires the Presence of Rust

Hormonal imbalance promotes the liver to manufacture sticky fats, high LDL cholesterol, high triglycerides, and a deficiency of HDL cholesterol (hormones and digestion sections).[1]

The opportunist mechanism contributes to blood vessel disease when either or both of the rust forming and hardness mechanisms also operate in an owner's life. The media stresses this mechanism. Most of the time, rust and hardening must be present before cholesterol begins the clogging process. This is evidenced by the fact that only fifty percent of all heart attack victims have elevated cholesterol levels. The rust and hardening processes need more attention if one is to lower the risk for blood vessel disease.

Blood Vessel Clogging and Cholesterol

Many physicians witness heart disease in patients with a relatively low cholesterol level. In at least fifty percent of heart disease cases there are some other factors that lead to blockage in the coronary arteries. The mechanism of rust operates in the majority of heart disease victims. Therefore, these mechanisms need a more complete consideration. These unidentified subgroups are at increased risk for developing diseased blood vessels despite normal cholesterol. The true mechanisms are important because these owners often possess a significant proportion of chemically reactive cholesterol and/or nutritional deficiencies.

Science has revealed safe and effective ways to avoid these processes. However, the ways one heals is knowledge that lacks profit potential so it is largely ignored. This knowledge will be gradually added back into the discussion and a rationale for treatment options will become possible.

Chemically Reactive Cholesterol and Rust

Cholesterol causes problems in the blood stream in three ways:

1. There are several different types of cholesterol-fat-protein particles. Each type is created for different purposes and possesses unique properties.

2. Cholesterol caused problems occur with excess gross volume of cholesterol in the blood vessels.

3. Cholesterol caused problem is contained in the amount of chemically reactive cholesterol in an owner's blood stream.

Cholesterol-fat Particle Chemical Reactivity

The types of fat making the cholesterol-fat particle determine the chemical reactivity. This reactivity quantifies the potential of certain types of cholesterol particles to attach to the inside of the arteries. Whenever cholesterol-fat-protein complexes attach to the inside of an artery the process to plug has begun. The previous step is the creation of a roughened area (rust or Velcro) for the sticky cholesterol to adhere to.

Rust produced on the cholesterol-fat particles circulating in the blood vessels creates a Velcro-like surface where the surface was shiny. These factors increase the clogging process.

The Body Needs a Specific Cholesterol Level

Every body has about one and a half pounds of cholesterol. It is an integral component of the cell membrane and makes up some of the package that holds the cell contents together. It serves as the building block from which all sex hormones, some salt and water regulatory hormones, and stress hormone are made. The balance between the hormones glucagon and insulin controls the amount of cholesterol manufactured in the liver. Processes that favor insulin will increase the liver manufacture rate of the bad cholesterol. Conversely, processes that increase glucagon lead to an improved cholesterol profile. High glucagon levels decrease the manufacture rate of cholesterol synthesis in the liver.

Types of Cholesterol-Fat-Protein Particles

Cholesterol is made in the liver and needed by all body cells. Cholesterol is transported by the blood stream from the liver to the cells. It cannot circulate alone because it is not water-soluble. Therefore, it circulates in the blood steam with water-soluble proteins. If the particle created by the liver has a higher protein percentage than the associated cholesterol, it is a high-density lipoprotein (HDL) or good cholesterol. Moderate alcohol consumption, regular aerobic exercise, female gender, low carbohydrate diet, adequate glucagon level, and taking cholesterol lowering drugs are common factors that raise HDL levels.

When cholesterol content rises on other transport proteins in the bloodstream, it is known as LDL and VLDL, or bad cholesterol. Sedentary lifestyle, male gender, high carbohydrate diet, high fasting insulin levels, low fasting glucagon levels, diabetes, low thyroid function and genetically bad luck are factors that raise this level.

Three Ways Cholesterol-Fat-Protein Particle Variables Can Harm the Blood Vessel

Friendly blood vessel fats include olive oil, salmon oil, and borage oil. Eating predominantly blood vessel protective fat helps keep cholesterol-fat-protein particles from oxidizing (rusting) regardless of the type. Conversely, if the LDL and HDL particles are derived from a fast food diet, the stage is set for blood vessel injury even though the cholesterol numbers look good. The worst oils are vegetable oils that are chemically altered by hydrogenation. Lastly, the worst scenario is when both of these harmful processes occur together. The cholesterol numbers look bad and the wrong types of fat make up the cholesterol and fat particles.

Cholesterol Particles made by the Liver are a Danger

The liver is a faithful servant to the directions it receives. Lifestyles that promote message content directed at the liver to make cholesterol and fat are a blood vessel risk factor. Conversely, some lifestyles promote message content directed at the liver promotes blood vessel health.

When the liver is directed to make sugar (carbohydrate) into excess fat and cholesterol, there is a potentially dangerous situation. The types of cholesterol-fat-protein complexes created by the liver differ drastically in their ability to be cleared from the blood stream by metabolically hungry cells. In contrast diet derived fat enters the blood stream packaged in a way that is readily accessible to the metabolically hungry cells. Liver manufactured fat and cholesterol is designed instead for the preferential absorption by abdominal fat cells (a much slower process). When certain conditions exist these liver made packages adhere to the injured areas of the blood vessels, inside the macrophages). In the genetically predisposed owner, these complexes tend to build up in the blood vessels within the macrophages at higher levels than are acceptable for the lining cells health. There is a difference between diet derived cholesterol-fat complexes and liver synthesized cholesterol-fat complexes.

Now that all three mechanisms of blood vessel injury have been introduced, it is time to develop how they become risk factors within their groups.

The three groups of risk factors are:
1. Rust promoting processes
2. Hardening processes
3. Opportunistic processes (including the three ways cholesterol can be harmful).

The Individual Risk Factors of Rust Promotion

Homocysteine

Homocysteine is a recent example where the lonely thinker lived long enough to expose a mainstream medical inconsistency. This particular medical inconsistency involves rust and is the story of Dr. McCully. While he conducted research at Harvard University, in 1969, he noticed consistent similarities between the blood vessels of patients with high homocysteine levels and in those with blood vessels that were clogged from atherosclerosis. He postulated that elevated blood levels of homocysteine were a significant risk factor for the development of blood vessel lining cell disease. He was promptly dismissed for his preposterous theories.

Several years ago in Finland, a large double blind study confirmed, in thousands of Finish men, that elevated blood levels of homocysteine are a powerful marker for predicting the development of blood vessel clogging pathology. Today, thirty years after Dr. McCully first discovered this association, homocysteine blood levels are one of mainstream medicine's official risk factors for identifying those who are at increased risk for the development of blood vessel disease.

Hormonal Fatty Acids as Determinants of Blood Vessel Health

The fact that small amounts of aspirin lower the risk of heart attacks emphasizes the importance of hormonal fats in the blood vessels. Dr. Barry Sears, in his book, ***Entering the Zone***, points out that aspirin does not lower cholesterol, blood sugar, or blood pressure.[2] Yet it is a powerful inhibitor of the tendency for a cardiac event.

Every time an owner takes an aspirin, they alter hormonal fats. This alteration diminishes the clotting process and increases the flow of blood over a diseased segment of coronary arteries. The increased blood flow increases the delivery of the repair molecules to the diseased section of the arteries.

Essential fatty acids determine what types of hormonal fats are possible. When owners make poor dietary choices, they make poor precursors to the hormonal fats that provide an important component of the lining of the blood vessel walls and on platelets. The anti-inflammatory hormonal fats act as lubricants for efficient flow of blood. Consuming the wrong precursors to the hormonal fats produces a destructive type of hormonal fat. In this situation, the ability to keep blood from inappropriately clotting diminishes. Clotting occurs when the hormonal fat precursors are activated to full-blown hormones. These hormonal fats are only in the blood stream for a few seconds, but during their brief existence they determine the production of clotting or lubricating mechanism in the blood stream. Lubricating hormonal fats are deficient when owners consistently make poor dietary choices causing the production of poor quality hormonal fat precursors. The quality of the blood vessel lining can be improved by encouraging the production of the lubricating forces. Unfortunately, most are poisoning the good and bad hormonal fats production by taking aspirin. Aspirin poisons the clotting forces slightly more than the lubricating forces.

What isn't being said about an additional class of inflammatory hormonal fats (leukotrienes) that aspirin inhibits less creates a problem. Leukotrienes are produced in the immune system and their manufacture is encouraged when substances like aspirin prevent the usual drain off of prostaglandin production. Aspirin often increases allergies and asthma conditions. These same inflammatory hormonal fats lead to progressive joint aches and stiffness.

Aspirin, consumed regularly, diminishes the production of the wrong types of inflammatory prostaglandins in the blood vessels. Consuming aspirin also increases swelling of certain tissues including lung, sinuses, and joints.

The work of Barry Sears examines the natural processes that encourage the formation of good hormonal fat precursors. Dr Sears has had experience producing optimal hormonal fat precursors in a variety of body types. His work provides a broader understanding of the importance of the essential fatty acids. His years of work have shown that owners can consume the right essential fatty acids, but other dietary factors sabotage their efforts. These factors cause the wrong overseeing hormones to be secreted and prevent the desired benefit.

Some foods cause high insulin production such as high carbohydrate diets (sections 2 and 3). This first dietary factor must be addressed if the owner is going to benefit from the manufacture of the beneficial hormonal fat precursors.

Some unfortunate owners do everything right by decreasing their insulin, but nutritional deficiencies cause them to fail in their health goals. These deficiencies are easy to remedy. If the owner fails to remedy these nutritional deficiencies, they are doomed to the frustration of becoming fatter, having clogged arteries, and high blood pressure. All of these health issues are avoidable with some simple nutritional intervention and counseling.

Heart Disease Resulting from Nutritional Deficiency

Often times, blood vessel disease is the direct result of varying types of nutritional deficiency. Most blood vessels will heal when nutritional deficiencies are corrected. The deficiencies injure blood vessels through rust promotion, hardening processes, or opportunistic mechanisms. Usually all three mechanisms are set into motion by nutritional imbalance.

Increased Blood Fat from Nutritional Deficiency

It has been asserted in the popular media that niacin supplementation may lower blood cholesterol. A more accurate statement would be to say that niacin is one of five nutritional cofactors that need to be present for optimal blood fat to occur. When all five of the cofactors are present, the body can absorb blood fat and burn it in the cellular power plants. When fat is processed this way, it creates the energy packets that are needed for cellular function. This combustion process ends with the release of carbon dioxide and water.

When the other four cofactors are not present, many owners are condemned to failed attempts at natural healing. These owners often return to symptom control medicine (the complex). The necessity of these factors is well documented in the medical biochemistry textbooks, but the discussion occurs in a convoluted fashion. Knowledge of these fundamental 'must have' nutrients provides another way to heal. Pantothenic acid, carnitine, riboflavin, and Co enzyme Q10 are required for fat combustion in addition to niacin.

Without these factors, there is the tendency for blood fat to rise (LDL cholesterol) despite efforts to optimize insulin, cortisol, epinephrine, thyroid,

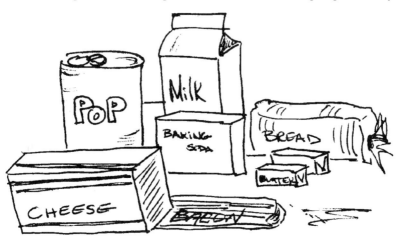

estrogen, IGF-1, and androgens (section 2). Owners who eat a low carbohydrate diet, exercise aerobically, and participate in stress reduction measures may not improve their health if one or more of the cofactors is absent. These motivated owners fail to achieve the desired blood fat and weight loss because no one has counseled them on these basic nutritional cornerstones.

Living in these nutritional 'traps' can be analogous to the creation of a smaller 'drain' for fat to exit once it has entered their blood stream. The drain is made larger when the cells have the nutritional mechanism to combust it. Optimal combustion of fat cannot occur without all of the cofactors. When fat is not combusted, it builds within a cell and eventually spills backward back into the blood stream. Increased fat is analogous to a drain that can no longer dispose of its contents. The contents of the blood stream are fat. The inclusion of these factors in the diet or in some cases receiving them intravenously will allow a 'bigger drain' to form. The drain in this analogy is the increased rate of fat removal made possible when the cells have the nutritional ability to process fat into carbon dioxide and water.

Owners who lack these five nutrients cannot properly access fat for the production of energy packets. This causes the cells to have power plant (mitochondria) problems because fat is the preferred fuel for many cel types.

Many owners do not receive sufficient amounts of these nutritional cofactors from their food. Multi vitamin pills may not solve this problem. When food is cooked and processed the five nutritional cofactors are destroyed. Absorption of nutrients is a critical factor in the health of an owner. Disease processes and medications affect what is absorbed and retained in the body. Empowerment comes from understanding why these factors play such a crucial role in the interrelationship between cellular power plants and extraction of energy.

Carnitine is made from the amino acid, lysine. Its synthesis also requires vitamin C, vitamin B6, and SAMe (S-adenosyl methionine). SAMe is critical to its manufacture and becomes rapidly depleted without adequate folate, vitamin B6, vitamin B12, serine and methionine, the methyl donor system (chapter three). For each carnitine manufactured, three SAMe molecules are used. Meat contains various levels of carnitine. Severe carnitine deficiency shows up as fatty liver disease and kidney hemorrhage and some forms of heart failure.

Carnitine is the carrier molecule that delivers fat to the cellular power plant furnace for combustion. The liver, kidney, and heart cells need tremendous amounts of energy to perform. The cells cannot use all of the potential energy contained in the fat molecules without transportation by carnitine. Endurance athletes supplement carnitine for increased performance.

Niacin (vitamin B3) is the second factor necessary to burn fat in the creation of energy packets. Two other cofactors, riboflavin (vitamin B2) and pantothenic acid (vitamin B5) need to be considered with niacin. These three cofactors must be present in optimal amounts just inside the outer furnace (mitochondria). When all three are present the combustion of fat traps energy packets (ATP). When any one of the three diminishes, there is progressive disability to trap energy. Heat is created instead of energy packets.

Pantothenic acid availability limits the rate of combustion of fat in the power plant. Fat can only be utilized when it is broken down two carbons at a time and attached to a pantothenic acid containing molecular machine, Co Enzyme A. This process cannot occur until carnitine has delivered fat to the outside compartment of the cell power plant. This acid is the essential ingredient for the manufacture of coenzyme A. Coenzyme A is the carrier molecule that allows the orderly combusting of fat energy, two carbons at a time. A deficiency in either carnitine or the cofactors disables the refining process to acetate. When fat is the raw material for fuel combustion, these cofactors are required or body fat will accumulate in the blood stream. Pantothenic acid deficiency leads to a marked slow down in burning fat calories.

The type of fuel that the mitochondria accept for combustion is restricted to one processed fuel type only. This is similar to power plants of the physical world. They can only combust one specific fuel type for operational purposes (natural gas, coal, radio active material, or fuel oil, etc). Whether raw fuel starts out as protein, fat or sugar, it needs to be processed into acetate before it can be combusted in the mitochondria. Acetate is the only fuel that the power plants can utilize aerobically. When acetate burns in the presence of oxygen, carbon dioxide gas and energy packets are created. The cell power plants only accept acetate for burning within the mitochondria.

Coenzyme Q10 (ubiquinone) is the last nutritional Cofactor. It is similar to niacin, riboflavin, and pantothenic acid, but Q10 allows for additional trapping of more energy (ATP) within the cell. Q10 is special in that it is made from the same enzymatic machinery as cholesterol. Without adequate Co enzyme Q10, the cells are compromised in their ability to generate energy packets and make more heat energy. This energy is waste. Without Co enzyme Q10 energy packet (ATP) formation diminishes.

Extreme energetic compromise occurs when the heart is without sufficient coenzyme Q10 because coenzyme Q10 constitutes a vital component, within mitochondrion. It is necessary to effectively trap energy within the power plant. This is a determinant of the performance of a cell. Lowered work ability leads to lower cardiac function. The heart has the highest needs of for coenzyme Q10. Huge amounts of energy packets are needed. Each heart cell has thousands of power plants (mitochondria) that need all five cofactors to maintain healthy cell function.

Popular cholesterol lowering drugs known as the statin class inhibit this crucial factors production. The presence of this factor is further compromised because coenzyme Q10 is unstable.

There is suspicion that people on these drugs tend to die at about the same rate as the untreated groups, but for different reasons. This is more alarming when adding in the suspected increase in cancer rates for owners who take these drugs.

The explanation could be from the fact that initially, cancer cells have a inferior ability to generate energy compared to healthy cells. When the body is healthy this is a major advantage within the immune system for destroying cancer cells at an early stage. Most immune systems continuously destroy cancer cells by generating high energy burst and targeting these packets at cancer cells. This exposes a link for why those taking statin drugs could be at increased risk for cancer. These drugs tend to deplete the body content of coenzyme Q10 and hence, cells like immune system cell types have diminished ability to out perform the cancer cell in energy generation.

This does not mean that statin drugs are never indicted for the prevention of heart disease. Many owners insist on taking a passive role in their disease process. For this group, their doctor has very few alternatives. Those owners willing to take responsibility for their health can use therapies without these side effects. These remedies can often times avoid statin drug usage and its potential side effects. The inclusion of high quality coenzyme Q10 would be a big help in the clinical situations where the statin drugs are needed. This need does not often occur in a motivated patient.

These factors need to be present nutritionally in order for fat to be utilized in the production of energy work packets. The utilization of sugar as fuel has other requirements.

Accessing Carbohydrate Energy for Cellular Needs

Carbohydrates can only be burned anaerobically (without oxygen) when any of five nutritional cofactors are deficient. This leads to massive increases in lactic acid production and fatigue. Fatigued cells have difficulty defending from rust and hardening processes. In the blood vessel lining cells this leads to an increase in Velcro formation.

When the five nutritional factors are deficient, the cell has no way of obtaining the necessary sugar fragment, acetate. This fragment can only be combusted in the presence oxygen.

In order to burn sugar (carbohydrate) to carbon dioxide and water, the cell needs five types of nutritional molecules in sufficient amounts plus adequate oxygen in the combustion chamber. Lipoic acid, riboflavin, niacin, pantothenic acid, and thiamine in the presence of adequate magnesium constitute these factors.

If the first part of sugar breakdown occurs without oxygen, a three-carbon fragment, pyruvate, is formed. Only when there is adequate oxygen and the five above factors can this molecule enter the power plant for further energy release. With a deficiency, pyruvate breaks down to lactic acid. The liver usually clears this acid from the blood stream, but when formation becomes excessive, it builds up in the muscles to prevent death.

The enzyme, pyruvic dehydrogenase and these five factors cut the head off (make a two carbon molecule, acetate) of pyruvate before it can form lactic acid and stabilize on the carrier molecule Co enzyme A (formed from pantothenic acid). The larger share of energy contained in a sugar molecule cannot be utilized unless all of the factors are present.There are many owners in pain and experiencing chronic fatigue only because their cells have a decreased ability to burn sugar energy in a healthy way. The smallest physical exertion condemns these owners to bed rest. Their tissues are full of lactic acid and this creates pain. These patients need to find a competent nutritionally oriented physician or they will continue to suffer. Not all chronic fatigue and muscle aches are from this cause, but a significant percentage is due to nutritional deficiency.

Amino acids can be used as fuel only after the liver converts them into sugar in a process called gluconeogenesis. All amino acids contain at least one nitrogen group (the amide). This group must be removed and eventually converted into urea in the liver for excretion by the kidneys. Adequate urea helps the kidneys concentrate their waste and conserve water. Cortisol, epinephrine, and glucagon hormones encourage gluconeogenesis. Epinephrine and glucagon have little effect without adequate cortisol. Insulin and growth hormone oppose gluconeogenesis. Amino acids are another source of raw fuel that needs refining to acetate before becoming combustible.

Male Gender – A Risk Factor

The risk factor of male gender is poorly understood. It was thought males lacked the protective effect that pre-menopausal females possess, secondary to their higher blood estrogen. Scientific data from postmenopausal females who took estrogen replacement therapy, fails to support this belief. Many physicians are beginning to be more cautious with estrogen replacement therapy because of estrogen's influence on increased cholesterol and triglycerides. Some physicians have reconsidered their prescription of estrogen therapy for supposed cardiac protection alone.[3]

There are many different types of estrogen that occur in nature each has unique bioactive properties. Some are strong stimulants that direct estrogen responsive tissues towards cell division. Too much message content from the various types of estrogen causes growth of uterine fibroids, breast cysts, breast cancer, increased body fat of the hips and thighs, increased insulin resistance, and interference with thyroid hormone activity. All available, patentable estrogen replacement prescriptions are not the right ratios or type of estrogen that the healthy female will produce.

Until further scientific research is available certain facts need to be considered. How the hormonal difference in pre-menopausal females confers the blood vessel protective needs to be clarified. There is good scientific evidence that the patentable prescription forms of estrogen increase the risk of developing heart disease. This may be due to the unnatural way that foreign estrogens stimulate the cholesterol and fat manufacturing machinery. When this is stimulated, the blood triglycerides increase (section two). Second, high estrogen also increases the risk of blood clots. Lastly, synthetic progesterone substitutes are not progesterone.

One type of progesterone is found in nature. This fact is important because many studies have used synthetic progesterone substitutes and later implicated real progesterone in the development of blood vessel disease. Progesterone has been unfairly implicated in the development of blood vessel disease. When examining the designs of these studies that purport a link to progesterone and heart disease, one discovers that the authors have confused synthetic progesterone substitute replacement therapies as equivalent to natural progesterone therapy.

Estrogen and progesterone types of hormones contain message content by virtue of their simple shape. In order to obtain a patent, synthetic hormones must contain an altered shape or mixture in an unnatural way. These alterations change the message content. Predictably, health consequences follow.

Smoking Facilitates Velcor Formation

Cigarette smoke injures the inner lining of the arteries. The damage is caused by several mechanisms. Cigarette smoke has high concentrations of carbon monoxide. Carbon monoxide binds to the red blood cell's oxygen binding sites about 200 times more tightly than the competitor, oxygen. Oxygen carrying ability in the average smoker is lowered by about 15%. Lower oxygen content is sensed and the bone marrow is stimulated to release more red blood cells. This raises the solid content of the blood to abnormal levels leading to an increased tendency for blood clots.

Second, carbon monoxide is an oxidizing agent. The presence of carbon monoxide causes rust in the inner lining cells of the waterways and lung tissue. In the lungs, oxidation of the numerous little balloons leads to rupture leading to emphysema. In the blood vessels, rust accumulation allows deposits of cholesterol in the blood vessel inner lining.

Finally, nicotine contained in smoke has the physiological effect of telling the artery muscle cells to contract in the extremities and skin. This decreases the available nutrition and oxygen delivery to those sites. Numerous patients no longer need high blood pressure medication once they successfully quit smoking. The penis qualifies as an extremity and is among the vulnerable sites. Imagine the Marlboro man's change in status if the public ever became aware of this interesting physiologic effect. It's a physiological fact that if one wants a smaller penis, he can smoke and someday the desired effect will be achieved.

Insulin and Blood Vessel Disease
Hormone Opportunist Mechanism

Hormone levels and life style choices can create a vicious cycle that results in unhealthy cholesterol levels. Scientific insights revealed that hormone levels affect behavior and behavior affects hormone levels.[4] The insulin trap is the first of several key hormone abnormalities that will be discussed in this manual.

High insulin levels turn on the fat and cholesterol enzymatic machinery (HMG Co A reductase) of the liver. Insulin promotes the type of cholesterol packages known as LDL and VLDL that is involved in heart disease. High glucagon levels, in the liver, curtail this type of cholesterol manufacture. A tug of war occurs in the liver between the message content of these two hormones. They are both secreted from the pancreas by different stimuli. Lifestyle choices that promote a healthy balance between these two hormones will naturally improve cholesterol content. Lifestyle choices that promote more insulin and less glucagon weaken the cholesterol profile.

A simple analogy to understand insulin is this; when driving into the gas station and filling the gas tank, a nozzle is used to connect the cars tank to the fuel pump. Insulin is like the nozzle that fills the cell's fuel tank. Without a nozzle there can be no fuel delivery.

The cellular fuel tanks are just like a car fuel tank. They can only hold a finite amount of fuel before it spills on the ground or back into the blood stream. Overly nourished owners spill cellular fuel (mainly sugar) back into the blood stream. When all the cellular fuel tanks are full, the liver must clear the blood stream of the excess fuel. The liver has a finite capacity to store excess sugar fuel. When the sugar fuel level exceeds the capacity of the liver to store it, at the direction of insulin, the liver begins to make this sugar into fat and cholesterol.

The newly manufactured fat particles (LDL and VLDL cholesterol) are excreted into the blood stream where they become fat cells in the belly area. Some of this 'yuck' sticks in certain owner's blood vessels when other Velcro factors exist. A technical indicator of this process is the beer gut.

Insulin directs the cells to take up the fuel building blocks (amino acids, fatty acids, and sugar) and store them as reassembled proteins, fats and glycogen. Insulin requires the help of insulin-like growth factor (IGF-1) for fuel uptake. Healthy owners have over one hundred times the IGF-1 in their blood streams as insulin. As owners become unhealthy, IGF-1 levels fall and insulin levels rise. Insulin preferentially facilitates the liver and fat cells in the uptake of nutrients from the blood stream. Conversely, IGF-1 facilitates the uptake of fuels by other cells. Many blood vessels related diseases have their origins in the fall of IGF-1 and the consequent need for excess insulin (sections two, three, and four).

Once the cellular storehouses are all full, insulin becomes a powerful and persuasive messenger to the liver. Insulin directs the liver to change sugar into fat and activate HMG Co A reductase which increases cholesterol production in the liver.

Insulin directed and manufactured fat and cholesterol is released into the bloodstream as the bad cholesterol-fat-protein particles (LDL and VLDL). LDL and VLDL are constructed in the liver for storage purposes. Storage of the various fuel groups is what the insulin message content does better than any other hormone. Consistent with this message, these particles are destined for storage sites. In certain genetically predisposed owners, the rate of removal from the blood stream is not fast and concentrations of theses particle rise. In contrast, dietary derived fat particles (chylomicrons) are easier for the body to eliminate from the circulation (section three). The more bad cholesterol (LDL and VLDL) the owner has in the bloodstream, the more the tendency there is for this sticky form of cholesterol-fat-protein complex to adhere to the arterial lining.

Fat cells in the abdomen area are directed by the same insulin message to take up liver manufactured fat. Macrophages that line the coronary arteries can uptake 30% of these types of liver manufactured fat-cholesterol-protein complexes. A sedentary lifestyle promotes these cells lining the blood vessels from accumulating more of this material. Eventually these cells grow into foam cells that are affixed to the inside of the arterial wall. This is the earliest recognized lesion in the development of blood vessel disease.

Earlier it was implied that the LDL cholesterol sticks to Velcro surfaces. Macrophages accumulate LDL cholesterol over time. This fact shows that it is slightly more complicated than that. Some authorities feel that the macrophages adhere to areas on the artery that are injured (Velcro has formed). Others feel that the macrophages serve a fuel storage role and the intent is to have ample fat fuel for cardiac and muscle cells the next time insulin levels drop or the owner exercises. In many owners the insulin level never drops to a level where the macrophage can release fat contents. In addition, sedentary lifestyles provide little opportunity for release to sedentary muscles and heart tissues.

In America there are many specimens of the high insulin states. Fast food establishments are full of these owners who have stuffed macrophages lining their coronary arteries and the accompanying expanded waistline. This excess fat creates trouble for the blood vessels because fat cells have a slow metabolic rate. The uptake of LDL and VLDL cholesterol occurs at a slower rate than the liver dumps it into the blood stream. The macrophage system is not designed to receive daily additions of fat to its cell population.

There is marked genetic variation in the rate certain owners can make LDL cholesterol in the liver and how fast it can be removed from the blood stream. In general, the higher the insulin level, then the higher the message content directed at the liver to increase LDL production. Certain owners have elevated cholesterol because their fat cells cannot remove the LDL cholesterol at the rate the liver is dumping it into the blood stream. This chronic situation allows ample time for some LDL cholesterol to be added to the macrophages that adhere to the Velcro patches that are created by the other risk factors.

Another useful analogy is a high volume faucet. The faucet flow is likened to the ability (directed by insulin) of the liver to manufacture LDL cholesterol. The drain is likened to the ability of the fat cells to clear this form of cholesterol from the blood vessels (the sink). Increased LDL cholesterol in the sink builds to higher levels when the drain is too small (fat cells in the abdomen area). The immune scavenger cells (the macrophages) ingest about 30% of these particles. They become laden and attach to places like the coronary arteries. Sedentary people have little stimulus for fat laden macrophages to release LDL and it continues to collect and grow into foam cells. This cycle repeats itself following each large meal. Foam cells are the earliest blood vessel wall change that leads to blood vessel disease. Genetics plays a role in how much carbohydrate it takes to over run the drain (fat cells).

Owners can't change their genetics, but they can change the stimulus (insulin level and sedentary lifestyle) and influence this type of heart disease.

Carbohydrate Overload and increased Insulin Affects the Appetite

High insulin message content, occurring with a high carbohydrate diet, is a powerful appetite stimulant. The higher the insulin levels in circulation, the more behavioral stimulation there is to satisfy the increased appetite. Reducing insulin levels has a dramatic affect on the appetite cravings as well as on amount of bad cholesterol. The effects of hormones on feeding behavior are substantial (hormone chapter). Carbohydrates also play a role in this process. Carbohydrate, in all forms, is by far the most powerful stimulant of insulin secretion in initiating this vicious cycle.

Gonads and Adrenals: Firing the Engines of Life

Poor gonad or /and adrenal function is a major risk factor that is often overlooked in the development of blood vessel disease. These glands have the ability to direct rejuvenation and healthful maintenance activities of the blood vessels. When optimal conditions prevail, they perform this task by secreting the appropriate types of informational substances. Optimal steroid mixture secretion is a prerequisite of good health. As this mixture diminishes, this imbalance reflects in the aging appearance of the body. When this happens in the blood vessels, rust that occurs fails to be repaired. The body tissues succeed or fail in this ongoing cellular infrastructure investment program (section two). Hormones made in the adrenals and the gonads are essential for directing rejuvenation.

Countering the Second Principle of Longevity: Loss of Flexibility

High Blood Pressure Causes Stiffness in the Pipes

High blood pressure ages the blood vessels by promoting progressive stiffness of the artery in the muscular layer in a defensive response to the elevated pressure. As the pressure increases, the muscle layer within the artery enlarges to accommodate the resistance. Resistance increases to counter the increased pressure in the artery. This process is somewhat analogous to the fact that the thicker a hydraulic hose is the stiffer they are. The same concept applies to arteries. The thicker arteries are less flexible and tend to have accelerated wear and tear. These changes result from the turbulent blood in the blood vessels that pummel the less elastic interior lining cells. This is the injury mechanism that results from all causes of high blood pressure.

Healthy arteries are flexible and this reduces the damage caused by the turbulent flow in the blood vessel. As the wear and tear occurs, weakened areas begin. Small breaks occur in vulnerable small arteries leading to leakage of trace amounts of blood into the surrounding tissues. These small bleeds continue until there is an irreversible loss in function in the affected organ. The most vulnerable sites to these silent small bleeds are the hearing apparatus, retina, brain, heart, and kidney areas. Injured blood vessels are another way of describing Velcro. The more Velcro there is, the more repair necessary to keep macrophages from adhering as temporary patch jobs against the injured blood vessel lining. Adding in the high insulin states, the macrophages uptake some of the extra LDL cholesterol manufactured in the liver and there is more acceleration toward blood vessel disease.

High blood pressure is a silent and symptomless enemy until late in the disease process. Patients in the early stage of this disease process insist that they feel fine and are less compliant with their high blood pressure medication. Most high blood pressure prescription medications work by poisoning an enzymatic process that results in a lowered blood pressure. Physicians justified the inevitable side effects because there was no better way.

Recently, an old scientific truth was reasserted. Magnesium is a powerful smooth muscle relaxant. Arteries generate pressure by contracting the smooth muscle layer. Some evidence suggests that intracellular depletion of magnesium content tends to make these smooth muscle cells contractile prone which leads to an elevated blood pressure. Adequate supplementation with magnesium can restore the natural balance and the blood pressure will come down without poisoning an enzymatic process.

Taking 500-700mg elemental weight of magnesium per day will significantly drop blood pressure readings in seven to fourteen days for some owners. Magnesium absorption is dependent on the manufacture of adequate stomach acid. Magnesium tends to open the airways and make the bowels more regular. The effect of magnesium on bowel movements varies with the ingestion of different types of salt. The most powerful salt form is magnesium citrate laxative. There are many different causes that lead to high blood pressure. Magnesium has a beneficial effect on some hypertensive owners. There are several other abnormalities that can lead to high blood pressure (chapter three).

Magnesium supplements come in the form of a salt. The weight of the salt pill is usually stated on the front of the bottle and is always more than the actual content of the weight of elemental magnesium (active ingredient). Usually in the small print on the back of the bottle is the weight of the elemental magnesium content per tablet. This amount ranges from 15-150 mg depending on the brand. All magnesium supplements are not equally effective. Some have a small amount of elemental magnesium per tablet and this requires ingesting a handful to receive what other brands contain in a single pill. There are some brands that are poorly absorbed and of little therapeutic value. Finally, some companies manufacture magnesium with salts of oxygen, which is unacceptable. Source Naturals, and some other manufacturers make an excellent line of magnesium products. Magnesium deficiency is only one example of how mineral imbalance can affect blood pressure.

Mineral Imbalance Can Cause High Blood Pressure

The larger problem of mineral imbalance is caused by a processed food diet. Processed foods have drastically altered mineral composition when compared to real food. Real food tends to be high in magnesium and potassium and intermediate in calcium content. Real food is usually low in sodium with the exception of calcium. Processed food has a reversed mineral content compared to real food.

The body is energized by an electrical system that is maintained by potential differences across trillions of cell membranes in the body. The body requires specific mineral proportions. A real food diet supplies these and a processed food diet does not. Around middle age cells begin to lose their electrical pizzazz. It is a miracle that the body can tolerate reversed electrolyte (minerals) ratio intake for as long as it does before it begins to fail.

The car battery electrolyte composition is an analogy that demonstrates the effect of mineral imbalance. Like the body cells that charge themselves by concentration differences around cell membranes, so to it is with car batteries. Car batteries are at maximum charge only when the different minerals are at maximal difference across the membrane. For this to occur, the battery manufacturer adds the proper minerals into the battery fluid. The chronic consumption of processed food is analogous to dumping battery fluid on the ground and reversing the proportion of electrolytes in battery fluid. Most owners would see this behavior as foolish. Yet, this is what they are doing every time they eat processed food. Around middle age the 'battery fluid' in the body begins to alter despite the best effort of the kidneys to compensate for the reversed ratio of mineral intake. This is the origin of many disease processes. One common disease that results from this imbalance is high blood pressure.

Most owners need about 4000 mg of potassium, 1000 mg of sodium, 1000 mg of calcium and 500 mg of magnesium every day. Profuse sweating increases sodium needs. Altered kidney and adrenal function will also alter these amounts. Most Americans obtain about 6000 mg of sodium a day and much less potassium than is needed.

Around middle age the cells have usually sacrificed much of their potassium to maintaining the blood potassium level. The cost to health when potassium is lost from cells is a decreased energy charge. This means that the afflicted cell do less work because of fatigue. Early fatigue is a sign of aging.

98% of body potassium is in the cells. This is the tank that sacrifices its potassium to the 2% tank in the blood stream. Many owners are misled when they have their blood drawn and the potassium result comes back normal. The blood test says nothing about the state of potassium content in the cells.

Potassium Deficiency and Sodium Excess and High Blood Pressure

Many owners have had the experience of receiving instructions from their physician about the benefits of a low salt diet. Very few are counseled about the importance of a healthy potassium to sodium ratio. The optimal ratio between potassium and sodium is a minimal of three-to-one. Most Americans are ingesting the opposite proportions between these two vital minerals. Food manufactures add many types of sodium to processed foods to preserve shelf life. Most of this added sodium does not taste salty. Sodium only tastes salty when it is in a salt of chloride (table salt). Monosodium glutamate, sodium aspartate, sodium benzoate, sodium nitrite, sodium alginate, sodium nitrate, and sodium sulfate are examples of added sodium. Sodium oxide is added to soften water.

Ways a chronic potassium deficiency will harm the body and raise blood pressure:

1. Kidney damage (sections two, three, four, five)
2. Insulin resistance (sections two, three, seven)
3. Increased cholesterol (sections two, three, seven)
4. The choice of normal testosterone and high blood pressure or a lower testosterone and normal blood pressure (chapter three, sections two, three, four, five, six, seven).
5. Irritable nervous system (sections five, six, seven)
6. Weakened cell force field (sections three, four, five)
7. Slower metabolism (sections two, three, six)
8. Loss of protein (sections two, three, four)
9. Chronic stress accelerates potassium deficiency (sections two, three, four, five)

The majority of high blood pressure problems are partially related to mineral imbalance. Potassium is the major mineral deficiency that is responsible for the high blood pressure of middle age. There are several other significant nutritional causes for high blood pressure.

These factors are proven mechanisms for the development of blood pressure elevation. Methyl donor depletion syndromes, nitric oxide deficiency, stiff red blood cells, a processed food diet, the wrong balance of essential dietary fats (hormonal fats), and inappropriate attention to the tug of war are occurring between the biogenic amines. All of these contribute significantly to blood pressure elevation and are rarely discussed (chapters 2 and 3).

A physician needs to oversee the transitional period. In this period, less hypertension medication will be needed after the implementation of magnesium or other methods and supplements. A sudden or premature cessation of prescription anti-hypertensive medications can produce dangerous rebound effects that place the owner at increased risk of complications.

There are disease processes that employ all three mechanisms on how it injures the blood vessel. Diabetes is such a process.

Diabetes Causes Rust, Hardening, and Usually has an Opprotunistic Mechanism

Diabetes

Diabetes diminishes health by injuring the blood vessels. Diabetes is a disease process that includes all three blood vessel injury mechanisms. High blood sugar injures the blood vessel lining cells and promotes Velcro formation. High insulin levels promote high blood pressure and stiffening mechanisms. High blood insulin also creates the abnormal amounts of LDL cholesterol, which is the opportunistic mechanism. All three combined together creates an accelerated path to blood vessel disease.

Until recently, medical approaches aimed at the prevention of blood vessel injury, from diabetes, were a disappointment. The treatment success of a diabetic is dependent on three variables. If these three variables are addressed squarely and honestly, the complications of diabetes are slowed down. In some cases, the complications can be avoided almost entirely. The first variable is "who" the diabetic patient consults for advice. The examples of Richard Bernstein, M.D., and Steven Gordon, N.D. demonstrate the significant results that can be achieved by the application of effective treatments.

A fresh scientific perspective is heard from Dr. Richard Bernstein, who developed diabetes at age twelve (***Diabetes Solutions***, Little and Brown Co.). When he was in his late twenties, he had many complications from the disease process including moderately severe kidney disease. His engineering background allowed him to approach his disease methodically and rigorously. He carefully noted his dietary intake and daily intake weight of the different food groups. He carefully followed any changes in his diet and the effects this had on blood sugar. He confirmed a simple concept and through rigorous dedication he reversed his kidney disease entirely. At the age of sixty-nine he is in better health than many of his peers. In this informative and well-written book he outlines a plan of healing from the potential complications of diabetes and the genetic tendencies to change carbohydrate into LDL cholesterol.

He discovered that since diabetes is a disease primarily of sugar metabolism then if one strictly curtails sugar (carbohydrate) the complications of diabetes are greatly diminished. Dr. Bernstein concluded that strict adherence to a low carbohydrate diet brings about a lowered insulin level and an optimal blood fat-cholesterol-protein complex profile that is one of the key predictors of blood vessel health. While Dr. Bernstein has insulin dependent diabetes (10% of diabetics) this program is equally beneficial for the adult onset diabetes patients (90% of diabetes patients). Even more exciting is that this program identifies a huge percentage of people on the road to developing heart disease because they have chronically elevated insulin levels. By following, Dr. Bernstein's program, these at risk owners can dramatically lower their heart disease risk.

This author was skeptical about Dr. Bernstein's findings. It was difficult to accept that eating high levels of fat and cholesterol could result in a dramatic reduction of those substances in the blood stream. Approximately five years ago the author observed different patients who had followed various versions of low carbohydrate diets. Some of them had heart disease, some had cerebral vascular disease, and some had diabetes. In most cases there was an agreement achieved about their obtaining a cholesterol profile at the start of the diet and then again in thirty days after trying their ridiculous diet. The author was shocked when the results began coming back thirty days later. With few exceptions, the cholesterol profiles for these disease types were dramatically improved. According to the mainstream medical dogma this should not have happened.

The author began working with a naturopathic doctor named Steven Gordon. Dr. Gordon persuaded the author to buy Dr. Bernstein's book and study it for a likely explanation why these contrary diets were working. Dr. Gordon began to treat his insulin dependent diabetes with a low carbohydrate diet and used the recommendations of Dr. Bernstein in his treatment program over the last five years. Dr. Gordon has reported immense benefits to himself and his patients.

The second variable that will predict the outcome of the diabetes treatment is the motivation of the patient to comply with taking an active and consistent role in changing his diet and lifestyle. Those patients willing to commit to positive changes have a high probability of treatment success. Patients who are unwilling to take responsibility for their lifestyle and insist on remaining passive in their disease process are condemned to symptom control medicine. These treatment modalities are littered with side effects and result in unreasonably limited outcomes.

The third variable that will predict treatment success is the classification of the type of diabetes. The minority of people has a type of diabetes that is not classified. The elevated blood sugar is measured, but the cause has not been established. Treatment modalities cannot be suggested when the cause of the elevated blood sugar is unknown. This group of diabetics will be identified in the liver chapter. It is important to have an accurate diagnosis that allows exploration of ways to heal.

There is an important common fact between most diabetes and heart disease patients. In the majority of these illnesses a high insulin level occurs. The difference between the diseases is that the adult onset diabetic's have reached a body mass that exceeds their genetic ability to make insulin. When this occurs blood sugar increases. In both heart disease and adult onset diabetics, high blood insulin is feeding fat accumulation in the arteries. By the time an owner develops obesity to the point of a rising blood sugar, their blood vessels are already diseased. The chronic elevation of insulin engorges their macrophages with fat.

The greater the body fat, then the more insulin required to sustain it. For those that may doubt this fact, consider how the opposite situation of childhood diabetes presents. Childhood diabetes presents with a rapid loss of body fat because insulin is deficient. Contrast this situation with the majority of adult onset diabetics who are obese. Obese diabetics have an excess of body insulin. However, their obesity has exceeded their genetic ability to increase insulin further.

Different genetic lines will have individualized upper limits of maximal insulin production. When body mass exceeds genetically determined insulin manufacturing ability the blood sugar will rise beyond normal and diabetes is diagnosed. This variability between different owners explains why in some owner's obesity is not extreme when they develop diabetes. In others, obesity is marked before their blood sugar rises and diabetes is diagnosed. High insulin is silently filling up these owner's vessel walls with fat before their pancreases failed to continue increasing insulin production. Some owners never reach the upper limit of insulin production despite becoming obese. Their high insulin levels will usually cause development of blood vessel disease at an early age. As a general rule, the greater the obesity, the greater the insulin level required to sustain this fat mass.

The association between increased insulin levels and blood vessel disease illuminates another important point. Mainstream medicine sometimes treats adult onset diabetes through raising insulin levels. While this approach will lower blood sugar, it is paid for with the price of further feeding fat to the blood vessel macrophages. This approach somewhat corrects the rusting processes, but raises the stiffening and opportunistic processes. The reader is cautioned to remember the group of diabetics that are neither type one or type two, but victims of some other abnormal hormone process.

This concludes the introductory level discussion of rust prevention and hardening processes. In the next chapter, how these same processes injure the red blood cells will be explored. Rusted and stiff red blood cells cause many complications in diabetes. In the blood vessels that have opportunistic processes in operation (high LDL cholesterol), the added insult of stiff and rusted red blood cells exaggerates the severity of the disease.

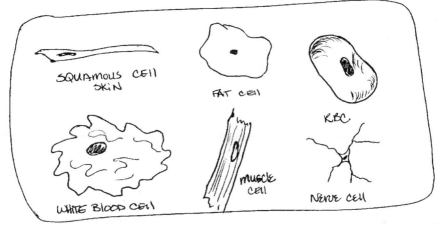

The Basic Unit of the Human Form is the Cell.

The numerous body cell types are analogous in some ways to the many different varieties of fruits and vegetables. The different cell types are composed of different textures of skin, color, shapes, sizes and consistency.

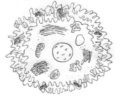

Extending this analogy one can envision the different skin types of these foods as analogous to the different types of environments that surround the cell types. Cartilage and bone cells that are widely spaced between the hard matrixes that they create are like coconuts. Red blood cells are like sponges in consistency (technically not a edible food, but the consistency and resiliency are accurate.).

Some owners have health problems because their cell types are like overly ripe fruit or vegetables. Fruits and vegetables have deteriorating qualities. The cell types also have deteriorating qualities that are observed in humans as the path to old age. The goal is to keep all the body fruits and vegetables in their most appealing state.

Almost all have a complete computer program (DNA), but only certain programs are active within a cell type. The programs that are active determine what a cell looks like and the

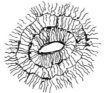

products that the different cell factories produce. The activity of the DNA program (genes) also determines the types and amounts of the different cellular machines (enzymes) that perform different assembly line activities. The cellular factories (Golgi apparatus, endoplasmic reticulum, etc.) need power to generate their activities. This energy is supplied by the cellular power plant (mitochondria). When a cell is healthy the energy packets (ATP) created by the combustion of fuel and oxygen are trapped in the cell. Many cells have additional waste incinerator facilities (peroxisomes). All cells have a cellular force field (plasma membrane). The cell membrane supplies energy for work, derived from available ATP, and shields the cell from harmful, foreign molecules. The supporting architecture for the cell's interior is called the cytoskeleton. The supporting architecture for the cell's exterior is called the extra-cellular matrix. When the supporting architecture diminishes the body assumes the flattened look of old age.

Chapter 2

Cells Traveling in the Blood Vessels

The previous discussion concerned the amount of stiffness and rust formation in the blood vessels. The cells that travel in these vessels (the pipes) are also a very important determinant of health. The cells that travel in the blood vessels can only be young and efficiently perform their purpose when they are flexible and without rust.

Many chronic degenerative diseases are made worse or arise completely from these two destructive processes that damage the red blood cells. Examples include: high blood pressure, fibromyalgia, complications from diabetes, peripheral vascular disease, brain deterioration syndromes, cardiac ischemia, kidney injury, and spleenomegaly. When the blood cells are damaged or diseased restoring flexibility and function can restore them to health.

The cells that flow through the blood vessels perform some of the body's most vital functions. First, no matter where in the body that oxygen is delivered (organs, muscle, bone, etc.), it is delivered by the red blood cells. The red cells deliver oxygen to the cells at the capillary level. The capillary is the level where oxygen is removed from the red cell. The red blood cells arrive at the capillaries and are literally squeezed by their passage through the narrow capillaries. This squeezing action releases the oxygen from the red blood cells into the body cells serviced by the capillary. This squeezing action occurs because the average capillary is slightly smaller than the diameter of a single red blood cell. When a red cell is healthy, the ability to deform and squeeze through the capillary is accomplished smoothly. After the red blood cell traverses the capillary the healthy red cell quickly recovers its shape.

The trillions of red blood cells within the body have the consistency of a sponge. At the level of the capillary, where oxygen is being unloaded, a stiff sponge causes problems. The red blood cell will tend to clog the capillary and will not compress sufficiently to deliver the oxygen, nutrients, etc which it is carrying. When the sponge re-inflates a vacuum is created. This vacuum causes the red blood cell to absorb waste molecules created by the body's tissue cells. These red blood cells are propelled through the blood vessel by a pressure wave, The pressure wave is created by the beating of the heart. It is the pressure wave created by the heart that propels these sponges forward through these tight spaces within the body tissues. When a red cell has become stiffened or rusted it has less elasticity to accomplish this important task of oxygen delivery in an optimal manner. An owner is more vulnerable to degenerative disease as the volume of sickly red blood cells increases within the body.

The analogy of the sponge describes a mechanism of high blood pressure. The heart is going to have to push harder to move stiff red blood cells through the tight capillaries. To accomplish this the blood pressure must go up.

This is why one of the most popular classes of blood pressure medicines is the calcium channel blocker. Calcium channel blockers make stiff red blood cells more flexible.

The red blood cells have unique energy requirements. The red blood cells are analogous to a man buried to his neck in the sand with flasks of water all around him. The water is analogous to oxygen within the red blood cell. The water content within flasks by the man's head cannot do the man any good because he lacks the appendages to get the water to his lips. The situation for oxygen usage within the red cells is similar. Even though they transport huge amounts of oxygen, they lack the machinery to combust oxygen for their energy needs. This is true because red cells lack mitochondria. Without mitochondria, red cells are unable to burn fuel aerobically. The red cell is forced to burn fuel anaerobically, which enfeebles their ability to do normal cellular work. Cellular work within the red blood cell is dramatically decreased because without oxygen there is less energy creation per gram of sugar consumed. Anaerobically consumed sugar creates a constant source of lactic acid as a waste product.

The fact that dead blood cells can still transport oxygen is important. This unfortunately happens in transfused blood because it's a difficult to keep blood alive for longer than about seven days. The practice of transfusing dead blood into post surgical patients may sometimes be responsible for the massive organ destruction that is commonly called DIC (diffuse intra-vascular coagulation). Problems arise with dead red blood cells because without life they are unable to generate the energy necessary to remain as flexible. Not all dead red blood cells plug the capillary, but with other dietary and lifestyle bad habits that are practiced by the donor of the blood the risk is increased. During the red blood cell's one hundred and twenty day lifespan it must remain flexible. Mainstream medicine sometimes offers prescriptions, like pentoxyphyline, that have a beneficial effect on red blood cell flexibility. However, these medicines are expensive and often have side effects. This is in contrast to known nutritional and life style choices that will positively affect the flexibility of red blood cells.

Factors that Determine Red Blood Cell Flexibility

1. Electrical cell membrane potential (strength of the force field)
2. High cellular magnesium content
3. Low cellular calcium content
4. High cellular potassium content
5. Low cellular sodium content
6. Adequate cellular zinc levels
7. Optimal ferrous hemoglobin with minimal ferric hemoglobin
8. Optimal blood sugar
9. Healthy dietary fat choices

10. Quality of steroids transported within the red blood cell
11. Quality of enzymatic machinery in the cell
12. The level of the completeness of the methyl donor system
13. Adequacy of vitamin C
14. Waste level within the blood stream
15. Thyroid status
16. Cholesterol status
17. Availability of glucosamine and galactosamine
18. Glutathione levels and other anti-oxidants
19. Level of exposure to oxidants, rust promoters, in the environment (ozone, volatile acids, inappropriate blood metals, smoking)

1. The electrical red blood cell membrane (the strength of the force field)

Red blood cells protect themselves and perform useful cellular work by the maintenance of an electrically charged membrane. However, unlike other body cells, the red blood cell is more vulnerable because its electrical charging ability is greatly reduced. Red blood cells are energetically weak. They cannot use oxygen and are therefore forced into anaerobic metabolism.

One of the determinants of the cell's flexibility is contained in the strength of their cell membrane voltage. Processes that weaken the voltage will make the red cell contents vulnerable to hostile invasion forces and also allow a loss of flexibility.

2. High inside the cell magnesium content

Adequate magnesium within the red blood cells causes the red blood cells to become more flexible. The blood pressure will be reduced as a result. Adequate magnesium within the red blood cell, past middle age in America, is unlikely if an owner eats a diet of processed food instead of real food.

Magnesium is also required by the red blood cells to create energy by the combustion of glucose in an anaerobic fashion. The red blood cell cannot create the energy packets (ATP and NADH, NADPH, etc.) to perform their work without adequate levels of magnesium.

The correct proportion of magnesium and potassium within the red blood cell creates the best possible energy content within the cell membrane. In contrast, there is the additional benefit of also having a low concentration of both calcium and sodium inside the red blood cell. The red blood cells require a constant level of energy supply in order to maintain the optimal ratios of these minerals. These four electrolytes concentrations are a powerful determinant to the health of any body cell. When one mineral within the red blood cell becomes deficient or excessive, then their proportional relationship with one another becomes altered. When the mineral relationships are altered within a cell, health consequences will occur (section five).

3. Low inside the red blood cell calcium concentration

Red blood cells contain less calcium than most of the other cell types in the body. This probably protects the hemoglobin content within the red blood cell or the enzymatic machinery that burns sugar for energy creation. As the magnesium content decreases inside the red blood cell more calcium can get inside. If the volume of calcium within the body cells is too high the calcium tends to injure the other cellular contents. This fact underscores the need for adequate magnesium relative to calcium content within the body.

4. Potassium, like magnesium, is needed within the red cell in high concentrations for many reasons.

Adequate potassium is necessary for proteins to remain stable. Red blood cells will often sacrifice their potassium content for the blood streams needs. The price paid for this donation is a weakened electrical charge of the red blood cell membrane. A weakened electrical charge means the red blood cell has less energy for both work (flexibility) and protecting itself from the invasion of hostile ions. However, the body prioritizes the potassium in the serum over the potassium in the red blood cell. Eventually, the deficient potassium situation recruits other body cells to sacrifice their potassium content, as well. The trouble here arises from, in part, that all body cells need adequate potassium in order to stabilize their protein content. In muscle cells potassium is needed to make larger muscle tissue. Muscle tissue is made up of protein. Therefore, owners that desire youthful vitality need adequate potassium within their red blood cells and other body cells.

Adequate potassium is necessary for insulin to effectively deliver fuel to the cells. High carbohydrate diets tax the potassium within the blood stream because as sugar goes inside the cellular fuel tanks it also must pull potassium with it (one to one ratio). The blood steam plasma must keep the plasma concentrations of potassium relatively stable. The red blood cell, in this situation, becomes forced to give up too much of its potassium. The red blood cell is first in line for donating some of its potassium, when potassium levels are low within the blood stream. Refined sugars come largely devoid of potassium content and therefore these types of meals can create this situation. As the problem becomes more chronic other body cells will donate potassium to prevent further drops in the serum potassium level.

5. Low inside the cell sodium content

Stress greatly increases the tendency for sodium content to rise inside the red blood cell. This occurs until the body is near death and then sodium content begins to fall off. The human body was not designed for chronic stress. Modern life can tend to be stressful. This fact will tend to increase inside the red blood cell sodium because stress causes sodium retention and potassium loss. The problem is exaggerated for those under stress when they chronically consume a processed food diet In these situations, the red blood cell is forced to compromise it's own well being in order to improve the way the blood plasma appears. This is why the blood test that measure serum potassium can be misleading as to the true inside the cell status for potassium content. Chronic stress and high sodium diets are another mechanism for the compromise of red blood cell integrity.

6. Adequate zinc levels

Adequate zinc is needed within the body cells types that make acid (hydrogen proton) or base (bicarbonate) from carbon dioxide gas. To do this they each need the enzyme carbonic anhydrase. Carbonic anhydrase needs zinc for activity. Red blood cells, stomach, pancreas, brain, prostate, kidneys and the testes all need to do this. In some tissues like the stomach, this enzyme splits carbon dioxide to secrete acid. In other places like the pancreas, the opposite reaction occurs in that it secretes bicarbonate instead. In other cases, carbonic anhydrase is crucial to prevent excessive body acid from accumulating and consequently damaging intracellular structures. Preservation of the red blood cell's architectural integrity is only possible when there is just the right amount of pH. This enzyme is fundamental within the body for pH balance. In the case of red blood cells it allows a continued oxygen carrying capacity. Owners' cells that lack adequate zinc levels are vulnerable to many harmful processes.

7. Adequate ferrous hemoglobin

The iron contained on the hemoglobin is necessary for the red blood cell to carry oxygen to the cells. When the iron contained on hemoglobin is oxidized (ferri hemoglobin) then it is of no use for the transport of oxygen to the tissues. The body has an elaborate and multi layered system to prevent this oxidation from occurring in more than nominal amounts. When this oxidation occurs in excessive amounts the body has multiple systems to remedy the problem. This fact is better explained below (the methyl donor system (13) below, vitamin C (14), and glutathione (19) levels).

There are medications that irrevocably damage the red blood cell's ability to bind oxygen. Medications like sulfa drugs, acetaminophen, nitroglycerin and phenacetin all have the potential to irreversibly form sulf-hemoglobin. Also mal-digestive states can allow hydrogen sulfide gas (rotten egg smell to farts) to become absorbed into the blood stream and combine with the red blood cell. When this happens hemoglobin will never carry oxygen again. If one is suspicious they can order a sulf-hemoglobin level and see what percentage of their blood is unable to carry oxygen.

8. Both a high and low blood sugar can injure the red blood cells flexibility

Uncontrolled diabetes (high blood sugar) has long been known to cause the red blood cells to become stiffened. This is a powerful mechanism for the etiology of the micro-vascular complications from diabetes. Conspicuous examples of the cell hardening are demonstrated when stiffened red blood cells become wedged in the capillaries of a diabetic's foot or retina.

Hypoglycemia has an adverse effect on red blood cell function. Low blood sugar renders the red blood cell vulnerable to penetration from ions like calcium. These ions will irreversibly bind with cellular contents such as proteins, causing deformation. Deformation of cell proteins causes diminished function. When the low blood sugar is severe enough, there is also the possibility of killing some of one's red blood cells off and therefore decreasing their flexibility permanently. It is important to realize that dead red blood cells can still carry oxygen. However, numerous hostile forces within the blood stream rapidly damage dead red blood cells.

9. Adequacy of healthy fat choices in the diet

The fats contained on and within the red blood cell are unique when compared to most other body cells. They are more similar to the brain's fat make up. These types of fats require huge amounts of the vitamins and nutrients contained in the methyl donor system (13 below). When these vitamins and nutrients are sufficient in supplies the fat content of the red blood cells is optimized. Optimized fat makeup is a powerful determinant of red blood cell flexibility.

When an owner eats processed foods around middle age varying levels of nutritional deficiency begin to occur. In many ways the red blood cell is more vulnerable than other body cells because it has a more limited ability to repair itself once damage has occurred. The red blood cell's limited ability to repair itself arises from three main sources. First, because it lacks a cell nucleus (DNA program) it cannot manufacture new proteins once protein damage occurs. Second, because it lacks a mitochondria energy generation becomes greatly reduced even in the best of circumstances. Reduced energy generation leads to less ability for the work of repairing damaged fat. Third, the blood stream is a hostile environment in many life situations and the red blood cell fat is therefore possibly exposed to these forces at a high rate of occurrence. Damaged fats on the surface of the red blood cell accumulate and compromise the flexibility of the blood cell. Certain dietary habits and nutritional deficiencies provide another mechanism to injure the flexibility of the red blood cells (sections two, three, four, and five).

10. The quality of the body steroids is a determinant of flexibility

Many of the body steroids are transported intermingled with the fats of the red blood cell membrane. High levels of cortisol tend to decrease flexibility while high levels of estrogen increase it. Many steroids rely on an interaction with the red blood cells as part of their delivery strategies to their target cells. In fact, enzymatic machines contained within the red blood cell convert the original steroid hormone to more powerful and different steroids. Estrogen provides one steroid example where this occurs.

11. The quality of the enzymatic machinery in the red blood cell

While the red blood cell was being constructed within the bone marrow, the cell's enzymes (cellular machines) were determined.

The construction phase is the only time that a red blood cell contains DNA. DNA is necessary to instruct the manufacture of proteins which makeup the red blood cell. The type and amount of the different enzymes that were made during this process are largely determined by the quality of the message content (types of hormones). The type of hormone message content determines the instructions, which the DNA program within the immature red blood cell receives. Message content directs the DNA program. The DNA program activity determines which proteins are made in a red blood cell. All enzymes are made from protein. Therefore enzyme content within a cell is determined by what hormones instructed its various DNA programs. This is the last chance a red blood cell will ever get, in regards to what it is equipped with, to perform metabolically, because it's own genetic program (DNA content) gets destroyed shortly after it is released into the circulation. This is in contrast to all other body cells that have the DNA program still present. Owners who have poor informational direction at the level of their bone marrow are cranking out inferiorly equipped red blood cells. The lack of genetic material within the red blood cell, after it is released into the blood stream causes it to have unique needs and vulnerabilities.

12. Adequate copper is necessary for an important enzymes manufacture in the bone marrow while the red blood cell is being constructed

One of the enzymes that are constructed while the red blood cell is being constructed within the bone marrow is called catalase. This enzyme protects the red blood cell from oxygen radicals by neutralizing them. Some owners are copper deficient and copper is a critical trace mineral that is needed to make the enzyme catalase. When this enzyme is deficient the red blood cell ages quickly and its flexibility becomes compromised.

13. The level of completeness of all the molecular components in the methyl donor system is a determinant of red blood cell flexibility

One billion times a second the body relies on the methyl donor system to prevent breakdown in molecular structure or improve biological messengers throughout the body.[5] Specialized fats in the brains and red blood cells require extremely high amounts of the nutrients that make up the methyl donor system. This is why people who do not eat enough fat in their diet tend to become deficient within this system. The low fat diet adherents use up tremendous amounts of their methyl donor system nutrients to manufacture these specialized fats. This quantity of these types of fats is routinely included in a more healthful diet. The depletion of the methyl donor system by the low fat diet causes a deficiency of these specialized fats as well.

Choline (lecithin building block) provides an example of the debilitating effect of the low fat diet. Choline is a specialized fat building block. Specialized fats are needed in high concentrations within both the red blood cell and nervous system. Choline synthesis requires three methyl groups for manufacturing it one time. These specialized fats are needed by the gazillions within both the brain and red blood cell. Eggs are nature's best source of choline. The methyl donor system depends on numerous vitamins and amino acids. Depletion of this system is sometimes the root cause of many degenerative diseases, like: high blood pressure, neuro-degenerative disease, and blood vessel disease.

14. Adequacy of vitamin C

When other anti-oxidants are deficient (glutathione, trimethyl glycine, and ergothioneine), vitamin C levels can become rapidly depleted. The vitamin C is required for the maintenance of ferrous hemoglobin within the red blood cell. This is the only form of iron that can transport oxygen to the body tissues. When vitamin C is used up in this fashion the total daily requirement increases tremendously. Some clinicians claim that the signs of scurvy (vitamin C deficiency) can develop when other anti-oxidants become deficient. The signs of scurvy occur because the rate of usage of vitamin C is many times greater than normal when other anti-oxidants are deficient. The major anti-oxidant within the red blood cell, that is needed to prevent the rapid depletion of vitamin C, is glutathione. This simple peptide is made from three amino acids. Certain prescription medications tend to deplete this important substance form both the red blood cell and the liver. Certain prescriptions and nutritional bad habits tend to deplete vitamin C more quickly (liver chapter). When these situations occur it is important to increase one's vitamin C intake. Ample vitamin C within the red blood cell will allow continued ferrous hemoglobin content. Ferrous hemoglobin is the only form of iron that can transport oxygen.

15. Waste level in the blood stream (discussion deferred until section four)

16. Thyroid status and red blood cell flexibility

The amount of thyroid message content (hormone level) affects the amount of cholesterol inside the red blood cell. Cholesterol within the red blood cell competes with the specialized fats. Specialized fats, like phospholipid, give the red blood cell the maximum of flexibility. Increased thyroid states tend to lower the serum cholesterol the same trend appears to be true with the red blood cell fat composition. High thyroid function increases the proportion of phospholipid relative to cholesterol in the red blood cell membrane. Conversely, low thyroid function retards flexibility. Thyroid hormone plays an important role within the body in facilitating waste removal activities from the cells, including red blood cells. The colon, immune system, kidney's, lung, skin and liver are dependent on adequate thyroid message content for their waste removal activities.

17. Cholesterol status (above and digestion section)

18. Availability of glucosamine and galactosamine to the red blood cell

The availability of glucosamine and galactosamine is one of the significant determinants of flexibility of an red blood cell. These substances promote the process of "gelation". This process is what allows the red blood cells to deform within the capillary. Jell-O is composed of both galactosamine and glucosamine. These are obtained from grinding up animal cartilage. The same molecules that give Jell-O its consistency also creates the flexibility of the red blood cells.

19. Glutathione levels

This important antioxidant keeps the preformed enzymes and oxygen carrying capacities intact for the life of the red blood cell. Prescription drugs could possibly deplete these anti-oxidants. One common medication ingredient, which requires glutathione for metabolism is acetaminophen. There are many other medications that deplete glutathione. Glutathione is found mainly in the liver and the red blood cells. Quality protein intake is necessary to increase production of this important anti-oxidant.

20. The level of exposure to oxidants (rust promoters) such as environmental ozone, volatile acids in smog, inappropriate blood serum levels of metals and minerals (aluminum, fluoride).

The more the blood cells are exposed to rust promoters then the greater the need for the anti-oxidants within the blood stream. (Ideally, one should also be thinking about ways to reduce chronic exposure to rust promoters.)

An increased blood fluoride and iodide levels will poison the energy metabolism of red blood cells. Increased exposure to these minerals will tend to jeopardize the red cells' energy production. Red blood cells whose energy production has been compromised are vulnerable to the rust and hardening mechanisms (#'s 1-20). Fluoride is a powerful rust (oxidizing agent) promoter ion within the body. This gives the average owner something to think about the next time while shopping for toothpaste and in deciding about iodized salt consumption.

The medical media's focus has been on blood vessels, but the cells within them are equally important to the pursuit of healthful longevity.

The sensationalism of what is for sale by the complex has largely excluded the important consideration of how flexible the red blood cells are within the pipes. The exclusion that regards the abilities of the trillions of microscopic sponges within has cost owners in America plenty. This is evidenced by both the quality of life lost and in the need for symptom control medicine with all it's side effects and diminished out comes.

When these microscopic sponges are pliable their ability to carry oxygen, nutrients, and deliver important body hormones is optimal. This process can be thought of as similar to when a sponge gets wrung from its water content. Like wise when red blood cells are at the level of the capillary and getting squeezed of their contents of hormones, nutrients and oxygen, their flexibility is a crucial determinant of how efficient one receives the molecules that are necessary for life to continue. Processes that stiffen the red blood cell predictably will lessen this life giving process and the owner will get a little bit older.

There is no need to worry about the details mentioned above because throughout the remainder of the book these will be better explained and ways to heal will also be discussed. In addition, the immune cells that are also within the blood vessel will be discussed in section five. It is included here so as to complete an introductory discussion of how rust and blood pressure elevation hardens more than just the vessels.

The goal of the next chapter is to offer pause when the diagnosis of high blood pressure arises. During the pause one needs to consider their level of motivation. Without motivation, symptom control medicine is all that is possible. However, when one truly is motivated to explore possible ways to heal the blood pressure elevation there is little risk with placing some attention on what may have led them to the pressure problem. Healing paths have no side effects. Many times when healing paths are explored there is no need for the complex's symptom control approachers are succeeding in limiting the thinking of healing possibilities available to western owners. This manual attempts to steer clear of religious belief systems proselytizing and allow the reader to choose their own understanding of why they are here on this planet and where they are going when they die.

Western scientific thinking often lacks understanding of the organizing energy contained within living systems. This limits healing opportunities. For this reason it is necessary to discuss in foreign scientific terms how energy moves in living creatures. If the reader allows this, what science has revealed about how emotional energies impact cells can be discussed.

This becomes important if one wants to see the inconsistencies that are revealed in mainstream medicine. When the energy contained in living things is infused in the discussion, often times the alternative treatment modalities begin to make more sense and seem less superstitious. Conversely, the much touted and publicized approaches pandered by the mainstream power complex begin to look frightening.

Chapter 3

High Blood Pressure

Mainstream medicine claims that more than ninety percent of all high blood pressure is from unknown causes. The implication usually leads doctors and patients to believe it is largely genetically determined. It is as if whenever the genetics get blamed the next step becomes how clever science is about their symptom control approaches. At the same time there is very little discussion of how the survival of the fittest led to the aberrant genes being selected through the ages. Healing paths open up when one begins to look at the outdated survival advantages, which owners who had these genetic tendencies possessed. The examples of insulin production and sodium conservation are both obsolete survival advantages carried over from the ancestors of primitive times. The case of insulin will be discussed at an introductory level here and more completely throughout the text. The case of sodium retention was introduced in chapter one and will be further introduced in this chapter.

The ancestor who could make insulin during times of plenty was at a big advantage during times of scarcity. A survival advantage occurred because insulin caused both a behavioral effect and a metabolic effect. Insulin stimulated within the owner a behavioral pre-occupation with food. This behavioral preoccupation focused the owner on feeding. Insulin's message content creates a preoccupation with the next feeding event. However, food scarcity never comes and owners with this survival trait tend to become fat and have high 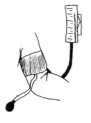 blood pressure, as well. The continued exposure to high insulin message content directs the liver to make fat and cholesterol. The old survival advantage has become a curse in today's world of high carbohydrate foods. This curse occurs in today's world because the owner who can make more insulin than the next owner will make extra fat, as well. One can heal their insulin caused high blood pressure problem when they are motivated and have a way to heal.

The second outdated genetic trait concerns the ability to retain sodium better than the next owner.[6] In prehistoric times sodium was rare. Natural food has many more times potassium than sodium. The owner during times of low sodium availability could conserve body sodium and therefore have a survival advantage. Today it is the curse of high blood pressure because processed food has a reversed mineral content from that of natural food. Natural food has high potassium and low sodium. However, processed food has very high sodium and much lower potassium content (sections two, three, four and five).

High Blood Pressure and Nutritional Remedies

The subject of this chapter is high blood pressure. The discussion will include the causes of high blood pressure, and some simple supplements and methods that can be used to reduce high blood pressure. The owner who uses these methods suggested may avoid the need for prescription medications and their unavoidable side effects. The earlier in the disease process that nutritional intervention is implemented then the higher the success rate for blood pressure reduction. When the owner addresses the nutritional cause of their elevated blood pressure, the need for prescription medication will decrease and further damage to their organs will diminish.

Chapter 1 described three common imbalances that cause an elevation of blood pressure (magnesium, sodium and potassium). Chapter two described how stiff red blood cells contribute significantly to blood pressure elevation. This chapter will describe other nutritional events that affect elevated blood pressure. The discussion in this chapter will rely on information provided in chapters 1 and 2. The information in chapters 1 and 2 will be discussed in light of the new factors that are introduced in this chapter. The goal of this chapter is to provide some additional insight of ways to heal from high blood pressure. The ways one can heal is the goal instead of the acceptance of symptom control medicine's paradigms.

When Adrenals Have Deficient Molecular Parts Blood Pressure Will Rise

Specific deficiencies in the adrenal gland can initiate the hypertension disease process. The owner using nutritional strategies can successfully treat these deficiencies. These nutritional strategies can reduce the owner's blood pressure and lover the owner's heart disease risk profiles, as well.

This first adrenal deficiency is called the methyl donor deficiency syndromes. Deficiencies of the various components of the important methyl donor system induce both high blood pressure and heart disease states.

There are differences in the message content between epinephrine and nor-epinephrine (both are known as catecholamines). When certain nutritional deficiencies develop epinephrine is the first to decrease and concurrently more nor-epinephrine is produced. This situation leads to significant physiological consequences within the blood vessel. The altered blood vessel performance then increases the risk for heart disease from the resulting high blood pressure.

The adrenal gland is divided into two components. They are the cortex and medulla. Biological, emotional, and environmental stresses are hard on both compartments of one's adrenal gland. Stress constantly triggers the steroid producing outer section of the adrenal gland. This causes cortisol to be secreted (among other steroids). Only when sufficient cortisol is in the blood stream can the cell receptors recognize epinephrine and nor-epinephrine message content.

Epinephrine and nor-epinephrine are also released by the adrenal medulla under stressful stimuli. This fact is important because without cortisol preparing the manufacture of the receptors for these adrenal medulla hormones (epinephrine and nor-epinephrine) their message content will go unrecognized (the hierarchy of hormones of section two). This subsection will only address the nutritionally induced imbalance between epinephrine and nor-epinephrine.

Normally the adrenal medulla secretes 90% epinephrine and only 10% nor-epinephrine. Epinephrine is preferred because it opens up the blood supply to the heart, skeletal muscles, and the liver. In contrast, nor-epinephrine does not do this. All other blood vessels, except the brain where blood flow is kept constant in the healthful state, are directed to clamp down when nor-epinephrine is the message (hormones contain message content). The net effect of epinephrine message content is a lowered peripheral vascular resistance because the muscle and liver blood vessel beds are so large. This effect is commonly referred to as a lower diastolic blood pressure. Epinephrine has this effect within the body even when the epinephrine level within the blood stream is relatively high. Epinephrine also increases cardiac performance, which may result in a slight rise in systolic blood pressure.

The effects of epinephrine within the heart, liver and skeletal muscle vessels are in direct contrast to the message that nor-epinephrine delivers to these blood vessels. Nor-epinephrine's message content directs the vessels to clamps down on everything except the blood supply to the brain. Nor-epinephrine's message causes the blood supply in all the vessels to constrict. In the brain the blood flow is kept constant. When blood vessels constrict without a corresponding dilation somewhere else blood pressure elevates. When owners are healthy the adrenal medulla (inner adrenal layer) manufactures 90% epinephrine and only 10% nor-epinephrine. However, when the adrenal medulla is deficient in certain vitamins and cofactors this ratio changes for the worse. A nutritionally caused inability to make epinephrine will tend to raise blood pressure when nor-epinephrine is secreted instead of epinephrine.

Both of these hormones act rapidly and effectively for the redistribution of blood flow. This effect causes the blood stream to maintain an adequate flow of blood in the brain during normal movement of the body. Without the outpouring of epinephrine or nor-epinephrine unconsciousness would result. For example, when an owner gets out of bed the forces of gravity cause the blood pressure to suddenly drop. When an owner is healthy their adrenal medullas make epinephrine in sufficient quantities to deliver a smooth machine that goes from lying flat to standing upright with grace and ease. Normally these hormones have a lifespan of about 2 minutes within the blood stream. Because of this very short lifespan of these two hormones there is a constant need for these hormones when one is either upright or under stress.

There is another process that occurs during body movement which effects blood pressure level. When an owner stands up or is stressed, there is a discharge of the sympathetic nerves. The endings of these nerves exist on the blood vessels. These nerves release nor-epinephrine only, onto the motor end plate of the smooth muscles of the blood vessels. The release of nor-epinephrine causes these muscles to contract and thereby constrict the affected blood vessels.

Nor-epinephrine released from the sympathetic nerves has a direct effect on the blood vessel muscles. Concurrently nor-epinephrine released from the adrenal medulla into the blood stream diffuses towards the same muscular layer but from the other direction. The additive effect between the sympathetic nerve activation that releases nor-epinephrine into the blood stream and the adrenal secreted nor-epinephrine has a powerful role in elevating blood pressure. The moderator of high blood pressure in these situations is epinephrine. Epinephrine increases blood flow to the heart, muscles, and liver. Adequate epinephrine release is therefore cornerstone in the prevention of high blood pressure.

Normally, this results in a tug-of-war between the full contraction and full relaxation of the blood vessel. Where a blood vessel ends up on the continuum is determined by the sum of the informational substances within the blood stream and the nervous tone instructions that reach this blood vessel. When a sub-optimal or unbalanced release of adrenal medulla derived epinephrine occurs then an increase in blood pressure becomes likely. When the owner is aware of this process a nutritional strategy may be implemented to reduce blood pressure and exacerbations of the symptoms of heart disease.

In order to obtain epinephrine the adequate molecular building parts and all of the nutritional cofactors must be present within the adrenal gland. These factors are a necessary pre-condition for the biosynthesis of epinephrine within the adrenal gland. Epinephrine and nor-epinephrine are derived from adequate supplies of the amino acid tyrosine. Tyrosine can be obtained from the amino acid phenylalanine.

The adrenal gland cannot convert tyrosine to epinephrine unless all of the nutritional cofactors are present within the adrenal medulla. Each step of the assembly line that eventually leads to the end product of epinephrine has a scientifically validated cofactor that must be present. If any one of these nutritional cofactors are missing, assembly stops and epinephrine synthesis becomes impossible.

The most common deficiency, which occurs in the adrenal medulla, involves the methyl donor system. The methyl donor system is needed for the conversion of nor-epinephrine to epinephrine. The last step in the assembly process is the conversion of nor-epinephrine to epinephrine. This last step cannot occur without a particular cofactor that is used with each epinephrine molecule that is made. This is one of the cofactors vulnerable to deficiency. This cofactor is called S-Adenosyl methionine (SAMe for short). SAMe is part of the methyl donor system. The SAMe cofactor donates its one methyl group to make one new epinephrine molecule. This spent cofactor has to be recharged. If it is not recharged it is called S-adenosyl homocysteine. This deactivated molecule will further degrade into adenosine and homocysteine within the blood stream.

Unless there is adequate SAMe available in the body, there cannot be adequate epinephrine biosynthesis. Insufficient epinephrine biosynthesis leads to an increased biosynthesis of nor-epinephrine. Increased release of nor-epinephrine will raise the blood pressure. There is an additional exacerbating factor for blood pressure elevation when SAMe is deficient.

When SAMe is depleted there is a marked decrease in the body's ability to clear both epinephrine and nor-epinephrine from the blood stream. Not only does the body have the wrong hormone being secreted (nor-epinephrine) because of the SAMe deficiency, but because of this same deficiency there is a decreased ability to remove nor-epinephrine from the blood stream! These hormones are cleared from the body when other SAMe's in the circulation methylates them. When nor-epinephrine has these types of methyl additions they become inactive and readily secreted from the kidney into the urine. The owner can become trapped in a vicious cycle of high blood pressure because the body is deficient in its ability to manufacture epinephrine and in the clearance of the sub-optimal nor-epinephrine. Without inactivation from other SAMe in the circulation this hormone is free to continue spreading it's message.

Nutritional attention for the ways to recharge one's methyl donor system (SAMe is one of the members in this group) often has the ability to heal the epinephrine deficiency and the nor-epinephrine excess. The correction of epinephrine deficiency is important because only epinephrine can oppose the clamping down of the sympathetic nerves during stressful times. When epinephrine output is deficient during adrenal medulla activation the blood pressure rises dramatically. The blood pressure rises dramatically because all information is contraction information at the blood vessel level. This is because only epinephrine moderates the contractile response. Epinephrine can do this because it has message content, which directs the liver, heart and skeletal muscles blood vessels to dilate. Conversely, nor-epinephrine cannot do this because it contains all contractile message content. All blood vessels in the body, except the brain, are being directed to contract, therefore, the blood pressure rises dramatically. The same deficiency that diminishes synthesis of epinephrine also causes the diminished breakdown of elevated nor-epinephrine. This is because SAMe is necessary for the inactivation of epinephrine and nor-epinephrine.

Only epinephrine has the special message property of opening up the blood vessels within the heart, skeletal muscle, and liver. When sufficient epinephrine occurs the body is directing blood into important areas and preventing dramatic blood pressure elevation. Blood pressure does not rise dramatically because the increased blood flow within these areas offsets the decreased blood flow elsewhere within the body. Within the rest of the body (excluding the brain) epinephrine directs the clamping down of blood vessels (constriction raises the pressure). Usually the net effect is a slight rise in the upper blood pressure value (systolic) and a slight lowering of the lower blood pressure reading (diastolic). This is called a widened pulse pressure. A widened pulse pressure indicates an increased cardiac output. In contrast, the stress response directed from the sympathetic nerves directs the constriction of all blood vessels except the brain. Adequate epinephrine release is crucial in times of stress to prevent the sky rocketing of the blood pressure. Sky rocketing blood pressure means that blood flow delivery to heart, muscle and liver is decreased. The sympathetic nerve activation coupled with the constriction effects of nor-epinephrine from the adrenal medulla will increase blood pressure, without adequate epinephrine.

The below listed cofactors are well documented in basic biochemistry textbooks as all being necessary for epinephrine to be manufactured. Basic medical physiology textbooks point out the marked difference between the effects on blood flow patterns and blood pressure between epinephrine and nor-epinephrine.

The synthetic sequence of catecholamines is tyrosine-dopa- dopamine-nor epinephrine-epinephrine. The necessary cofactors that are needed in the synthesis sequence of tyrosine to the end product epinephrine are: tetrahydrobiopteran (made from folate), pyradoxil phosphate (vitamin B6), vitamin C, and SAMe.

There are many necessary additional cofactors and vitamins which are needed for the recharging of SAMe. These cofactors and vitamins which are needed to recharge SAMe are called the methyl donor system. The molecules that make up the methyl donor system are: methionine, serine, vitamin B6, vitamin B12 and folate. These factors are involved in the remanufacture of SAMe once it has been degraded to S-adenosyl homocysteine. The methyl group is needed to convert nor-epinephrine to epinephrine. All of these cofactors, which are involved in recreating SAMe, are known collectively as the methyl donor system. Depletion of this system has predictable consequences but paradoxically has been largely ignored by mainstream medicine in the clinical setting. It should be emphasized that the consumption of extra methionine without proper attention to the adequacy of the other methyl donors will lead to elevated blood homocysteine levels because of the inability to recharge SAMe after each epinephrine is made.

Summary of vitamins and cofactors for the conversion of tyrosine to epinephrine

Tetrahydrobiopterin (made from folate)
Vitamin C
Vitamin B6
SAMe

A real food diet will provide most of these cofactors and the methyl donor group, especially if one eats eggs. Eggs are rich in methionine. However, a processed food diet will likely lack one or more of these vitamins and cofactors. Many B-vitamin formulations are often deficient in folate content. Without adequate folate the methyl donor system will not function. All members of the methyl donor system need to be present or SAMe levels fall and homocysteine levels will rise.

The rise of blood homocysteine levels has been documented to signal a powerful risk factor for blood vessel disease (chapter one). However, if one applies basic biochemical principles to the analysis of homocysteine's role in the development of heart disease it reveals it to be an unlikely agent in the direct injury of blood vessels. Rather it is more probable that it is a biochemical red flag that something is wrong within the owner's nutrition status. When blood homocysteine rises epinephrine synthesis will decrease proportionately.

Elevated homocysteine levels denote a malfunction within the methyl donor system that leads to decreased epinephrine production and increased nor-epinephrine production. Elevated blood homocysteine levels may reflect a convenient biochemical marker to identify a depleted methyl donor system. One of the pathologies of a depleted methyl donor system is it causes high blood pressure to develop (among other things). Elevated blood pressure and diminished blood flow to the heart muscle will result whenever nor-epinephrine occurs in the blood stream in higher than normal amounts compared to epinephrine. Dr. Steven Gordon of Whitefish, Montana, points out that finding an elevated blood homocysteine level may provide high blood pressure's etiology and it's solution as well.

When one appreciates the fundamental role that both a highly functional and interrelated methyl donor system plays a way to treat blood pressure becomes possible. When this approach is considered in disease prevention strategies it begins to make sense why the adrenal medulla nutritional state is important.

This brings up the beauty of healing paths versus symptom control medicine. Prescriptions are all about symptom control and contain all the inevitable side effects as well. Healing does not have negative side effects. This is because once a problem is fixed it is over with.

None of these cofactors is more risky than if one takes of a multiple vitamin, in the general population. Each of the above listed cofactors has proven biochemical necessity in the synthesis of the epinephrine hormone. Healing involves working with the body to correct unbalanced states. When a given owner is healthy their adrenals predictably contain optimal amounts of each of these cofactors and produce adequate epinephrine to maximize bodily function.

The caution is to avoid allergic reactions, which some owners have to the fillers and trace contaminants in certain brands of nutritional supplements. In general one should choose the best brand and quality (pharmaceutical grade).

Once in a while there will be an owner who is allergic to vitamin C. Obtain the advice of a competent physician who will work on natural healing of the adrenal function and reduce the blood pressure naturally.

It turns out that the sympathetic tone is often increased in hypertensives and this central nervous system effect contributes greatly to the observed increase in blood pressure. The neurotransmitter involved in this case is nor-epinephrine. What is often under appreciated with regard to blood pressure is the tug of war between the sum of the hormones' message content within the blood stream and the message content delivered by the central nervous system. This dynamic equilibrium provides insight into the consequences of epinephrine deficiency.

Nor-epinephrine is a more powerful messenger when delivered within the nerves to the blood vessel, these nerves end in the muscular layer and when active direct contraction. However, when nor-epinepherine is acting within the blood stream it has less ability to raise blood pressure at a given concentration of secretion. Only within the nerves does it have powerful contraction effects. This is a subtle but important point. Epinephrine deficiency can cause blood pressure elevation merely because there is an insufficient counter balance to the powerful nerve message contained in the presence of nor-epinephrine.

Epinephrine has powerful vascular effects starting at 50pg/ml, but nor-epinephrine doesn't exert its vasoconstrictor effects within the blood stream until 1500pg/ml. Nor-epinephrine's ability to raise blood pressure is mainly through its affect as a neurotransmitter within the sympathetic nervous system. Epinephrine is a counter response to the sympathetic nervous system's tendency to raise blood pressure.

The second deficiency syndrome that leads to high blood pressure

The second deficiency syndrome, often overlooked in many owners that suffer from high blood pressure, is nitric oxide deficiency. The lack of nitric oxide gas in certain situations can raise blood pressure. Nitric oxide is manufactured in the blood vessels. This gas is a powerful artery and vein relaxant. Healthy owners produce nitric oxide in the right amounts and locations. This needs to happen to keep the blood flow optimal.

A deficiency in the production of this powerful and locally acting messenger gives the green light to many nasty blood pressure raising substances. These blood pressure raising substances in the presence of adequate nitric oxide otherwise would not be manufactured within the blood vessel lining cell. Nitric oxide is a powerful blood vessel wall relaxant. Nitric oxide is also a powerful suppressor of the insulin-induced manufacture of the blood pressure raising hormone, endothelin. Both nitric oxide and endothelin are informational substances that act exclusively locally (they are type 4 informational substances in the hierarchy of hormones, section 2). The enzyme, nitric oxide synthase, which makes nitric oxide gas from the amino acid arginine needs four cofactors or it cannot perform this task. The absence of any one of these cofactors causes a nitric oxide deficiency and the blood pressure rises.

The enzyme that makes nitric oxide is called nitric oxide synthase. It needs the presence of the cofactors arginine, Thiol, tetrahydrobiopterin (made from folate), flavin mononucleotide (FMN), and flavin dinucleotide (FAD) in order to produce nitric oxide. FMN and FAD are made from riboflavin (vitamin B2). A deficiency of any one of these cofactors, within the numerous cells that line the body's waterways, causes diminished nitric oxide production. Diminished production tips the antique weight scale in the direction of unopposed blood pressure elevation.

The menu of cofactors required for the production of nitric oxide is one of the reasons that garlic is given credit for lowering blood pressure Garlic contains thiols, which is one of the cofactors necessary for the production of nitric oxide. The other four cofactors are also obtained from nutritional sources. Tetrahydrobiopterin is obtained by consuming royal bee jelly or is manufactured within the body from folate. FAD and FMN are obtained by having adequate riboflavin (vitamin B2) in the diet. Lastly, arginine is an amino acid that needs to be adequately consumed in the diet or made from Krebs cycle intermediates. Krebs cycle intermediates are mostly found within the mitochondria of cells.

In some instances oral replacement is not adequate for these types of deficiencies. There are some cases where owners for one reason or another lack the ability to absorb optimal vitamin nutrition orally. When this is the case it would warrant the extra precaution of intravenous or intra-muscular vitamin replacement therapy.

Most of the above vitamins and cofactors are contained in conventional chelation protocols. Perhaps this is a partial explanation for their continued devotees in the face of the ongoing mainstream medicine criticism. The addition of thiols would complete the supplementation of the above necessary cofactors needed by nitric oxide synthase. In the case of methyl donor deficiency, mentioned in the previous subsection, the addition of folate, methionine and serine would possibly prove of benefit in the chelation setting.

Prescription medications that raise nitric oxide levels, but it is a secret

There is an additional insight about nitric oxide production and it's relationship to a popular blood pressure lowering medication called, the angiotensin converting enzyme inhibitors. These types of medications affect the histamine like content of the body, which also powerfully lowers blood pressure. The mainstream textbooks say very little about this powerful association. Instead, they discuss in great detail the blood pressure lowering effects as being the result of lowered angiotensin two levels.

It is really quite a shock to most physicians when they begin to see evidence that the touted mechanism for a drugs action is not always the only way that they have an effect on the body. The ACE inhibitors are such an example. The drug literature focuses almost exclusively on the supposed powerful role that angiotensin plays in tightening up the blood vessels directly. However, very little of this literature discusses the well-documented fact that inhibition of this very same enzyme raises the total body content of a histamine like substance, bradykinin. This explains why a dry nagging cough is the number one side effect. In addition, bradykinin is well known to lower blood pressure but it is paid for with the price of increased leakiness of the capillaries in areas like the lungs and kidney. May be there was a marketing problem if this mechanism was related to an increased histamine like substance content within the body. No one will probably ever know for sure. Nonetheless, it is instructive to see a possible bigger problem with other drugs in how the physician gets 'groomed' into thinking about how these drugs work.

Because these drugs increase bradykinin within the body they also increase nitric oxide production as well. Increased bradykinin is a powerful stimulant for turning on the enzymatic machinery within the endothelial cells lining the arteries. Bradykinin and histamine share the same receptors in the body. They also act in a similar manner. They contain similar message content. Once bradykinin becomes elevated it then tends to stimulate the mast cells to release histamine, as well.

The other touted benefit of these angiotensin converting enzyme inhibitors (ACE inhibitors), is there documented benefit in the preservation of kidney function. To understand that this benefit is both a circuitous and expensive solution in many cases one needs to recall four things. First, ACE inhibitors conserve body potassium and this has a known kidney protective effect on the tendency to become potassium deficient. This medication then lowers blood pressure despite the elevated sodium in the body by the less realized mechanism of increased bradykinin's within the body. Second, bradykinin increased presence also lowers blood pressure by being a powerful stimulus for nitric oxide production.

Third, if a given patient was correctly counseled about a real food diet instead of a processed food diet, before kidney damage occurs from a chronically low potassium, blood pressure medication in these cases would no longer be needed.

The fourth fact to understand about the consequences of decreased angiotensin two production is the affect this has on the adrenal glands. Rather than get all lost in the inconsistent evidence that these ACE inhibitors have on aldosterone levels it becomes more instructive to look at the consistent evidence. The evidence is consistent that decreased angiotensin two will directly correlate with a decreased ACTH output. A decreased ACTH output will decrease the stimulation to the adrenal glands to release aldosterone, cortisol and DHEA.

This little detail has powerful implications for another mechanism for how these medications lower the blood pressure. It also has powerful implications for why diseases like autoimmune disease are made worse when these owners take these types of medications. Owners are made worse with autoimmune disease because they already have a wounded adrenal system (section two). The addition of an ACE inhibitor will only exaggerate the diminished adrenal function, which operates in these diseases. This also provides a clue as to why these same types of owners will be at increased risk for Neutropenia and lymphocytosis (section two).

Now it is time to turn the analysis on its head. The biggest road block mentally is in the realization that people who consume high potassium and magnesium diets relative to total sodium intake are also going to have a high aldosterone. Increased potassium intake will powerfully stimulate aldosterone release. However, in these cases a diuresis will ensue because total body sodium is not excessive. Stress or ACTH alone will tend to raise aldosterone secretion and in this situation, of a high sodium diet, this is inappropriate. When this happens blood pressure will rise. The point to consider is that perhaps a little effort spent counseling an early hypertensive on how to change their mineral intake ratios by eating 'real foods' (section three) would have some merit before condemning them to medication with all it's side effects.

ACE inhibitors have been shown to improve a patient's clinical situation while in heart failure. What is not said is that histamine like substances have a powerful strengthening action on heart muscle performance. This effect is obviously one benefit of these medications. The increased histamine like content within the blood stream will increase the effectiveness of the heart pumping with each beat.

Steroids have a role in blood pressure

Certain steroids increase the calcium concentrations within the cells and therefore alter cell functions. The trigger to synthesize nitric oxide within the cells lining of the blood vessels is the increase of calcium concentrations within those blood vessel lining cells, the endothelium. Low insulin levels, high bradykinin levels, and high levels of certain steroids all lead to increased calcium within the cells that line the arteries, the endothelial cell.

The ability of certain steroids like progesterone to increase cell calcium content is well documented. When sperm encounters the progesterone molecule, within the cervical mucus, this promptly triggers the rise in intracellular calcium. High intracellular calcium will disable a sperm. This is one of the reasons that high progesterone levels prevent pregnancy.

This is routinely occurs within the central nervous system, as well. Progesterone affects the nerve cell's intracellular calcium concentration and also changes the neural cell's operational properties. In fact, progesterone, at very high levels produces anesthesia. At more physiologic levels there is a calming effect. Nerves become calm when they can charge up their membrane (increase the voltage about the membrane). Generally, nerves are less irritable when the membrane voltage is increased.

DHEA is at the highest concentration of any steroid within the blood vessels in the body. Because certain steroids increase cellular calcium it is not too far fetched to speculate that they are also one of the triggers that increase calcium concentrations within the endothelial cell. No one has specifically studied which steroid does this within the blood stream. However, it is probably progesterone or DHEA.

The emerging data suggests that steroids play an important role in blood vessel health. The effect that certain steroids have on cellular calcium concentrations will probably turn out to be another way that the body controls blood pressure. The ability of steroids like progesterone or DHEA to encourage nitric oxide formation could be a powerful determinant in blood vessel longevity. If the data proves to be accurate it would be another method of encouraging blood pressure back to optimal levels.

Syndrome X

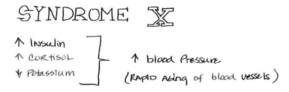

Another consequence of a low potassium diet concerns the fact that when potassium intake is low then more insulin becomes necessary to do the same job (insulin resistance). The increase of insulin and the consequent destructive hormonal cycle is made worse when chronic stress is included, as well. High insulin also is a powerful stimulant to fat cell growth. Lastly, that concerns the increased insulin, is how these people can often be thought of as the typical Syndrome X types.

Gerald Reaven, M.D., of Stanford University, coined the term, Syndrome X. This term describes those owners who are on an accelerated path for blood vessel rust production. Dr. Reaven believes that Syndrome X is secondary to having high blood insulin. He explains the clinical signs of this syndrome as the result of the high insulin state. His opinion of the clinical signs of the high insulin state are: increased abdominal fat, high blood pressure, increased blood triglyceride level, elevated LDL cholesterol, increased skin tag growths on the neck and under the arms, increased blood clotting tendency and an accelerated rusting (oxidation) rate within the blood vessels. This author feels that the signs of high blood pressure and increased rusting rate are better explained by two additional factors. One is the chronically elevated production of cortisol caused by a hectic lifestyle. The second is that these owners consume a processed food diet.

The syndrome X owners are on an accelerated tract to an old body. Their fundamental defect is both elevated insulin levels and a setting of increased stress (section two). Increased stress will accelerate potassium loss. Low potassium and low magnesium diets with elevated sodium intake will increase the disease activity (chapter one). In many ways a high stress hormone output could help explain how Syndrome X patients age so quickly and have high blood pressure as well. This is better illustrated by the fact that chronically elevated cortisol is like telling the body that there is always an emergency. When the body perceives an emergency (real or imagined) the body's energy gets redirected into survival pathways. In syndrome X owners the survival pathway is the norm instead of rejuvenation activities.

When body energy is chronically directed into survival pathways, the wear and tear changes will become more likely. Wear and tear changes become more likely secondary to the lack of cellular repair activities. This helps to explain why Syndrome X owners tend to age so quickly. Not only do they tend to have high insulin derived disease but also high cortisol derived disease. Cortisol directs body energy into catabolic pathways. Too much catabolism within the blood vessels leads to wear and tear changes.

The severity of the Syndrome X is exacerbated by the consumption of processed foods.

Dr. Reaven is right about insulin having some role in the blood pressure elevation of these owner types. One of the reasons that elevated insulin raises blood pressure is that it is a powerful stimulant to the blood vessel lining cells production of endothelin. When endothelin production increases blood pressure then rises. High insulin levels also diminish the ability of the blood vessel lining to produce nitric oxide. The diminished production of nitric oxide further reduces the body's ability to maintain an appropriate blood pressure level.

Large amounts of insulin within the blood stream require large amounts of cortisol to effectively counter insulin's behavior of moving every last sugar molecule out of the blood stream. Cortisol counters the effect of insulin by increasing the blood sugar levels. Cortisol, however, directs body energy and molecular building parts into survival pathways and out of repair and rejuvenation pathways. Anti-oxidant synthesis and blood vessel repair are deferred with a chronically high cortisol level. The stress effects exacerbate the effect which insulin has on cortisol levels. When the owner experiences chronically high levels of cortisol release, the body energy is directed away from cellular rejuvenation activities. Syndrome X causes the inefficient use of molecular building parts for repair activity by the body. The correction of this dysfunctional process begins when the healthy and appropriate ratio of cortisol and insulin is restored within the blood stream. This can be substantially accomplished by nutritional rather than symptom control treatment plans. Before a description of those strategies is provided a syndrome closely related to Syndrome X will be described. This syndrome can be treated by very similar nutritional strategies used for the treatment of Syndrome X.

The description of syndrome X provides an insight into the tendency for people with Type A personalities (hard driving and aggressive types) to develop heart disease. One, or both, of two different processes, could cause this tendency. The first process is the predictable increase of cortisol that occurs when the owner experiences the stress to perform and achieve during her/his daily activities. The increase in cortisol will direct the blood sugar to rise as part of the survival response. The increase in blood sugar demands a corresponding rise in insulin levels that facilitate the uptake of blood sugar. This elevated blood insulin, caused by type A behavior, has the identical effect on the body as the elevated blood insulin caused by dietary and nutritional behaviors. One consequence of increased insulin is the increased production of fat and cholesterol in the liver.

The second process, found in Type A personalities and Syndrome X is the development of blood vessel disease. There is evidence that the blood vessel disease is caused by the continued demand for more epinephrine secretion. Epinephrine secretion is normally increased as part of the stress response. The excessive demand for epinephrine can increase both the blood pressure and blood sugar raising tendencies. Blood pressure will tend to rise when the adrenal stimulation becomes chronic. When the adrenal stimulation becomes chronic, in the setting of nutritional cofactor deficiencies, the blood pressure raising nor-epinephrine begins to get secreted instead.

Keeping the above two considerations in mind add understanding of how exercise may benefit hard driving and over achieving types (type A personality) undo some of the metabolic aberrations mentioned above. This is accomplished in part by utilizing the blood sugar released by the direction of increased stress hormones, both cortisol and epinephrine (section 2). In addition, attention to rebuilding nutritional vitamin and mineral status will help alleviate the nutritionally derived causes of high blood pressure.

Finally, in order to complete the introductory discussion of syndrome X, the importance of IGF-1 levels needs mention. Healthy owners predictably have high normal IGF-1 levels. IGF-1 is synthesized within the liver in response to DHEA. Growth hormone release causes the IGF-1 stored within the liver to be released. Normal owners have at least one hundred times the IGF-1 in their circulation as they do insulin. IGF-1 acts like insulin for the cells outside the liver and fat. High IGF-1 levels lower the amount of insulin needed within the body. IGF-1 levels provide a mechanism for fuel uptake by cells outside the liver and fat cells between meals. In contrast, insulin is designed to facilitate the liver and fat cells to remove fuel out of the blood stream following meals. Troubles start around middle age in sedentary and stressed owners. These two lifestyle traits combine to diminish IGF-1 levels (section two, the muscle chapter and the liver chapter). A lower IGF-1 level means that insulin secretion must rise to abnormally high levels in order to attempt to offset the decrease in IGF-1 levels. This detail explains why Syndrome X types present with elevated fasting insulin levels. Healthy owners have greatly diminished insulin levels in the fasting state. Insulin has a half-life of ten to twenty minutes. Fasting insulin therefore is a pretty good marker for diminished IGF-1 levels (excluding diabetes). The primary health effect when IGF-1 levels fall and insulin levels rise concerns the activation of the fat and cholesterol making machinery within the body. The consequences of this fact are explained in the next chapter.

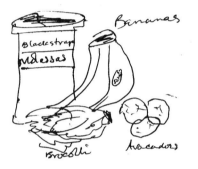
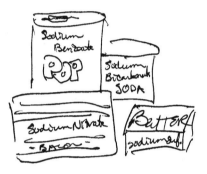

Mineral Table

Breads, etc.	Amount	Na+	K+	Cal	Mg++	Ca++
White Bread	1 slice	142	29	76	0	32
Rye Bread	1 slice	139	36	61	0	20
Whole Wheat Bread	1 slice	132	68	61	0	20
Biscuit	1 (2"dia.)	185	18	104	0	0
Cornbread	2 1/2 sq.	263	61	178	0	133
Pancake	1 (6" dia.)	412	112	164	16	60
Waffle	1 (7" dia.)	515	146	206	13	143
Graham Cracker	2(2 1/2" sq.)	95	55	55	14	12
Brown Rice	1 c + salt	550	137	236	86	20
White Rice	1 c + salt	767	57	223	26	24
Bran Flakes	1 cup	207	137	106	108	26
Corn Flakes	1 cup	251	30	92	16	6
Oatmeal	1 c (cooked)	523	146	132	57	22.5
Pufffed Rice	1 cup	148	33	140	0	10
Wheat Flakes	1 cup	310	81	106	108	100
Wheat Flour	1 cup	130	0	499	0	0
*Egg Noodles	1 cup	3	70	200	31	19
*Macaroni	1 cup	1	103	192	20	8
*Spaghetti	1 cup	1	103	192	0	0

Beverages	Amount	Na++	K+	Cal	Mg++	Ca++
Coffee, Instant	1 Tblspn	3	87	3	*80	*50
Coffee, Regular	1 cup	2	65	2	10	3
Beer	12 oz	25	90	150	46	36
Gin, Rum, Vodka	1 oz (80 proof)	0	1	65	0	0

Sweets	Amount	Na++	K+	Cal	Mg++	Ca++
Angel Food Cake	1/6 cake	340	106	322	0	88
Brownie	small	50	38	97	0	0
Chocolate Bittersweet	1 oz	1	174	135	30	6
Chocolate, cupcake	1 piece	74	35	92	0	0
Choc. chip cookies	10 (2.5" dia.)	421	141	495	0	32
Chocolate Syrup	1 oz	20	106	92	24	3
Gelatin, sweet	3 oz	270	0	315	0	1
Honey	1 Tblspn	1	11	64	0	1
Jelly	1 Tblspn	3	14	49	trace	4
Sherbert, Orange	1 cup	19	42	259	16	104
Sponge Cake	1/6 cake	220	114	196	0	42
Sugar, Brown	1 cup	44	499	541	0	187
Sugar, White	1 cup	2	6	770	trace	trace
Sugar, powdered	1 cup	1	4	462	trace	0

Fruits	Amount	Na++	K+	Cal	Mg++	Ca++
Apple	1 (2 1/2" dia.)	1	116	61	6	10
Apricots, Fresh	3 medium	1	301	55	8	15
Apricots, Dried	5 lg halves	6	235	62	11	10
Banana	1 medium	1	440	101	33	7

		Na++	K+	Cal	Mg++	Ca++
Blackberries	1cup	1	245	84	28	46
Cantalope	1/2 (5" dia.)	33	682	82	28	28
Cherries, Sweet	10 count	1	129	47	8	10
Dates	10 count	1	518	219	29	27
Figs	1 piece	1	126	52	8	18
Grapefruit	half	1	132	40	10	13
Grapes	1 cup	3	160	70	3	9
Honeydew Melon	half (6 1/2" dia.)	90	1881	247	9	8
Orange	1 medium	1	290	66	15	56
Peach	1 (2 3/4" dia.)	2	308	58	6	5
Pear	1 (2 1/2" dia.)	3	213	100	5	10
Pineapple	1 cup	2	226	81	22	12
Plum	1 (1"dia.)	0	30	7	<1	1
Prune, Dried	10 medium	5	448	164	51	58
Raisins	1 tablespoon	2	69	26	3	5
Raspberries	1 cup	1	267	98	22	28
Strawberries	1 cup	1	244	55	16	22
Tangerine	1 (2 3/8" dia.)	2	108	39	10	12
Watermelon	1 cup	2	160	42	18	14
Avocado	1 medium	21	1097	324	70	19

Fresh Vegetables	Amount	Na++	K+	Cal	Mg++	Ca++
Asparagus	1 cup	3	375	35	22	30
Beans, Lima	1 cup	3	1008	191	126	54
Beets	1 cup	81	452	58	28	22
Broccoli	1 cup	34	868	72	38	72
Carrot	1 medium	34	246	30	11	19
Celery	1 stalk	50	136	7	4	16
Corn, Sweet (no butter, no salt)	1 ear	0	131	70	34	2
Cucumber	1 large	18	481	45	33	42
Eggplant	1 cup	2	300	38	10	30
Lettuce, iceberg	1 head (6" dia.)	48	943	70	48	102
Onion	1 cup	17	267	65	16	32
Peas	1 cup	3	458	122	34	62
Potatoe, Baked	1 medium	6	782	145	55	20
Potatoe, Boiled	1 medium	4	556	104	30	7
Radishes	10 large	15	261	14	4	9
Spinach	1 cup	39	259	14	158	244
Sweet Potatoe	1 medium	15	367	272	32	70
Tomato	1 medium	4	300	27	13	6
Watercress	1 cup	18	99	7	8	40

Canned Vegetables	Amount	Na++	K+	Cal	Mg++	Ca++
Asparagus	14 1/2 oz can	970	682	74	22	34
Beans, Green	8 oz can	536	216	41	18	36
Beans, Lima	8 oz can	1070	1007	322	94	50
Beets	8 oz can	535	379	77	40	34
Carrots	8 oz can	535	272	64	22	62
Corn, Creamed	8 oz can	585	241	203	44	8
Peas	8 oz can	569	231	159	22	44
Spinach	8 oz can	519	550	42	132	194

*Tomatoes	8 oz can	36	273	88	13	6
Dairy Products	**Amount**	**Na+**	**K+**	**Cal**	**Mg++**	**Ca++**
American Cheese	1 oz.	322	23	105	6	174
Blue Cheese Dressing	1 Tblspn	164	6	76	0	0
Cheddar Cheese	1 oz.	147	17	84	8	204
Cream Cheese	1 oz.	80	25	110	2	23
Cottage Cheese	1 cup	580	144	172	14	154
Parmesan Cheese	1 oz.	208	42	111	14	390
Swiss Cheese	1 oz.	70	29	105	10	272
Butter (salted)	1 stick	1119	26	812	2	27
Butter (unsalted)	1 stick	<1	<1	812	2	27
Buttermilk (cultured)	1 cup	319	343	*88	27	285
Skim Milk	1 cup	127	355	*88	28	302
Whole Milk	1 cup	122	351	159	33	291
Evaporated Milk	1 cup	297	764	345	60	658
Heavy Cream	1 Tblspn	5	13	53	1	10
Ice Cream (no salt)	1 cup	84	241	257	9	88
Hot Chocolate	1 cup	120	370	238	24	93
Hot Cocoa	1 cup	128	363	243	0	0
Egg Yolk	1 medium	8	15	52	1	23
Egg white	1 medium	42	40	15	4	2
Egg Broiled	1 medium	54	57	72	5	25
Yogurt, Plain	1 cup	115	323	152	26	274
Meat and Poultry	**Amount**	**Na++**	**K+**	**Cal**	**Mg++**	**Ca++**
Beef						
Corned Beef Hash	1 cup	1188	440	398	14	9
Frankfurter	1 medium	627	125	176	6	7
Heart	1 oz	29	66	53	0	0
Hamburger	2.9 oz	49	221	235	5	2
Liver	3 oz	156	323	195	0	0
Rib Roast	6-9 ribs	149	680	1342	22	11
Flank Steak	3 oz	45	207	167	26	7
Porterhouse Steak	11 oz	155	680	1400	28	9
Sirloin Steak	11 oz	173	793	1192	32	12
T-Bone Steak	11 oz	152	660	1431	28	9
Lamb						
Chop	1 medium	51	234	341	27	28
Roast	3 oz	60	273	158	36	16
Pork						
Bacon	1 slice	123	29	72	<2	<1
Chops	3 oz	47	214	300	15	6
Ham, baked	3 oz	770	241	159	18	5
Roast	3 oz	698	218	281	0	0
Spareribs	2 pieces	65	299	792	0	0
Veal						
Loincut	3 oz	60	570	220	9	10
Roast	3 oz	57	259	229	21	23

Chicken

Broiled	4 oz	75	310	154	28	19
*Light Meat	4 oz	60	240	120	25	18
*Dark Meat	4 oz	45	100	180	27	19

Turkey

White Meat	4 oz	70	349	150	29	29
Dark Meat	4 oz	42	169	87	26	26

Fresh Fish & Seafood

Bass, striped	3 oz	0	0	168	27	69
Clams	4 clams	144	218	56	12	52
Cod	3 oz	93	345	144	36	16
Crab	1 cup	0	0	144	0	78
Flounder	3 oz	201	498	171	27	15
Haddock	3 oz	150	297	141	33	27
Halibut	3 oz	114	447	144	72	37
Lobster	1 cup	305	261	138	80	138
Mackerel	3 oz	0	0	201	63	9
Oysters	3 small	21	34	19	45	39
Salmon	3 oz	99	378	156	29	180
Shrimp	3 oz	159	195	192	30	45

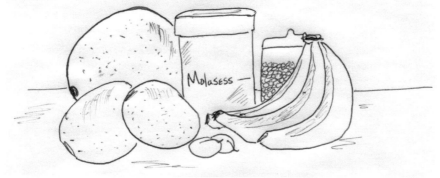

SECTION II

THE HORMONES GIVETH AND THE HORMONES TAKETH AWAY

Principle 3

Balanced hormones equal a youthful state of being. Imbalance results from either an excess or deficiency of individual hormones. Imbalanced hormones accelerate cellular deterioration, which leads to an old body. Western medicine overlooks this fundamental truth causing dietary failure, brittle bones, blood vessel disease, changes in body stature, diminished organ function, decreased mental ability, loss of muscle and joint function, immune dysfunction, refractory depression, and shriveled or flabby skin. The alert reader needs to be aware of the discrepancies often missed by the conventional approach to hormonal imbalance.

Mainstream medicine has numerous treatment strategies. These treatment strategies only address the consequences of hormonal deteriorations in a peripheral way. Many physicians focus their medical treatment on the 'symptom control' paradigm. Symptom control has little to do with how one heals and always has side effects and toxicities. This leads to more medicines and procedures. Blindly following the symptom control complex leaves the typical owner with copious amounts of medicine and many procedural scars.

Medications and a history of medical procedures are often poor attempts for regaining lost quality of life. The quality of one's hormones most substantially impacts the owner's health and ability to age gracefully. The holistic approach to degenerative processes includes the medical data necessary

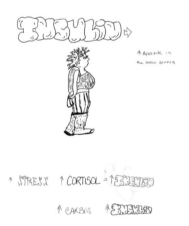

to restore hormonal health. By addressing the owner's hormonal status and utilizing a holistic approach to hormonal health, the possibility of healing many chronic-degenerative and age-associated diseases becomes possible.

Mainstream medicine also possesses the medical data necessary to restore hormonal health. Unfortunately, traditional medical texts present this medical data in a disintegrated format. This creates substantial consequences. First, incomplete scientific holisms cause many unnecessary chronic-degenerative diseases. Many physicians are not trained to relate the more complete and congruous scientific data. Second, supplementing one or two deficient hormones with a synthetic or altered mixture leads to side effects and toxicities. In both common methods of practice, hormonal imbalances or inferior replacement hormones, the owner ages more rapidly.

Science provides data to accomplish an effective and appropriate hormone balance in an owner. This natural process occurs when hormones achieve an improved quality and proportionate relationship. Imbalance reflects the quality of life lost by not adhering to improvement of the hormone status.

Before hormone quality can be understood, one needs a workable and concise definition of what qualifies as a hormone. Each hormone, by virtue of its unique shape, carries a message through the blood stream to specific cells.

This precise shape activates change within a range of receptors when it is delivered to the cell. Very slight changes in the shape of the hormone change the message content. The messages direct the cell on how to spend its cellular or behavioral energy.

The quality of the hormones determines the efficiency of the message content. The message content determines how a cell will spend its available energy. With this in mind, confusion can be avoided in medical literature. Medical literature is uniformly disorganized in making it easy for doctors and patients to grasp the hierarchy between the different hormone classes. As one becomes more knowledgeable about the hormone hierarchy, they will be less gullible when they read a sensationalized version of the latest scientific discovery.

Chapter 4

Obesity

Obesity Can Be Cured When Hormones Are Optimal

With sensationalism in mind, obesity serves as a constant example of medical strategies that fail. By addressing hormonal factors, restoring and maintaining appropriate proportions and quality, obesity can be healed.

Inadequate attention is given to the influence hormones have on regulating body weight. Each diet addresses some of these issues, but ignore others. Nutrition experts counsel those with large weight to frame ratios of the need to reduce caloric intake. Most approaches ignore the role hormones play in feeding behaviors. The seven main hormones imbalances, which perpetuate obesity, can be thought of as a Torture Chamber effect.

An effective weight loss strategy must include a method of obtaining and maintaining the proper relationship between the body's hormones. The strategy must also include a method to affect the behavior caused by the hormones.

Though there are seven main hormones, initially the focus will concentrate on the first three as they relate to obesity - insulin, cortisol, and androgen. Insulin contributes most to making fat. Cortisol sabotages dieters by increasing insulin under stress. Androgens counteract the ability of insulin to make fat.

Consider the biggest fat maker – insulin. When this hormone is elevated beyond healthful levels, a vicious cycle of failed diet attempts and progressive weight gain occurs. Progressive obesity requires a high production of insulin. Insulin contains a powerful message to activate the appetite center within the brain. Once activated, the desire for the next feeding event becomes excessive. The tendency toward obesity is the direct result of elevated insulin levels causing an excessive compulsion about food.

Insulin is the hormone of abundance. In prehistoric time, abundant insulin allowed the owner to store energy as fat when food was available. Erratic food supply made this primitive body design essential for the survival of the species by focusing the body energy on feeding. Conversely, in times of scarcity there is little need for insulin because all available fuel is needed to survive. The predictability of the modern world food supply made this original body design feature obsolete.

The molecular configuration of insulin plus the bound receptor creates specific message content. The different receptors possessed by different cells determine the final message that a cell receives.

Insulin uniquely directs the different fuel types into cellular storehouses. When all the cell cupboards are full, the liver is told to make carbohydrates into fat. Insulin further facilitates and assists in the storage of fat in the belly area. Abdominal obesity stands out as a good clinical marker for owners who have high insulin levels. Conversely, insulin deficiency, which occurs in juvenile onset diabetes, presents itself with a loss of body fat.

Cortisol sabotages those who attempt to diet under conditions of chronic life stress. High stress leads to higher stress hormone secretion. Increased cortisol levels lead to the amplification of the insulin message. The amplification of the insulin message is another obsolete feature in the original human design.

The intent of the original human design was to survive the physical stresses of the prehistoric world. Survival of a physical stress requires ample body fuel availability to increase the physical strength. Cortisol increases body fuel availability dramatically by directing the liver to dump both sugar and fat into the blood stream of the stressed owner.

Cortisol causes other hormones to amplify fuel availability also. Modern stress is usually mental stress. The body cannot tell the difference between mental or physical stress. The body recognizes the unused fuel released by mental stress as an inappropriate elevation of blood fuel (sugar and fat). Since the fuel cortisol directs into the blood stream isn't needed, there is an increase in insulin.

The extra fuel created by mental stress requires insulin because without a physical challenge the extra blood fuel has nowhere to go. The increase in insulin causes an increase in the message content to direct the manufacture of body fat. This commonly overlooked fact further stacks the odds against dietary success in the unaware owner. Cortisol levels will increase without consistent habits that either reduce or counter stress. Without a plan when one is under stress, the tendency toward obesity will increase.

Carbohydrate consumption, in relation to protein or fat, stimulates a powerful insulin release. When the appetite center is stimulated, a feeling of hunger follows the increase in insulin.

Thus, a vicious cycle is started. The obese owner consumes carbohydrates. Excess insulin created by the carbohydrates creates the message of ravenous hunger. Hunger creates the desire to eat more carbohydrates that are turned into fat. This can be thought of as the torture chamber effect.

As the obese owner grows, in size, his body secretes even more insulin for each unit of carbohydrate. There are more fat cells given the message to take more fuel out of the blood stream. When mental stress increases, the problem compounds due to the elevation in blood sugar. Unlike physical stress, mental stress does not require an increase of blood fuel for survival. Insulin secretion becomes necessary to remedy the abnormal amounts of blood fuel when the body realizes it has been fooled. Considering ways to optimize insulin and cortisol levels will greatly increase the odds of a continued and sustained weight loss.   Four additional hormones contribute to obesity.   These four will be discussed after the first three are discussed at an introductory level.

There are specific fat making hormones, which direct the body energy either toward or away from fat production.   Consider androgens – the anti-fat hormones.   The tendency toward fat diminishes when androgens are present in optimal amounts.

This group of hormones contains testosterone, DHEA, androstenedione, and possibly progesterone.   These hormone types reach their peak in early adulthood in both sexes and decline a little each year after age twenty-five.

Before endorsement from the 'certified experts' for these hormone's replacement protocols is sanctioned, the complex will need to allow adequate study. Despite the long known age related decline in this class of hormones, experts often demand expensive double blind controlled studies and the need for further tests. They know this research could potentially affect the more lucrative symptom control measures. They tenaciously suppress research about real hormones and funds are often difficult to get for further study.

Smoke and mirror techniques of the press releases often hold back forward thinking. The complex controls the life-blood of various media sources through generous advertisement expenditures. Some physicians are beginning to develop a healthy level of skepticism regarding this arrangement between the media and the 'scientific' community.

The androgens, with varying degrees of potency, counteract the ability of insulin to make fat.   This much has been well documented by numerous scientific studies and included in basic medical physiology textbooks. This high level of androgens helps explain how adolescents can indulge indiscriminately in a high carbohydrate intake without gaining body fat.   Adolescents have higher androgen levels than those who are older.

High androgen levels further correlate why adolescent boys consuming the same junk food diets as adolescent girls, tend to gain less fat.   Adolescent boys have higher androgen levels than their female counterparts. There is less fat manufactured with a higher total androgen message.   As male and female gonads and adrenals age, total androgen production falls.   The reduction of androgen content compels the body to be more responsive to the effects of insulin and cortisol.

Increased androgen that occurs during puberty on prepubescent and obese boys, usually expresses itself as a profound loss of body fat.   Muscle mass increases simultaneously.   The tendency to lose body fat is secondary to the increased androgen countering the effects of both cortisol and insulin.

A supplementation program of androgens can have serious side effects and even result in death from inappropriate use. Understanding the competitive and complex interrelationship of hormones becomes an advantage for the owner to avoid side effects. However, there is no substitute for first improving behavioral, emotional, and nutritional efforts. When all of these approaches are implemented the body will begin to heal.

Hormone physiology can become complicated if one includes the numerous hormones, their inter-relationships, counter regulatory responses, cascades of successive release, and fast and slow feedback loops. This manual is about owner empowerment not about becoming a scientist.

Owner empowerment can help one understand the basics of the treatment options given to them. Viewed in this way, one can begin to appreciate that the hormones occupy a central role in regard to the numerous degenerative diseases. However, the hormone role here is largely eviscerated from the mainstream treatment strategies today. If one adds the importance of balance to the hormones within, a fundamental defect in the practice of medicine today will be corrected.

With hormone balancing in mind, the owner begins to appreciate the inner turmoil that confronts a large weight to frame individual. Obesity is caused by increased body insulin and cortisol with a fall in androgens. A superficial explanation for a medical condition often misleads and can be potentially destructive to the healing process. How can an earthling ever begin to lose weight when their hormones scream for them to shovel in the food? When one has the hormone setting within that directs behavior toward feeding, they are in the torture chamber. One cannot step out of this torture chamber until their hormones allow it. Hormones direct behavioral and body energy.

Popular diets available are incomplete for various reasons. Successful weight loss requires consideration of all seven fat related hormones - insulin, cortisol, androgens, estrogen, insulin-like growth factor type one, thyroid and epinephrine. Inappropriate feeding behaviors are the result of inappropriately proportioned relationships between hormones. Weight loss becomes prevented and fat production becomes promoted when theses seven hormones are out of balance.

This subsection has been about an introductory discussion of the first three hormones that commonly prevent weight loss success. Each of these first three hormones will be better explained later. For now, just begin to get a feel for how imbalanced hormones trap one in obesity. While considering the ways that obesity is perpetrated, the common failings of popular diets need explanation.

High protein diets, like Dr. Atkins' *Diet Revolution*, improve the probability for weight loss by partially addressing hormone imbalance. Eating protein instead of carbohydrates reduces insulin – the fat maker. Using this principle also turns down the appetite center in the brain.

High protein diets often fail by creating a mineral imbalance between sodium and potassium. When mineral imbalances occur, weight lose is prevented because the body then requires increased insulin secretion for sugar intake. In this case, the failure rate is secondary to overlooking the importance of mineral balance.

Other popular high protein diets fail to manipulate all seven hormones that are a determiner of obesity. A successful diet must affect the hormone-based urge to consume food. The power of these hormones is an important concept for weight loss and other health successes.

The weakness in the high protein diet turns out to be the strength of some of the other diets. The high fruit, vegetable, and unprocessed grain diets often have superior mineral balance content. These diets fail because of the other hormonal imbalances they perpetuate.

> The ideal diet combines the best of each diet and eliminates the part that sucks the owner back into the torture chamber. Understanding how the seven different body hormones either help or hinder weight loss is essential. Later in this section and in sections three and four the mineral needs of the body will be explained. Implementing these interrelating factors allows ways for obese owners to get on healing paths.

Seven Hormones to Consider When Healing from Obesity

The general development of the seven obesity hormones includes cortisol, insulin, and the androgen class (testosterone, DHEA, androstenedione, and progesterone). Thyroid, epinephrine, insulin-like growth factor type one (IGF-1) and estrogen complete the main hormones contributing to obesity. Some words of encouragement and an acknowledgment concerning the pitfalls in thinking spread by the certified medical experts need to be addressed.

The American Dietetic Association (ADA) perpetuates the popularized "Torture Chamber Diet". Most owners on a high protein diet find the first week, while insulin levels decline, to be the hardest. Why? - Because they are stepping out of the torture chamber. The torture chamber results from dietary and behavior lifestyles that keep the owner preoccupied with their next feeding event. When the owner sticks to low carbohydrate intake and begins a committed exercise program, they begin to notice a marked decrease in their appetite. Decreased carbohydrate was considered medical heresy over 20 years ago when physicians like Dr. Atkins began to advocate this approach towards weight loss.

High protein and low fat diets are only part of the solution to the obesity problem. Each human body has unique needs and abilities. A cookie cutter diet will fail. This book empowers the owner to unravel his own personal weight dilemma.

The ADA's diet will not work for the vast majority of obese owners. The ADA still advocates that almost 60% of total daily calories come from complex carbohydrates. This may be effective for owners who have minimal stress hormone (cortisol) and adequate androgen to counteract insulin's fat building message. This ADA diet will only work for those owners who are already at their optimal weight. The more obese owners will require a more demanding program. Demanding programs are necessary to reverse the hormonal imbalance created by a high carbohydrate and mineral imbalanced diet. Hormonal imbalance creates the torture chamber. When an owner is in the torture chamber, longterm weight loss becomes difficult to achieve.

Hormonal imbalance in the Torture Chamber will be the emphasis in this section. Other missing components of popular diets will be addressed later.

Stress and the Torture Chamber

An elevated level of blood cortisol traps the owner in the torture chamber and plays a powerful role in making fat. It makes the modern owners fat by programming an obsolete survival response.

Prehistoric man survived physical stress assisted by cortisol. Both mental and physical stress leads to the dumping of sugar into the blood stream. However, only mental stress necessitates an increase in insulin levels. Physical stress requires a physical response thus consuming the increased blood sugar to provide physical energy. Mental stress does not use the extra sugar because no physical response is required. The body cannot distinguish between mental and physical stresses. The consequence here is that the same stress hormones are secreted in either case.

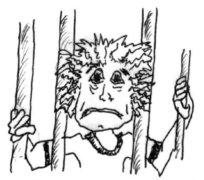

When under mental stress, exercise counter acts the high sugars created by stress hormones. No one knows how many minutes one has to exercise before insulin is secreted into the blood stream to mop up the high blood sugar. By using extra blood sugar, exercise counteracts the need for insulin.

The stress response activates the blood sugars elevation to provide fuel for a perceived physical threat. Modern mental stress is a powerful roadblock to weight loss. Following a low carbohydrate diet very closely can still fail to achieve weight loss in situations of chronic mental stress. Mental stress raises total insulin output. Increased insulin accompanied by lack of physical activity causes blood sugar to convert to fat. The old adage 'walking it off' is wise because the solution is exercise.

A Deeper Understanding of Insulin, Cortisol, and Androgen

An extremely low carbohydrate diet is critical for the obese owners to lower insulin levels. A reduction in their insulin level is essential for reducing the message content to feed. Less food consumption naturally follows.

Clinical situations demonstrate the powerful role insulin plays in feeding behavior. A high insulin level, which occurs in adult onset diabetics, is one example of how high insulin levels become physically demonstrated. Diabetologists observed that insulin supplements, given to most adult onset diabetics, have an undesirable side effect of increased appetite and weight gain. Where this is not the case, there is some other cause for the adult onset diabetes (liver chapter). The higher the insulin levels in an owner, the more body fat that they will have. Insulin is the body's premier fat maker and is second to no other hormone.

If a diabetic owner adheres to a low carbohydrate diet, they will require less medication to keep a normal blood sugar level. This is true whether they ingest oral medication or use insulin shots. Many adult onset diabetics following this program lose their need for insulin shots.

A low carbohydrate diet reduces the insulin level – a situation that must be monitored to control the blood sugar level. The insulin modulator or supplement that is prescribed is based on the initial insulin levels needed in the blood. When these levels of need are reduced, the amount of the insulin supplement then becomes too high. The owner should be in close consultation with competent medical counsel during this transition.

Insulin is the growth factor for fat cells. Body fat cannot be produced or maintained without it. Obese owners always have higher insulin production than non-obese owners. Insulin levels increase due to mental stress, sedentary lifestyles, abuse of carbohydrate consumption, low IGF-1 levels, and deficiency in the androgen class of steroids. In most obese owners all five of the above mechanisms are in operation. All five of these processes lead to increased insulin levels. Their roll in reducing or increasing insulin's fat production will be examined and discussed.

Cortisol

Elevated blood cortisol enhances insulin's fat producing roll. The adrenal glands manufacture cortisol, which needs to be normalized to achieve weight loss. The owner's level of physical activity forms one determiner of the resultant cortisol mediated insulin level.

In healthy individuals, normal amounts of cortisol are analogous to the oil that the tin man needed in the *Wizard of Oz*. Healthy joints need cortisol to decrease the physical inflammatory stimulation caused by the stresses and strains of physical activity. Cortisol binds to joint cells' receptors creating inflammation suppression. The inflammation suppression message results from the combination and precise shape of cortisol and the unique shape of the joint cell receptor. Different tissues have different receptor shapes. The way a specific hormone combines with different receptor sites determines the message content.

This helps explain the variability of message content that results when a simple molecule like cortisol binds with different types of receptors. The introduction of this additional detail deters one from thinking of cortisol as a villain. Many diseased states arise from a cortisol deficiency (adrenal chapter).

When the body experiences stress, increased amounts of cortisol are released. Energy is then redirected toward survival activities and away from cellular maintenance. Part of the survival response directs adequate fuel into the bloodstream for surviving physical stress. If physical stress is met by a physical challenge, the exercising muscles will use the extra blood sugar. Extra insulin is not required. However, with mental stress the extra fuel in the blood stream has nowhere to go. Mental stress causes the release of more insulin to remove the blood sugar from the blood stream turning it into fat. This scenario demonstrates how elevated cortisol can help make one fat. However, it is always insulin that makes fat. Cortisol helps only when its presence causes the release of increased insulin.

Insulin and cortisol cause dysfunction to the body's health when there is no physical challenge. Lack of physical activity creates another part of the vicious cycle in the torture chamber. Unhappiness found in the Torture Chamber arises due to out dated hormonal responses to modern day mental stress.

Under mental stress, cortisol secretion inappropriately elevated the blood sugar and insulin must be secreted to bring the blood sugar level to normal. Exercise is the path out of this torture chamber. Physical activity reduces blood sugar without the need for increased insulin. Sooner or later, the body realizes it has been fooled into raising the blood sugar inappropriately. The need for extra insulin corrects the body's erroneous elevation in the blood sugar.

Cortisol also affects the amount of androgen that is available to the body. Excess cortisol directs the gonads to release and manufacture less androgen. When cortisol is released, the release of another hormone, prolactin, follows. Prolactin directly inhibits testicle and ovary production and secretion of their steroid hormone products.

When owners are under chronic stress, the diminished androgen reduces the body's ability to eliminate or use fat. Diminished androgen production amplifies the effect of the insulin message. Without adequate androgen, there is not a sufficient counter response to fat development.

When cortisol increases above normal, there is more potential for fat development. Cortisol affects fat development by the imbalances it creates with androgens and insulin. Cortisol is the primary hormone used in the stress response. It directs how energy is used during stress. Prolactin is important, but its role is initiated and directed by superior hormones such as cortisol.

Life processes are all about energy. The stress response is just one of many expressions of body energy. All hormones message content concerns the direction body energy will flow. Healthy owners have the right hormone milieu. The right hormone milieu is only possible when the hormones are balanced. The right hormone balance causes the wise use of available body energy. Conversely, unhealthy owners have unbalanced hormones. Unbalanced hormones direct the body energy to be spent unwisely. Unwise use of available body energy eventually displays itself in the body form.

For example, a common body form effect of excess cortisol is moderate fluid retention. Owners usually look puffy in the face after staying up all night because an excess of cortisol was secreted. In addition, there are numerous other far-reaching effects due to the chronic over production of cortisol. These will be explored more thoroughly later in this chapter and throughout the remainder of this manual. For now its important to understand the basic synergism, mentioned above, between insulin and cortisol. In this regard, these two hormones act together to prevent an optimal weight goal achievement. In addition, androgen levels can be adversely affected by abnormal amounts of either insulin or cortisol. This is the third hormonal aberration briefly mentioned above. One of the main body androgens is DHEA. DHEA, when one is healthy, occurs at higher amounts than any other body steroid.

DHEA - the Introduction to Androgen

DHEA is a major body steroid and the major androgen hormone manufactured in the adrenal gland. The androgen steroid designation means it builds up the body form. This is in contrast to cortisol, an adrenal steroid of the catabolic class. The catabolic class of hormones consumes body structure for fuel needs. In addition, the catabolic class of steroids directs body energy into survival activities. The androgen class of steroids directs body energy into rejuvenation activities.

DHEA is also the most predominant androgen in the body. Both DHEA and cortisol are manufactured in the adrenals that sit on top of the kidneys. DHEA levels steadily increase, starting at age 7 and continue to climb until age 25. A steady decline to about 10% of their peak value occurs in the last year of life. DHEA has been implicated as the messenger that directs numerous rejuvenation activities within the body. DHEA in many ways is the oppositional hormone to the message of cortisol for these reasons.

Paradoxically, the same stimulus that increases cortisol release also simultaneously releases DHEA. A healthy owner releases about twice the amount DHEA as cortisol. With this ratio, energy never gets too far into catabolic processes as DHEA opposes cortisol direction of energy. It takes both optimal cortisol and DHEA amounts to balance the message content of where the body spends its energy.

Clinicians tend to ignore DHEA levels importance within the body because it is a relatively weak androgen compared to testosterone. However, it is important not to forget the power of peripheral conversion of the weaker steroids, like DHEA, to testosterone in places like muscle. Adequate androgen that opposes cortisol becomes necessary for muscle maintenance. Higher than normal cortisol, compared to androgens, creates a marked increase tendency for fat development in place of muscle.

This clever body design feature allows women to obtain the benefits of androgen within their muscles without the masculine side effects. Women get message content to their muscle cells telling them to rejuvenate with adequate DHEA levels. Masculine side effects occur when testosterone increases in the blood stream. The female body has the ability to side step this problem unless DHEA levels are too high. DHEA appears to serve important functions in the brain and nervous system because the concentration is at a level five or six times that found in the blood stream (brain chapter).

Some believe that DHEA is the androgen most responsible for blood vessel maintenance. In health, the body's adrenals make just the right amount of both DHEA and cortisol in the proper proportions. Ratios facilitate an optimal harmony between cellular rest and rejuvenation activities. Imbalance in this ratio is emerging as an additional risk factor for the development of blood vessel disease (Syndrome X). There are additional consequences, other than obesity, to health when the ratio of DHEA to cortisol becomes imbalanced (adrenal chapter).

The adrenals, while still healthy, make both adequate DHEA (strength hormone) and cortisol (anti-inflammatory and stress hormone). The first hint of obesity related old age begins to occur when the proper balance in the content of the adrenal secretions between these two hormones deteriorates.

Both a loss of muscle mass and an increased tendency to gain weight demonstrates the imbalance between DHEA and cortisol. The physiological responses are predictable due to their fundamental nature.
DHEA signals muscle restoration and building. Cortisol directs body fuels away from the restoration process and into a stress response activity. When these two antagonistic hormones are out of balance, an owner's physical form diminishes and the body will not lose weight.

Androgens Oppose Cortisol and Insulin

The importance of DHEA to women concerns the maintenance of adequate muscle and bone mass accomplished by the process of peripheral conversion. The details of peripheral conversion are beyond the scope of this owner's manual. Once the DHEA arrives in the muscle or bone cell it converts to the more powerful testosterone. Testosterone, by virtue of its shape, contains a more powerful androgen message content. The more powerful androgen message directs more rejuvenation activity within the target cell than a weaker androgen would. The additional benefit of this design in the female owner prevents masculinity. Masculine traits would occur if testosterone was initially released into the blood stream because of message content.

The adrenals manufacture another relatively weak androgen, androsteinedione, which, like DHEA, peripherally converts to testosterone within the muscles. The ovaries secrete androstenedione hormone that also converts peripherally into the more powerful steroid, testosterone. The reader only needs to be aware of this introductory example for how there is some overlap between one's ovaries and adrenals in the production of androgen. Androgen levels are one hormonal determinant of how fat one will get.

Some owners want to know how they can get their cortisol levels down and begin to facilitate their adrenals and gonads (ovaries or testicles) ability to increase the manufacture of these critical androgens. This is a case where one has to accept the painful truth before healing can begin. Owners who have high insulin, high cortisol, and less than optimal androgens from both the adrenals and gonads, hate to exercise. Trust the doctor on this one.

The same hormone imbalances that drive the appetite also reduce the owner's physical energy level. They are not lazy. Their energy declines because their hormones are out of balance. In the beginning, a daily walk, swim, bike ride, or whatever aerobic exercise the owner chooses will be driven by sheer will power. When the owner initiates and maintains a moderate exercise program, cortisol and insulin levels will begin to fall. The androgen output, from both the adrenals and the gonads, will begin to rise. Moderate exercise contributes to the restoration of an appropriate balance between cortisol and androgens. When normal hormone messages are played, the desire for exercise increases. In this way, exercise provides a powerful way to realign the balance of the first three fat maker related hormones. Androgens tend to increase when physical work or the blossoming into adolescence occurs.

The beneficial effects of high androgens on body form are exemplified during the teenage years. The transition from childhood to adolescence carries out a dramatic change in the body hormone milieu. Behavioral changes during the teenage years are only one manifestation of changing hormones. The surge in androgen production during the teenage years causes a marked loss of body fat and a concurrent increase in muscle and bone mass. Conversely, leaving out the deleterious hormonal changes that accelerate the sedentary attitude only perpetuates the torture chamber.

The torture chamber is a physical status where hormones are imbalanced. This imbalance creates the vicious cycle of physical decline. The behavioral effects of hormones cause the urges that lead owners to become parents. Hormones also cause owners to make those minute-to-minute, day-to-day, poor decisions that lead to an old body prematurely. The owner who intends to slow the rate toward an old body needs to focus on their hormone status.

The torture chamber effect also leads to obesity through imbalanced hormones. Message content falling off contributes to the torture chamber effect. To assess their ability to counter the fat making hormones, the contribution of both the adrenals and ovaries as independent sources of androgen must be considered.

If female owners knew the truth about patentable estrogen and synthetic progesterone substitutes shortcomings, they would probably rise up and prevail in a successful class action lawsuit. Often the pursuit of profit wins over what is reflected in a more complete scientific understanding. Natural hormone replacement therapy is not patentable and hence not as profitable for the pharmaceutical companies. The common practice of pandering hormone replacement therapy today doesn't stand up under the rigors of scientific scrutiny. The complex spends enormous resources grooming the way physicians think and this practice starts in medical school. Because of this, many physicians continue these inferior hormone replacement strategies. This occurs despite good scientific evidence to the contrary. The opposing medical opinions are found collecting dust.

Physician's access to this information is eliminated through the heavy hand of the advertising dollar. The advertising dollar is maximized in operation in the numerous popular medical journals. In addition, the ability to fund pertinent research to these natural hormone replacement methods is further controlled by a government that benefits when health care costs increase. Expensive health care increases the total taxation revenues more than it increases medicare and medicaid costs. Lastly, the tried and true technique of the complex funding a poorly run study puts fear into owners regarding treatment alternatives. These sensationalized studies 'leak' to the press where they become maximized.

This is commonly called the 'smoke and mirror' tactics. Life is too short to get all worked up about the way the complex keeps owners thought patterns 'inside the box'. It is worth considering the next time one picks up mainstream reading material or listens to media sources. When these common sources of information start sounding too good to be true, they probably are. The latest what-is-for-sale item needs the media as well. Increasingly, the media lines with the financial interest of the complex.

In addition to DHEA output from the adrenal glands, functional ovaries fight fat when they contribute to the female androgen output. Intact ovaries produce androgen hormones when in the healthy state. Androgens produced by the ovary are testosterone and androstenedione. This function of androgen production helps the adrenals elevate total androgen message content within the female body. When this function is sufficient, the rejuvenation message content increases. Conversely, when rejuvenation message content diminishes, the body cells begin to deteriorate.

Two other steroid hormones produced by the ovaries are estrogen and progesterone. Many female owners fail to receive adequate androgen replacement after surgical removal of their ovaries. The lack of androgen replacement when the ovaries are removed is one of the common side effects of conventional hormonal replacement. Another concern regards the lack of real hormone replacement in these situations.

The tremendous influence of the complex constantly collides with how ovarian hormones contribute to the healing of the obese owners. In this regard, it is necessary to briefly touch on the hormonal workings of the intact ovary. The healthy ovary manufactures three types of estrogen during the first half of the menstrual cycle in larger amounts - estriol with less estradiol, and estrone. During the second half of the cycle the female body produces increased amounts of progesterone to counter-regulate estrogen's cellular effects. The term counter-regulate means to denote the common body theme of balance. All hormones in the body need balance by opposing hormones. Estrogen opposes progesterone.

There is a cyclical rhythm that occurs within the healthy female. The message content of estrogen needs to be effectively counter balanced by progesterone later in the month. Optimal types and amounts of these three estrogens exist in a healthy female. These two counter regulatory hormones create a rhythm.

The chapter on ovaries contains a complete discussion in regard to how the ovaries contribute to female health. It is important to focus on how sick or removed ovaries can contribute to obesity. In addition, there is the obesity created from synthetic or altered hormone replacement that will be briefly discussed below in the next subsection. Lastly, it is important to remind the reader about the ovaries role in androgen production. Adequate androgen production within the ovary powerfully deters weight gain.

The healthy ovary manufactures androgen primarily in the form of androstenedione. The ovary also manufactures and releases testosterone. Androstenedione manufacture becomes powerful when it becomes peripherally converted to the more powerful testosterone. Many clinicians do not understand this fact and therefore mistakenly feel that since androstenedione is a relatively weak androgen compared to testosterone its supplementation is unnecessary. The same line of reasoning prevails in regards to the fall of DHEA production within some owner's adrenals. Again, what these clinicians forgot is the concept of peripheral conversion in specific body tissues, to the more powerful testosterone-like hormones. This becomes critical to female owners having a biological mechanism to achieve the benefits of androgens message without masculine effects. Adequate, but not excessive, androgen is the goal within the female body. Only in this situation can the female body preserve muscle mass and minimize fat development.

Surgical removal of the ovaries accelerates the tendency to gain weight. Weight gain occurs due to the reduction of androgens. This leads to an increased ability of insulin and cortisol to exert a more powerful combination message to create body fat. The fat making message increases because the adrenals are the only androgen producing glands left within these owner's bodies. This is not the only powerful aberration working insidiously to alter body habitués for the worse.

With the removal of the ovaries, the risk of androgen deficiency from a new source develops – the doctor. The tendency to gain fat is equal between synthetic hormone replacement therapies and removal of the ovaries. Conventional medical practitioners routinely prescribe synthetic female hormones.

One of the early pioneers, John Lee, M.D., began to understand the superiority of natural (real) hormone replacements - like progesterone. He pointed out years ago that there is only one progesterone found in nature. Dr. Lee also pointed out that natural progesterone is not patentable. It needs to be chemically altered in order for drug companies to have a patentable substance. Patents allow profit by conferring a marketing advantage for a number of years. This occurs because patents allow the sole rights to both the manufacture and distribution of the patentable substance. Drug companies exist to make money.

Effective marketing of these progesterone substitutes does not mean that the best science is being practiced. Owners in America need to realize that they live in a profit driven health care system. Whatever sells is sensationalized and marketed in the same manner as any other capitalist business enterprise. Side effects are minimized and benefits are exaggerated whether it's a car, a pill, or toothpaste. In addition, when considering tax revenues, the government often becomes analogous to the fox guarding the hen house. With reality in mind, it becomes more believable that there are numerous examples where good scientific understandings gained through rigorous hard work and brilliance continue to go unnoticed or are ignored because the results affect profit.

The inferiority of synthetic hormones, which include progesterone and estrogen, is explained relatively easily. Steroid molecules are simple in the world of hormone message content. The exact shape in a simple message carrier is important. If the shape of a hormone changes, then the message content changes. The shape of a synthetic hormone varies from the shape of a natural hormone. Therefore, the message also varies. When a physician prescribes a synthetic hormone for hormone replacement therapy, the change in the hormone message has a profound effect on the woman's health.

For over forty years, the knowledge that a change in the angle of one bond on the estrogen molecule, estradiol, makes the message thirty times more powerful to direct cells to divide. This results in estrogen sensitive cells, like breast cells, receiving the message to divide by an increase of thirty times. Stronger synthetic estrogen contributes to obesity problem as well.

The estrogen bond angle change refers to the difference in potency between alpha-estradiol and beta-estradiol. The weaker type, beta-estradiol occurs naturally in humans. The version that is thirty times more powerful, alpha-estradiol, does not occur naturally in humans.

The creator probably has a good reason for this. This type of estrogen is found to exist in the urine of pregnant horses. There is a new way to make this from wild yams or soy, but it still contains alpha-estradiol that has been chemically manufactured instead of collected from horse urine.

Later in this chapter, when the health of the ovaries is being discussed, a more complete review of the different synthetic estrogens and the side effects will be undertaken. Briefly, a very slight change in the shape of natural estrogen changes the message content. Conversely, no patent is available unless the estrogen shape is changed. Being cognizant of this reality helps simplify what is really going on with women's health today.

The reason synthetic estrogen contributes to obesity will be explained shortly. The introductory example exposed how estrogen replacement, through unnatural means, could entirely change the message content. The next example shows how progesterone substitutes also change the message a cell receives. Progesterone substitutes may diminish the manufacture of other steroids. Instruction comes from examining likely reasons why progesterone substitutes mean trouble for owners.

Progesterone serves as the basic building block for many other steroid hormones manufactured within the adrenals and gonads. Adrenals and gonads need adequate levels of natural progesterone to manufacture critically needed testosterone, cortisol, androstenediones, and a large percentage of the estrogens. However, synthetic progesterone substitutes don't serve as building blocks for biosynthesis of other steroids.

There is an additional suspicion. Synthetic progesterone is not close enough in structure to natural progesterone to serve as a building block within the enzymatic machinery designed to process natural progesterone into other needed steroid hormones. The consequence to the body is that the enzymatic machinery cannot convert synthetic progesterone, because of its structure, into essential steroids as natural progesterone does.

The presence of these unnatural substitutes within ones enzymatic machines leads to a decreased cellular productivity of the other vital steroids. For this reason, synthetic progesterone usage is associated with obesity. It is important to separate how synthetic progesterone and estrogen, each in their own way, contribute to the obesity problem. In the case of synthetic progesterone, it is through the mechanisms described above. The additional contribution of high amounts of estrogens to obesity is described below.

High Estrogen Levels Can Promote Obesity
The Fourth Hormone to Achieve Normal Weight

When estrogen rises beyond normal levels there is a varying tendency to promote two of the hormonal factors creating obesity. The ability of estrogen to raise insulin and lower androgens in certain females becomes apparent.

Three main clinical situations promote estrogen induced weight gain. Not all female owners will express these tendencies equally. This variability may have a genetic basis. Not all women with an increased estrogen state tend to gain weight equally. However, high estrogen states tend to promote weight gain in many female owners. This fact will be the focus of this subsection.

The first clinical example for estrogen induced weight gain is from birth control pills. They predictably increase insulin in the body. The mechanism for this situation arises from a hormone tandem that results when estrogen is high.

First in the hormone tandem of successive release is the stimulation of growth hormone. This occurs in the increased estrogen states of birth control pills. Growth hormone will initially raise blood sugar. It is the second hormone in this tandem, that estrogen simultaneously inhibits, which alters the normal pattern of events.

When estrogen levels are optimal, the release of growth hormone directs the simultaneous release of insulin-like growth factor, the second hormone in the tandem. Insulin-like growth factor has powerful insulin-like blood sugar lowering message content. This message content tends to lower the blood sugar that the growth hormone initially elevated.

This tandem hormone effect provides an effective way for the cells to receive fuel from the blood stream without raising insulin levels. High estrogen states, although initially stimulating growth hormone release, counteracts the normal tandem by inhibiting insulin-like growth factor release. The normal hormone tandem is interrupted because high estrogen involves the simultaneous inhibition of insulin-like growth factor release.

Insulin-like growth factor (IGF) is an insulin-like hormone that acts normally out in the cells. Its presence lowers the amount of insulin needed by the body. The IGF released assists insulin by taking sugar out of the blood stream. When IGF levels diminish, the growth hormone directs increased sugar to be released into the blood stream. More insulin has to be secreted from the pancreas. The more insulin secreted, the more message content there is to make body fat.

The second clinical situation of estrogen-caused obesity involves increased prolactin levels caused by the increased estrogen state of birth control use. Prolactin inhibits ovarian hormone formation and release. This hormone-induced mechanism, associated with obesity, is generally not operational in pregnancy because of this physiologic state has the growing placenta. The placenta manufactures androgens even though the ovaries become relatively dormant by the fifth month of pregnancy. When a female owner takes birth control pills the body thinks it is pregnant. During birth control pill usage, prolactin levels rise because estrogen levels approach pregnancy levels.

Potential obesity problems occur because, like pregnancy, the birth control pills increase prolactin levels. Unlike pregnancy, there is no placenta (hormone factory) to correct the inhibition of steroid production. The potential for problems compound due to the fact that the birth control pill does not contain androgens, only estrogen and progestins (synthetic progesterone substitutes). Androgen production can fall within owners and their adrenals are left all alone for this task. Some female's adrenals are not up to the challenge of increased androgen production and obesity ensues.

The third clinical situation of high estrogen-induced obesity is beyond the level of this discussion. For those who are curious, it involves the dramatic increase of sex hormone-binding globulin that high estrogen levels direct. The little bit of androgen, that may be produced by the ovary in high estrogen statesa gets trapped on a carrier protein in the blood stream at ninety eight percent of the efficiency level. This is all that needs to be known for now about the fourth hormone type, estrogen (ovary chapter).

Thyroid Function and Weight Gain
The fifth Hormone to Consider When Achieving Normal Weight

The fifth hormone type to consider for weight loss strategy is the thyroid hormone. Thyroid turns up the 'furnace flame' in the trillions of mitochondria within the cells. The more heat produced in the mitochondria, the more calories burned. More calories burn because more fuel is required in these microscopic power plants. Just like in the physical world of power plants, the cells burn more fuel when the energy generation increases. Thyroid hormone facilitates the cells ability to burn more fuel. Owners who lack sufficient thyroid message content will not be able to burn fuel at high levels. A lower fuel usage promotes fuel storage as fat.

The problem in the clinical setting is the standard practice of making diagnostic decisions based on a laboratory analysis of a blood sample. The blood sample represents one instant in time - the moment of the blood draw. Basic hormone physiology teaches that hormones fluctuate widely throughout the day, with various states of activity, environmental temperatures, and emotional states. Somehow, the standard of care regarding the testing for hormones levels, like thyroid, is in direct violation of these basic scientific observations. How can a doctor diagnose - or reassure - with confidence without testing for the condition in as accurate a way as possible?

Scientifically, testing for the amount of thyroid hormone detected with a 24-hour urine sample is appropriate. A period of 24 hours is sufficient to average out the peaks and valleys of amounts of hormones. This average gives the physician a more accurate picture of a patient's true hormone status.

This concept will be discussed in more detail in the chapter regarding the 100,000 mile examination and later in this section where the thyroid glands contribution to health. Be alert to the fact that there are owners with diminished power plant flames. Diminished power plant flames lead to slower metabolism. Slower metabolisms burn fewer calories. When fewer calories burn, energy for life diminishes and vulnerability for weight gain increases.

It is important to relate the interdependence between thyroid hormone and the sixth hormone, adrenaline, in the prevention and healing from obesity. One of the messages that thyroid contains when it binds to certain nuclear receptors (DNA programs) is the go ahead for the manufacture of adrenaline receptors throughout the body. Cortisol also contributes message content that is equally crucial for the adrenaline receptor synthesis to be finished.

If sufficient amounts of cortisol and thyroid hormone are available when adrenaline is released in the blood stream, there will be mature receptors present. Mature receptors are necessary in order to receive the adrenaline message. The adrenaline message directly stimulates fuel combustion within the mitochondria by making fuel more available to cells. When more fuel is available to cells, metabolism increases.

Adrenaline
The Sixth Hormone to Consider When Achieving Normal Weight

Adrenaline carries out the receptor activation initiated by both cortisol and thyroid message content. Adrenaline activates the receptors manufactured by these two more powerful hormones. Only when there are sufficient receptors can adrenaline's message be heard by the target cells. When adrenaline releases under these normal circumstances, metabolism increases. When metabolism increases, fuel consumption increases.

Some owners suffer from various forms of adrenal insufficiency. It is of little use to manufacture sufficient thyroid hormone and cortisol when the body experiences inadequate adrenal function through lack of adrenaline. The manufacture of epinephrine by the adrenal gland takes place in the adrenal medulla. The manufacture of cortisol takes place in the adrenal cortex. When the cortex fails, the diminished ability to make one or more adrenal steroids becomes the problem. Adrenaline manufacture is needed to follow up

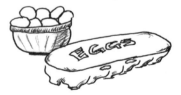

on what both the thyroid and cortisol message started in the creation of adrenal receptors.

Overtaxed adrenal glands can often masquerade as a thyroid problem. These owners walk like a thyroid problem and talk like a thyroid problem, but they are not a thyroid problem. Patients feel lousy and intuitively sense something is wrong. These owners' standard fatigue work-ups come back normal at their doctor's office. A superficial inquiry leads to superficial platitudes and the statement that nothing is wrong. Some of these owners end up on antidepressants. How can this be?

A common example is revealed when one understands where adrenaline (epinephrine) is derived. There are twenty different amino acids that, when arranged uniquely in sequence, type, and amount become the various proteins. The body manufactures most of these de novo. Eight essential amino acids must be obtained in the diet. The egg is the only food source that contains all eight. All other protein sources are deficient in one or more amino acids. Adrenaline is derived from the essential amino acid phenylalanine.

The above discussion explains the importance of attaining adequate phenylalanine in the diet, but there is a subtle and often overlooked reason for adrenaline deficiency.

Protein disassembly requires adequate stomach acid and digestive juices if essential amino acid supply lines are to be maintained. Owners who lack sufficient stomach acid and/or digestive juices tend to become deficient in essential amino acids necessary for the reactions of life. Deficient adrenaline manufacture is one of the problems that can ensue due to ineffective disassembly of protein.

Another cause of adrenaline deficiency is failure to obtain the necessary molecular building blocks for manufacture. Most adrenaline is made from phenylalanine or the closely related amino acid, tyrosine. Many physicians understand this much. Vitamins and cofactors, which are necessary to make either one of these amino acids into adrenaline, often go unnoticed. Deficiency of any one of them halts this critical hormone's biosynthesis. The nutrients necessary for the manufacture of adrenaline are tetrahydrobiopterin (folate derived), vitamin C, vitamin B6, vitamin B12, folate, methionine, and SAMe (S-adenosyl methionine). The most common deficiency arises from a deficiency of SAMe which is clinically evidenced by an increase of blood homocysteine levels. SAMe is part of the important methyl donor system and will be better explained in section three.

A deficiency in one or more vitamins and cofactors results in health problems. These additional health problems develop because the adrenal secrets partially manufactured adrenaline (dopamine or nor-adrenaline) into the blood stream. When this occurs, deficiencies of one or more vitamins exist. Dopamine and nor-adrenaline have different shapes, therefore a different message. A different message results when altered molecules bind to the adrenaline-like receptors.

When elevated amounts of nor-adrenaline enter the blood stream instead of adrenaline, a drastic tendency toward high blood pressure occurs. A single, simple vitamin deficiency can physiologically be the cause of elevated blood pressure. Some of these hypertensive owners may prefer taking vitamins. In this case, vitamins instead of blood pressure medicine, lead to healing without the predictable side effects.

> When was the last time a mainstream medical doctor inquired about these possibilities before prescribing medication? Please note, it is not the intent of this discussion to cast disparaging remarks on the many caring and kind physicians practicing today. It has been quite shocking to this author, while researching this work, the numerous holes in physicians (and this author's) educational exposure addressing healing versus symptom control. It isn't usually the physician who is to blame, but rather, the way that simple concepts are continually corrupted. The motive is money.

A more complete explanation of adrenaline insufficiency follows later. The sixth example of hormonal mechanism leads to obesity. Without an adequate adrenaline response, metabolism slows because fuel combusts slower. Less fuel combustion leads to lower food intake tolerance before becoming obese.

Insulin-like growth factor type-1 (IGF-1)
The seventh hormone to consider for healing obesity

IGF-1 occurs at levels one hundred times insulin levels when an owner is healthy. IGF-1 acts like insulin outside of the liver and fat cells. The more IGF-1 in circulation, the more cells outside of the liver and fat can procure fuel and nutrients. Growth hormone release promotes normal liver to release IGF-1 into circulation. In this way, when an owner is healthy, it is the ample IGF-1 circulating in the blood stream that keeps cells filled with nutrition.

As long as there are sufficient amounts of IGF-1 manufactured and released by the liver, there will be less need for insulin release. Insulin release in healthy owners falls to very low levels between meals. However, unhealthy owners will tend to need massive increases in their insulin levels because IGF-1 levels have fallen. When IGF-1 levels fall increased amounts of insulin are needed outside of the liver and fat so that other body cells can receive nutrition. The trouble with insulin levels increasing, to make up for the nutritional message deficit, regards its role as fat maker. Unlike IGF-1, insulin delivers a powerful message in the liver and fat cells to uptake fuel and make it into more fat. Healthy owners gain weight less readily because their cells, like muscle and heart cells, can receive nutrition with the help of IGF-1. It is the high insulin level that makes an owner fat. Normal insulin levels store just the right amount of fat and sugar within the liver and fat cells to get the owner from meal to meal.

The liver chapter explains the particulars of how important a high IGF-1 level is in regard to health. Here, it is only important to understand how when

IGF-1 falls then the insulin level needs to rise. Insulin on the rise means fat making will also be on the rise. When IGF-1 levels are at healthy levels then muscle and organ development are facilitated.

Seven Types of Hormones that can Condemn One to Obesity

The individual seeking guidance on optimizing his insulin, cortisol, androgen, estrogen, thyroid, IGF-1 and adrenaline levels has a weight loss advantage. Weight loss advantage occurs from ways that behavior and metabolism favorably influence cells to receive good information.

In the sections that follow, ways to optimize the health of glands that produce these seven types of hormones will be reviewed. In addition, many other diseases that arise from failure or excess within the hormone producing glands will be addressed. There will also be development toward understanding how these glands become injured.

Oral Hormones and the Liver

The "first pass" effect, in the liver of orally ingested steroids complicates steroid hormone replacement. Oral supplements are required to pass through the liver once they have been absorbed by the digestive tract. On average, about 70-80% of an ingested steroid is removed from circulation following oral administration. The ingested steroid remains inside the liver.

There are two important concepts regarding the liver first pass effect. First, the liver itself is rich in steroid hormone receptor sites. Failing to comprehend this can lead to a powerful message to liver cells altering their function (including liver cancer in some cases). Second, sometimes synthetic steroids are not well metabolized. Poor metabolism of certain steroids within the liver leads to sequestering of these hormones. When steroids sequester within the liver, they promote liver congestion phenomena.

Some physicians have substantiated this congestion phenomenon clinically. The observation that a large percentage of blue eyed females who chronically take birth control pills witness a gradual change of their original eye color to green. The Chinese medical theory associating liver health with eye color makes this clinical observation acutely disturbing.

In summary, taking steroid hormones orally, without thinking about liver health, is potentially dangerous. Safer alternatives are available in the forms of patches, creams, and injections in some cases. These routes bypass the liver first pass effect allowing the liver to use its energy for more constructive tasks, like disarming environmental toxins.

Chapter Five

Adrenal Glands

The adrenal glands sit on top of each kidney. They are about the size and shape of an acorn. The 'seed' makes the adrenaline and is directly wired into the sympathetic nervous system. This sympathetic nerve connection facilitates the release of adrenaline. Adrenaline conveys an overall body message of both alertness and increased metabolism. The 'cap' makes the adrenal steroid hormones (aldosterone, DHEA, progesterone, androstenedione, and cortisol) from cholesterol. Aldosterone is a key hormone in the regulation of salt and water balance. DHEA and cortisol can be thought of as regulatory opposites.

As cortisol levels rise, the message that directs cellular energy into survival pathways increase. This redirection of cellular energy occurs whenever cortisol levels rise beyond a very low threshold. In the healthy state, low levels of cortisol (below the threshold) provide anti-inflammatory, cellular rest, fluid retention, and maintain blood vessel responsiveness to adrenaline's message.

DHEA and androstenedione are from the androgen class of hormones that direct body energy into cellular infrastructure investment activities that lead to cellular rejuvenation. The role of progesterone within the adrenal also seems to counter the salt and water retaining effects of cortisol and aldosterone.

There is a 'tug-of-war' between the adrenal androgen and cortisol message content. Modern life complexities often cause chronic stress that increase cortisol levels. Typical modern stress comes in the form of deadlines, job insecurities, complex multiple task responsibilities, and incessant noise, to name a few. If one adds increased consumption of carbohydrates, which increases the need for more cortisol, gland exhaustion becomes possible. Increased cortisol is needed to balance the effects of increased insulin in the blood stream. One gains insight about this modern day problem if consideration is given to the counter-regulatory response necessary to keep all this extra insulin behaving.

Low blood sugar is often the first clinical sign that adrenal glands are beginning to fail in the output of cortisol (stress hormone). When the cortisol level becomes inadequate, the first symptom is often 'brain fog' - a warning sign that something is wrong with the hormonal balance. The loss of balance leads insidiously to an amplification of the mental problem.

Balanced hormonal responses create a cellular communication harmony that underlies the healthful state. As the adrenals lose the ability to respond to the demands for balance, 'brain fog' ensues.

The androgen class of steroid hormones in the adrenal glands is DHEA and androstenedione. While DHEA is only made by the adrenal gland, androstenedione is made by the ovary and adrenal gland. DHEA only will be discussed here, but the reader can also extend this as applicable to androstenedione. Different body tissues prefer to interact with different androgens.

DHEA is particularly important in females as it displays the utility of peripheral conversion into more powerful androgens, like testosterone, once inside the target cell (muscle, ligament, bone). Peripheral conversion spares females the masculine effects of dumping straight testosterone into the blood stream. DHEA (and androstenedione) are much weaker androgens than testosterone. DHEA, like other androgens, directs cellular energy into cellular infrastructure investment activities. Regular infrastructure investment is necessary for continued health. This approach leads to a diminished masculine message carried within the blood stream.

As the adrenal loses the ability to keep up with the demands for hormonal products, DHEA manufacture can be the first to drop off. This imbalance is often missed clinically. At this level of dysfunction, there are only subtle clues. Females are more vulnerable to the ravages of diminished DHEA production as there is less androgen output from the ovaries, relative to the male testes. These patients tend to experience increased fatigue and the earliest signs of deteriorating musculoskeletal structures.

As stress continues, the adrenal glands cease to make adequate cortisol to counter balance insulin's blood sugar lowering message and causing 'brain fog'. 'Brain fog' often indicates adrenal imbalance has continued long enough for moderate cellular damage to occur. Cellular damage occurs secondary to the prolonged survival message that directs energy away from rejuvenation.

At a cellular level, the lack of rejuvenation leads to old cellular components - factories (organelles), machines (enzymes), and cellular charge (the battery) – plainly, old age.

The body has a backup system in the gonads for specific steroid type hormones (not cortisol or DHEA). The amount of DHEA produced in the healthy adrenal gland can be a thousand times the amount of testosterone produced in the ovary. The amount of androstenedione production within female ovaries, under the best of circumstances, approaches one-fifth the adrenal amount of DHEA normally produced. The ovary has no ability for the manufacture of DHEA. Internal havoc is probable when the adrenal becomes wounded. The wounded adrenal gland led to the description of diminished adrenal reserve over fifty years ago.

Diminished Adrenal Reserve Syndrome

In the 1950's, John W. Tintera, M.D., pioneered the concept of adrenal exhaustion. He noted that adrenal exhaustion often results from prolonged stress and added this to the previously accepted causes. Some of the other causes were various infections, hemorrhage, genetic defects for certain adrenal steroids manufacture, and medication side effects. This focus is on how stress leads the way to diminished adrenal function. This will tend to manifest low blood sugar episodes.

In 1955, he published a paper in the New York State Journal of Medicine that included over 200 cases of patients with sub-optimal adrenal function. Almost all of these patients suffer low blood sugars. He called this state of sub-optimal adrenal function, hypo-adrenal-corticism. Dr. Tintera noted that the chief complaints in patients who suffer from diminished adrenal function were similar with low blood sugars (hypoglycemia).

Years later, it was established that cortisol, secreted from the adrenal gland, was a powerful counter-regulatory hormone to the blood sugar lowering effects of insulin. As the adrenals in these patients began to fail in their ability to counter the message of insulin, these patients would present with low blood sugars.

The body design included a system of counter-balanced hormones. When secreted, a given hormone was always counter-balanced by a response from an opposing hormone or group of hormones. The balancing hormones directed energy expenditure, so energy never moves too far in any direction.

In these cases, insulin desires to remove every last sugar from of the blood stream while cortisol moderated the effect of insulin. The balance between these two hormones avoided going too far in any one direction for energy expenditure. Disease results when this balancing system becomes impaired. Dr. Tintera correctly deduced that when prolonged stress depleted the ability of the adrenal to respond as a counter-balance to insulin, blood sugar regulation diminished. Patients with impaired adrenals were unable to secrete sufficient cortisol so their blood sugar became unstable. These patients were more vulnerable to the threat of hypoglycemia.

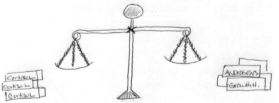

Hormones always need opposition from counter hormones to maintain balance. It helps to understand balance if one envisions an antique weight scale. In general, whenever there is a hormone secreted (weight), there should be an adequate counter-hormone response (counter weight) or health cannot be maintained. Healthy owners have balanced 'weight scales' that secrete a given body hormone in the optimal amount. The counter-response hormone is also secreted in the optimal amount and with appropriate timing.

Improved laboratory testing, developed over the last 40 years, has led to more accurate testing of patient's hormone profiles. Unfortunately, owners in America live in a profit driven health care system. The profit motive results in a $25,000 solution receiving press coverage while the $1,000 solution collects dust. The basic knowledge of what science has revealed empowers an owner who suffers from diminished adrenal function. This approach opens options that can lead to healing instead of symptom control. This knowledge allows awareness of some inconsistencies perpetrated by the profit motive of the industrial medical complex.

Diminished adrenal reserve steps off the path of health. The body wants to heal from adrenal insufficiency. The adrenals of some owners will never fully recover. After understanding some basics, the owner has arrived at a place to begin on a journey towards renewed wellness. A competent, loving physician or health practitioner can coach the owner in this next step. This problem lends itself to a change in one's lifestyle and nutritional habits and often a need for temporary pharmacological hormonal support. Real hormones are the only treatment that leads to healing. Synthetic hormones alway have side effects and toxicities. This critical difference will be explained in this chapter. This case history will serve as an introductory example of how one begins to heal.

Case History

Julia, a 55-year-old female, complained of extreme fatigue, gloom, easy weight gain, dry feeling and painful joints, brain fog, hot flashes, insomnia, and excessive weakness. For many years she consulted numerous physicians in an attempt to obtain relief. Her ordeal led her to take thyroid medication with only modest improvement. Estrogen patches resulted in minimal effects on the hot flashes. She obtained a 24-hour urine test to check her adrenal steroid output. DHEA levels were not detected. Cortisol output was in the mid-normal range. A fasting blood insulin level was taken later and proved very high.

Julia had no medical insurance, but provided an intriguing association between the on set of her symptoms with the use of birth control pills (which contain high doses of estrogen). High doses of estrogen promote blood vessel clotting. The adrenals are anatomically vulnerable because their venous drainage system has only one outflow vein. Obstruction of this vein can occur on high dose estrogen resulting in injury to the adrenal gland.

Julia began taking extremely low doses of pharmaceutical grade DHEA (10 mg - two times a day - excluding weekends). This regimen was further supplemented with high quality panax ginseng extract at 2500mg a day. As often happens with high insulin states, Julia's blood pressure ran a little high. In transition of learning how to live on a low carbohydrate diet, Julia was prescribed 500 mg of magnesium (elemental weight) and liberal amounts of Energen brand garlic. Both of these lower the blood pressure.

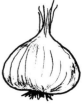

Julia's education was directed toward convincing her that by adhering to a low carbohydrate diet, her insulin levels would fall. A decrease in insulin levels leads to lower blood pressure and unlocks fat stores from insulin's grip. High quality, pharmaceutical grade progesterone cream was also prescribed at a rate of 2 ounces a month with one week off every month. Real progesterone is regenerative to most post-menopausal females (ovary chapter). In the weeks that followed, dramatic improvement was noted in all areas.

The confusion over what ginseng will do for aging adrenals is instructive to the deceptive scientific duplicity of different vocabulary hiding common concepts. For years, as this author studied the peculiar biochemistry of ginseng, he came upon the names of the active ingredients - saponins and sapogenins. He read Dr. Lee's progesterone biochemistry text only to discover that some of the saponins and sapogenins were only a few molecules away from progesterone contained within a 'package'. The conceptual roadblock lifted. The explanation for all those fertile and gracefully aging Asians regularly taking ginseng began to make sense.

The duplicity of scientific vocabulary surfaces when one realizes prescription related drugs are referred to as plant glycosides. In contrast, when they are considered herbal substances, they are referred to as containing saponins. When a curious physician inquires into the molecular makeup of the saponins, he finds a scientific roadblock. Once he becomes aware of the duplicity, he can access a whole wealth of data. For example, the plant glycoside, digitalis is related to testosterone in a package. If a curious physician ever got this far in the analysis, he would see how ginseng and digitalis share similar powers in their ability to provide the body with steroid precursors within a 'package'.

It's probably time to explain the side effects from regularly taking quality ginseng. This will also explain why quality ginseng is one of the hardest herbs to obtain. Asians don't want Americans looking as good as them so they keep their secret to themselves and sell mostly inferior grade ginseng in America.

Ginseng stimulates gonads and adrenals in the aging body by virtue of providing ample progesterone as the critical steroid building block. If there is any life in the gonad, libido rises considerably - as does male prowess. This is probably due to increased testosterone production. Without certain nutritional factors being present in adequate supply, an owner will see little effect from ginseng. There are additional considerations involved when one desires a return of optimal steroid synthesis.

Some authorities feel that ginseng has an effect on stimulating the master hormone gland, the pituitary, in a beneficial way. This makes sense. Chinese medical theory purports that ginseng is an 'adaptogen' in the face of life stress. It may be that when the master gland (located at the base of the brain) activates, there will be multiple benefits to the endocrine glands throughout the body. Examples would probably include thyroid, adrenal, gonads, and –

possibly - the thymus. Ginseng is worth considering when adrenals begin to fail. Ginseng may act on the body at other locations beyond the adrenal.

Hormone Mimics

Hormone mimics diminish the health of adrenals and gonads. Pervasive and insidious effects of hormonal mimics surface in the worldwide phenomenon of falling sperm counts in men. Androgen levels are the primary determinant of a man's sperm count. Hormone mimics surface from environmental and nutritional sources. Around the world chemicals like DDT and Agent Orange have been implicated in the estrogen mimic effect. These mimics compete with men's androgen tone, causing sperm counts to drop increasingly each decade.

The numerous common chemicals that exert a biochemical message effect, along various degrees of estrogen mimicry sounds fantastical. When one considers that all estrogen mimics share a similar molecular shape with their estrogen counter part, it becomes conceptually consistent. The common shape in the 'key' of estrogen is technically called the aromatic ring. Trouble starts because these diverse chemicals all contain the estrogen 'key' shape and once inside the body they lead to an unnaturally high estrogen message content.

In many ways, estrogen and estrogen mimics are counter-regulatory to the effect of androgens like testosterone. The most frightening aspect of turning up the estrogen message, in men and women is the powerful cell division message that certain estrogen and estrogen mimics deliver. This can cause abnormal growths in the prostate tissues of some men - a prime cause of benign prostatic hypertrophy (BPH). In women, estrogen dominance (relative to progesterone) leads to an increased tendency towards developing fibrocystic breast disease, uterine fibroids, breast cancer, PMS, and others.

Saran wrap, plastic food containers, and the liners inside canned foods all contain estrogen mimics. As a general guide, the higher the fat content, the greater the tendency for hormone mimics to migrate into the food. Prime environmental hormone disrupters are DDT, PCB's, and dioxin. DDT (a suspected 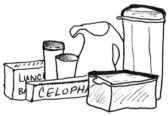 carcinogenic in mammals) is an environmentally persistent insecticide that causes fragile and broken eggshells in wild birds. Estrogen-like substances stimulate cell growth in estrogen sensitive tissue.

Though banned in the late 1970's, PCB's used in transformers and other electrical components still persist throughout the environment. The list of detrimental effects includes severe birth defects, cancer in animals, as a link to intellectual deficits in children. These mimics clearly stimulate cell division inappropriately.

Dioxins have been shown to cause cancer in animals and humans and have acted like estrogen in animal studies. In 1979, the environmental protection agency banned some herbicides because they were contaminated with dioxins. There are still numerous additional sources including paper bleaching facilities, polyvinyl chloride factories, and trash incinerators. The EPA modified industrial practices with some success, but it has proved difficult to eliminate them all.

Plasticizer compounds may leech from landfills into the environment, but do not seem to linger in human bodies. Two types of plasticizers suspect in causing problems are phthalates and adipates. In lab animals, phthalates cause liver cancer and testicular damage. Adipates in animals studies link to shortened life spans and decreased fertility. Bisphenol A, a building block of plastic manufacture, used in dental sealants and food can liners, causes enlarged prostates in animals.

There are several low cost strategies to avoid ingesting estrogen mimics. Reduce consumption of suspect compounds by avoiding plastic containers and wrappers. Consider using alternatives to pesticides and insecticides on both lawn and pets. Wash fruits and vegetables thoroughly or buy organic foods. Limit consumption of suspect fatty foods where these compounds accumulate in the food chain. Watch for local fish pollution possibilities. When reheating food, don't use plastic. Heat accelerates transfer of the hormone mimics into the food.

Adrenal Health Determines Immune Systems Appropriateness and Readiness

Many owners in America wake up tired, catch colds and coughs frequently, and deal with stress poorly. Many have diffuse aches in their muscles and joints. The depressed majority has lost their zest for life. Most have allergies or asthma that worsen with prolonged stress and fatigue. In the more severe cases of diminished adrenal function, chronic degenerative diseases like rheumatoid arthritis, systemic lupus erythematosus, ulcerative colitis, Crohn's disease, fibromyalgia syndrome, and colitis surface. Many of these ailments appear to be from divergent sources. Often, each of these afflictions traces back to a poorly functioning adrenal system.

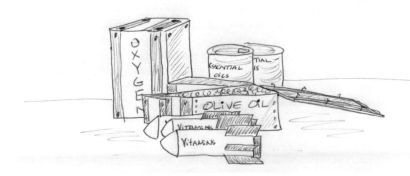

The science behind the dysfunctional adrenal gland system conflicts with the symptom control medicine approach. The complex panders the symptom control medicinal philosophy. Many physicians have no idea that a deeper understanding of adrenal function can often lead to considerable improvement in the disease. They have been groomed to think of the adrenals in a very superficial and piecemeal way.

Medical textbooks are curiously deficient in the discussion of interrelated consequences of a diminished adrenal reserve. Instead, their discussion focuses on the most extreme examples of adrenal dysfunction. Examples of these extremes are Addison's disease (cortisol deficiency) and Cushing's disease (cortisol excess).

A peripheral discussion may skim the surface of cortisol's role in the prevention of hypoglycemia. Cortisol is the major player in the prevention of hypoglycemia. Most discussions concern hormones within the adrenal gland, but fail to unite the other hormones. Most medical textbooks completely ignore the concept that some owners may have diminished adrenal function under conditions of stress. These owner's levels of dysfunction are not as severe as those of an Addisonian patient.

Doctors are taught to think about disease of the adrenal in a piecemeal fashion. Cushing's disease exemplifies this. A hallmark of this disease is losing muscle and gaining body fat. The reason body fat goes up is not directly related to the markedly elevated cortisol levels that are present with this disease. Cortisol initially promotes muscle and fat loss. Increased body fat is secondary to elevated blood sugar. The elevated blood sugar results from the high cortisol message content which then directs the liver to release sugar into the blood stream. The body eventually realizes that the blood sugar is elevated inappropriately. Excess insulin releases into the blood stream to counter this situation. Increases in insulin required to make the blood sugar normal leads to the increased making of body fat. Lost protein is due in part to the elevated cortisol, but prolactin also increases when cortisol is elevated. Increases in prolactin levels then inhibit the gonads to counter the high level of insulin. The inhibition of the gonads is often left out of the discussion. Also left out is that a slight elevation in the blood sugar will inhibit growth hormone release. Diminished growth hormone release will lead to a diminished ability to hold onto body proteins (liver chapter). This specific disease example points to the incongruous discussion between the various hormone abnormalities and the way physicians learn to think about adrenal disease.

The examples of Cushing's and Addison's disease are extreme examples of adrenal dysfunction. Cushing' disease produces extremely high cortisol production rates. Conversely, Addison's disease has an extreme deficiency of cortisol. The deficiencies are so significant that viability can only be maintained by taking cortisol supplements.

What about owners whose adrenal abnormality lie somewhere between these two extremes of adrenal dysfunction in stressful situations? Both of these situations have health consequences. Mainstream medicine most often recognizes the extremes of adrenal dysfunction. The consequence of this is that there are owners suffering, but not in immediate danger of death. This common medical practice is analogous to only consi dering thyroid dysfunction if it is on either extreme and puts the patient at risk of death.

Science could help owners with the above disease improve their adrenal systems function. Curiously, this is not the case. Medical educations do a better job at alerting physicians to the subtleties of altered thyroid function and the diseases that follow. Before ways to heal from these diseases are discussed, there needs to be a discussion about two important facts. First, steroids have a powerful nature when compared to other body hormones. Second, different disease presentations result from the same common deficiency of cortisol and/or DHEA. Much is known about the first fact. Very little is understood about the second fact and that awaits further scientific investigation before a plausible explanation can be given. Be aware of this current mystery.

The common property of the steroids vitamin A and thyroid hormone must be introduced. These hormones are the most powerful of all hormones. These steroids include testosterone, estrogen, DHEA, androstenedione, cortisol, progesterone, and aldosterone. There are others of less importance. The power of this group lies in the fact that only these hormone types carry their message directly to all DNA programs throughout every cell. No other hormones directly influence the DNA program.

These hormones interact with the genetic program. They directly determine which genes are turned off and on. Gene activity determines which body proteins are manufactured. Healthy bodies have the exact amount of protein types. The only way to get the right amounts of protein types is to have the right amounts of these powerful hormones giving directions. The quality, type, and amount of these powerful hormones determine how wisely available energy is spent. These hormones carry their message by virtue of their unique and precise shape. The steroids vitamin A and thyroid differ from other hormones by binding directly with many DNA receptors. They have access to every body chamber.

The unique property of these hormones allows them to be the determinants of which DNA programs are being activated or repressed. Owners that have the proper quality, amounts, and timing of these hormones are given a tremendous health advantage. The effectiveness of these hormones is related to the quality and amounts of the lesser hormones. These hormones are the most critical of all hormones. Ways to heal begin with considering their quality within an owner.

The power of these hormones lies in their control of the genetic program. An excess or deficiency provides an abnormal message content to the DNA of the cells. When the wrong DNA programs are activated or repressed, the cell spends energy unwisely. Energy used foolishly on the wrong proteins, wrong repair to rest ratios, wrong immune activation level, wrong amount of cell product, etc. describes a disease process.

Though diseases have predictable results, identical excesses or deficiencies will initiate different diseases in individual owners. This is only partially understood and the understood portion is complex.

Any of the six links in the adrenal system chain will cause disease when it becomes defective.

In today's world of harried physicians and managed care, the owner needs to be aware of the six levels where the adrenal system can fail. Erroneously, most attention toward adrenal health inquiries have limited the focus to one or two levels only. Consequently, many owners diagnosis are incorrect and/or they receive symptom control treatments. Thus owners miss out on ways to heal themselves. The next subsection explores the six levels of the adrenal system and how any one of these being defective leads to the above-mentioned adrenal system related diseases

Uniting high stress and a defect within the adrenal system make any of the adrenal system diseases worse.

1. Allergies
2. Asthma
3. Colitis

4. Systemic lupus erythematosus
5. Rheumatoid arthritis
6. Crohn's disease

In this subsection the reasoning will be explored. Attention will be given to why many physicians who look for a diminished adrenal system function fail to find it. They have not been trained to evaluate all six links in the adrenal system. The chain in the adrenal system includes:

1. Hypothalamus in the brain.
2. Master control panel gland for hormone glands, the pituitary, which hangs on the underside of the brain.
3. Healthy adrenal gland function.
4. Blood stream transport system.
5. Complete and intact characteristics of the DNA receptor waiting for something to do within the target cell.
6. The result of DNA program activation is the manufacture of certain protein-composed receptors for the 'lesser' hormones.

A defect at any of the six levels behaves clinically as if the adrenal system isn't functioning properly. Most physicians have not been educated in evaluating the integrity of the entire system. The profit in treating symptoms of the above diseases overrides the incentive to educate physicians about the other side of the story. Some lonely thinkers clunk along with some really good healing insights while the complex supports effective ways of marginalizing these scientific discoveries.

One of the heroes in the lonely thinker/scientist category is William McKenzie Jefferies M.D. Dr. Jefferies, the author of *Safe Uses of Cortisol,* 1996, brings over 45 years of clinical insight to the discussion of illness secondary to a malfunctioning adrenal system. His career in Endocrinology included professorships at both Case Western Medical School and more recently at Virginia Medical School. All of the above diseases are discussed and reviewed in his book. This book is a must read for an owner with any of the listed diseases secondary to a poorly functioning adrenal system. Education is necessary to step beyond symptom control and into healing.

Many physicians have been effectively taught to fear cortisone treatments over the long haul. This training has been so well performed that many physicians are automatic in their response to hearing the word cortisone or steroid. The typical response confuses physicians and the public by failing to differentiate cortisol in physiologic doses versus higher doses.

These diseases arise from an adrenal deficiency. Each unique deficiency has different proportions of the various adrenal steroids that are not getting to the afflicted owners DNA programs.

The six links in the adrenal health chain follow and this discussion will elaborate on why this occurs. Without complete inquiry into all six links, these diseases continue to smolder until they erupt. Diseases that erupt require symptom control and symptom control has side effects.

The media campaigns have persuaded physicians and owners into fearing even small doses of the natural body manufactured cortisol. This is despite the fact (evidence to be discussed shortly) that the diseases mentioned before have a deficiency of cortisol function in common. These diseases often directly result from a failure of the DNA program to receive adequate adrenal steroids.

An extension of Dr. Jefferies' work addresses the emerging realization that healthy, activated adrenals secrete a mixture of steroids in preformed ratios. This optimizes the message content of a healthy owner whenever the stress response activates. Only giving cortisol in all instances of the above diseases results in the potential for a lessened healing response. A lessened healing response results from the exclusion of the other adrenal steroids that are normally produced.

To understand how the adrenal system becomes compromised, a brief review of the break down mechanisms in any of the links will be explained. Keep in mind that other adrenal steroid imbalances may contribute significantly to a disease process.

First Link - Hypothalamus - the top of the Adrenal System

Almost fifty years ago, autopsies were performed on victims of various flu epidemics.[7] A revealing analysis of the adrenal glands proved that victim's adrenal tissue was unstressed and even looked inactive in some cases. This pathological discovery contradicts all other known diseases. A normal adrenal will damage itself trying to combat a disease process if that is required. In all other stress producing infections that lead to death, there are signs, at autopsy, within the adrenals of extreme adrenal depletion and hemorrhage (except flu and mononucleosis).

Strong evidence today shows that some viral illnesses diminish the ability to activate the hypothalamus. When the hypothalamus isn't being activated, the entire adrenal system fails to activate. The hypothalamus is the first link in the chain of adrenal health. Nothing starts in the survival message release, cortisol and other steroids, until the hypothalamus is activated. Viral illnesses, like the flu, damage this ability in the first link.

The symptoms of flu are commonly: fever, chills, malaise, body and joint aches, weakness, anorexia, and a general grouchiness. These happen to be the same symptoms of cortisol deficiency in the acute state. Some physicians have found support for administering low dose cortisol when the flu first appears. The flu symptoms quickly abate and the illness often retreats. It is important not to misdiagnose a bacterial infection as the flu because this treatment will make the infection worse.

One current thought - there are some owners with autoimmune disease that originates from a viral illness. The viral illness somehow damaged their hypothalamus from turning on the adrenal system properly (the first link in the adrenal chain of health). In some, the decreased direction from the hypothalamus only becomes evident during times of extra stress. Extra stress increases the body requirement for cortisol. When the hypothalamus fails to deliver the message to the second link, the pituitary, the increased production of cortisol becomes impossible. The impossibility arises because the first link is inactive and therefore all successive links are inactivated.

This example demonstrates how a virus can decrease the ability of the hypothalamus to perform its function and activate the successive links in response to an illness or stress. When the hypothalamus is diminished, stress can cause one to exceed the level of adrenal gland functional ability. It may be prudent to supplement these owners with adrenal products during times of increased stress or disease activation.

Second Link - Pituitary - Hangs Off of the Underside of the Brain

This pea-sized gland has hormone secretions that stimulate the growth of many endocrine glands and the release of their hormone contents. In a healthy state, it releases adrenocorticotropic hormone (ACTH). ACTH is derived from a larger precursor hormone called proopiomelanocortin. This hormone cleaves into numerous fragments producing ACTH, the body's natural opium (endorphin), and pigment producing hormone (MSH). The natural pigment-producing hormone increases in people with poor health of the adrenal glands and they tend to get pigmentation changes on their skin. The pituitary increases the message content that directs the adrenals to activate their secretion ("whipping" the injured adrenal to produce more steroids). In these situations, the pituitary releases all three hormones. This leads to increased skin pigmentation.

Link Three - Adrenal Health Determines the Mixture and Amounts of Adrenal Steroids

The adrenal gland makes six types of steroid hormones:

Cortisol	Aldosterone
DHEA	Androstenedione
Estradiol	Progesterone

Steroid production within the adrenal glands depends on many different vitamins. Unless all the needed vitamins are present, steroid production is compromised. The adrenal gland contains the highest concentration of vitamin C in the body. Steroid biosynthesis critically requires Vitamin C. B vitamins are also needed. Vitamin A is necessary to activate the adrenal glands DNA program properly for the products of its manufacture. The need for large amounts of vitamin C might explain why this vitamin seems to be so effective in activating the immune system.

Several factors influence the ability of the adrenal gland to produce steroids. The level of aldosterone is a powerful determinant of the body's steroid synthesis rate. Several genetic defects lead to a diminished ability to produce one or more steroids.

Aldosterone levels determine the rate of all the other adrenal steroids production. Steroid production rates within the adrenal are controlled by aldosterone because it controls the rate-limiting step of steroid biosynthesis. This step is the conversion of cholesterol to pregnenolone. Aldosterone activates the enzyme that performs this conversion, side chain cleavage enzyme.

High potassium intake (live food diet instead of dead food) relative to sodium intake will increase aldosterone levels. Blood pressure tends to remain normal when the sodium content in the diet decreases. Aldosterone, a steroid hormone, activates the DNA programs within the adrenals and gonads for increasing steroid manufacture within these glands. When the DNA program activate in this way it directs the manufacture of side chain cleavage enzyme. Medications that decrease aldosterone levels will tend to cripple steroid production (sections three through five).

Certain owners have genetic weaknesses causing an excess or deficiency of adrenal steroids. Physicians who can piece together clues allowing a specific diagnosis can supplement with the deficient steroid and the excessive ones will return to normal. Enzymatic deficiencies cause diseases such as: polycystic ovary syndrome, adrenogenital syndrome, salt wasting hypotension, cystic acne, hirsuitism, and menorrhagia to name a few.

Fourth Link – Adrenal Steroids Within the Blood Stream

Once the adrenal receives the message from the pituitary, link two, its preformed steroids dump into the blood stream. Adrenal steroids transport within the blood stream in three different ways. The first mode of transportation is free within the liquid component of the blood stream. The second is within the red blood cells and the third is attached to carrier proteins. The proportions of each of these ways to transport steroids have powerful effects on the availability of the adrenal steroids to the cells DNA programs.

American laboratories completely ignore the amount of steroid transported within the red blood cells. In addition, the amount of steroids bound to the carrier protein is sometimes poorly evaluated. These two common errors lead doctors to falsely reassure their patients that their adrenal gland functions normally when it doesn't.

The adrenal system level most commonly evaluated is the blood stream. This incomplete mainstream approach overlooks what is actually known about the steroids in transit within the blood stream.

The majority of certain steroids are transported within red blood cells. This is a powerful mechanism for these dominant hormones getting squeezed into tissue at the capillary level. Relying on serum (the liquid component of the blood that is devoid of cells) for determining one's level of active hormone is wrought with difficulty. It is now known that steroids within the red cell are actually more representative of the 'steroid pressure' driving their message into cells.

When the body needs cortisol, the blood stream supply depletes rapidly. Dr. Jefferies noted Dr. Ingle's demonstration (from the 1940's) that cortisol levels in the blood stream did not rise when extra amounts were given during times of stress. Stress created a rapid movement of cortisol into the tissues when needed to survive. The increased need for cortisol is not measurable in the blood stream.

The clinician must consider, while measuring the cortisol level of those with the potential for diminished adrenal reserve, some patients tend to have deceptively normal blood cortisol levels while low stress prevails. However, during stress their adrenals' production of cortisol diminishes. In these cases of diminished adrenal reserve, blood testing or a twenty-four hour urine test for cortisol production can be deceptively normal. Some of these patients will require an ACTH challenge test before their diminished reserve shows up on laboratory tests.

The ACTH challenge test measures the ability of the adrenals to increase cortisol production when stimulated. Since ACTH is the actual hormone that stimulates the adrenal to release cortisol, a challenge with this hormone should increase cortisol within thirty minutes. A normal response is two times greater than the level before the adrenals were challenged with ACTH.

Many owners, with diseases related to adrenal deficiency; fail to achieve this increase in cortisol production. Many of these diseases intensify when an owner is stressed. Stress increases the need for cortisol within the cells. The cell DNA needs cortisol to survive various stresses of life. The above diseases come about when certain cell DNA programs receive defective amounts of the adrenal steroid message. If any of the six links of the adrenal system are broken, a deficiency can result. A broken link causes a defect for all levels below it. All six links need to be intact or the above types of diseases begin to manifest.

Physiologically, the ability to handle stress depends on adequate increases in cortisol. Adequate increases in cortisol direct energy into survival pathways. Surgeons see first hand the importance of cortisol production in the ability to survive the stress of surgery. Following the stress of surgery, a patient will die if their adrenals are incapable of increased cortisol production. When cortisol release skyrockets into the body, potassium loss increases. Consequently, these two facts are routinely provided for post operatively. Potassium and cortisol are administered in the post-operative period. This precaution prevents severe complications in case a post-surgical owner's adrenal glands are not up to the task.

One of the best ways to screen for defects in the first four links of the adrenal health chain is in obtaining a twenty-four hour urine test. The urine test misses the last two links in the adrenal health chain. Unfortunately, very few physicians can interpret the complex issues that arise from the results of this test. Also, the standard method on which the twenty-four hour urine test is calibrated is to give the patient instructions regarding a normal stress day. This raises the question about missing those patients that only become adrenal compromised during times of stress (when there is an increased need for cortisol that they cannot provide).

Fortunately, there are valuable clues that will show a deficiency in the adrenal system (all six links in the 'chain'). These clues can occurs within the blood stream whenever a white blood cell differential is performed. If the eosinophils, (a type of white blood cell), are elevated, the adrenal system may be deficient. If neutrophils decrease and lymphocytes increase, another red flag of adrenal insufficiency should go up. When either clue occurs, the physician should thoroughly check the six levels of the patients adrenal system. A cortisol deficiency will allow abnormalities of these white blood cell types. All of the diseases (listed at the beginning of this section), have a high likelihood of increased eosinophils in their clinical picture.

Another valuable clinical discovery indicates that patients with an adrenal system deficiency consistently wake up tired. This is especially true when their disease process is active. This contrasts to the low thyroid patient who tires in the afternoon.

Occult infections and hidden malignancies can present with some of the same clinical findings as adrenal deficiencies. As a precaution, rule these out before initiating a treatment plan for an adrenal problem.

Fifth Link – DNA Associating Nuclear Receptor Must Be Complete and Undamaged or No Message Can Be Delivered

For a steroid to deliver its message content to a cell, there must be a receptor to receive it. The resulting shape of the receptor plus the exact shape of the steroid creates a message within the DNA to activate or repress the bound gene. If no receptor is present then no message can be delivered. Owners who suffer from this problem will have a deceptively normal lab test. At times they can have normal eosinophils and neutrophils in certain clinical situations. Sometimes a disease behaves like an adrenal problem, but the lab values come back normal. The lab values only check steroids to the fourth link. Although level five and six are often suspected when one looks at the white blood cell abnormalities, they are not always accurate.

No one knows how many patients suffer from this type of defect. When a level five defect happens, there is the right hypothalamus input, the right pituitary input, the appropriate adrenal response, and the proper transport within the blood stream. Cortisol, without a preformed nuclear receptor, does not activate the DNA properly, which causes the problem.

Nuclear receptors differ for different steroids. Thyroid, vitamin A, and optimal steroids are all necessary to make each other's DNA receptors.

Unless a physician is aware of this fact, even the 24-hour urine tests will look deceptively good in some cases. What the physician tests for isn't the level of the problem, when link five is the culprit for adrenal system disease.

There is much to be learned about the fifth link of adrenal system malfunction. Recent scientific insights have the potential to help solve the 'why' for receptor defects within the DNA. These results point to the increased understanding that many of these 'big daddy' hormones depend, in an interconnected way, for activation and manufacture of their various DNA receptors. There is agreement that vitamin A, thyroid, and cortisol all contribute to the manufacture of certain receptors. Since many Americans are vitamin A deficient, this could be the cause of some of these diseases.

It is worth some investigative work to try and assess the status of these powerful hormones by means of a well-run twenty-four hour urine test. If the clinical situation is suspicious then a careful trial of some of these hormones is warranted as long as there is frequent follow up and the patient is properly motivated.

Link Six – Result of DNA Program Activation is the Manufacture of Specific Receptors for the Lesser Hormones

When a steroid activates a DNA program (gene) protein synthesis results. Protein synthesis is determined by the DNA sequence that was activated. Some of the steroid message directs certain DNA programs to produce receptors for the lesser hormones. Lesser hormones are all hormones not included with thyroid, vitamin A, or steroids. How the hierarchy works between hormones will be explained at the end of this section.

The bodies of some owners make antibodies to the 'secondary' receptors that are made by the message of the steroids DNA program. Antibody complexes with these receptors essentially deactivate the lesser hormones ability to bind their receptor. These receptors for the lesser hormones comprise the sixth link of the adrenal chain of health. Caution should be taken not to confuse the previous nuclear receptor (link five) with these secondary receptors (link six). The nuclear receptors can only bind thyroid, vitamin A and steroids. Only when the steroids bind to the DNA programs (level five), can the manufacture of the next level of receptor be directed. A level six receptor occurs as a result of the message content of the steroid hormones.

The steroid message results in synthesis of specific receptors for specific 'lesser' hormones that follow within the blood stream (hierarchy of hormones). The integrity of these 'lesser' hormone receptors needs consideration, the sixth link for adrenal health. Problems at this level of the adrenal chain can cause or contribute to disease. Like level five problems, the lab tests can look deceptively normal.

This has probable merit in the production of adrenal system related disease due to finding antibodies to various 'lesser' hormone receptors. In these cases even though these 'big daddy' hormones designate the receptors be built they are inactivated by the immune system.

All hormones need their receptors to be intact if their message is to be delivered. To understand the message content, receptors that are on the cell surface need to function properly. 'Lesser' hormones receptors tend to be on the cell surface. This contrasts to the 'big daddies' hormones. Their receptors are near the DNA program.

When antibodies disable the 'lesser receptor' before the 'lesser hormone' (i.e. adrenaline) arrives, that cell can't receive the hormone message content. This creates adrenal deficiency in the clinical situation, even though the first five 'links' in the adrenal system are intact. These unfortunate patients will almost always have normal blood values for adrenal steroids and normal twenty-four hour urine values for those steroids involved. Their disease results from the message not being able to activate when the lesser hormones arrive. The lesser hormone cannot activate its receptor when the immune system has disabled it. In these cases the steroid directed and manufactured receptor has been disabled by the immune system.

The antibodies to the cortisol directed manufacture of the adrenergic B2 receptor (adrenaline) demonstrates this. Antibodies to these receptors have been found in patients with asthma and allergic rhinitis (hay fever). The development of an antibody test for B2 receptors would help to identify some of these patients who suffer these two diseases. The inclusion of testing for antibodies to the nuclear steroid receptors is also appropriate as it would evaluate antibody production against either a level five or a level six problem as well.

The accuracy of this last suggestion needs to be confirmed by further research. Until then, it will be up to their physician to follow both the owners steroid hormone profiles and the clinical presantation for signs of excess or continued deficiency.

The six links in the adrenal health chain are a way to conduct an initial inquiry as to the status of an owner's endocrine function within these glands. Many additional diseases result from an imbalanced interrelationship between adrenals and ovaries.

The next chapter introduces this interrelationship. Like the adrenals the ovaries can be best understood by understanding the multiple levels (links in the chain of ovary health). The testicle chapter is also similar and will be found at the end of this section.

Chapter 6

Ovaries
Modern Females Dilemma

A defective ovary system can show similar clinical pictures to that of a defective adrenal system. However, the origins of the diseases differ because of different defects in the 'chain links' of the ovary system of health. If the physician fails to evaluate all six links in the 'chain' then the disease will be treated in the symptom control paradigm. Female owners interested in healing need an education in how these glands work and what they need at all six levels within the ovarian system.

Healthy females have highly functional ovaries and/or highly functional adrenal glands. Around age thirty-five, many female owners begin to experience various levels of hormonal decline. The clinical clues are there, but the physician needs to know how to look for them.

Prescribing synthetic replacement hormones cause problems. They do not contain the intended body message content that female owners require. Since the aberrant message content directs DNA programs in unnatural ways, these patentable versions always have side effects. This chapter contains scientific revelations on this subject. Other pertinent information relates how natural female hormones keep middle age at bay. Both declining natural hormones within and unnatural synthetic or altered substitutes end up with diminished outcomes. Diminished outcomes predictably occur whenever the body cells natural message content is disrupted.

Message content disrupts because synthetic hormone replacement alters the shape of the hormone. Natural hormones are altered to gain a patent. Without a patent, no financial advantage ensues. Financial advantage has nothing to do with healing. How one heals revolves around replacing the lost message content by nutritional, lifestyle, and real hormone replacement. This chapter is about the problem of symptom control, why real hormones are better, how nutrition affects the ovaries health, and the six links in the ovary chain of health.

Introduction to the Imbalanced Hormonal States of Female Owners

The general imbalance in pre-menopausal female owners today is from too much and the wrong types of estrogen. Too much estrogen occurs relative to the availability of the counter regulatory hormone, progesterone. For post-menopausal females the imbalanced hormone situation can be more variable but progesterone deficiency is always present.

The important difference between natural progesterone and the synthetic progesterone substitutes (commonly called progestagens and progestins) is not widely understood. Lack of this knowledge has lead countless female owners to suffer from unnecessary and chronic disease. Natural progesterone plays an important role in maintaining female health.

Estrogen and progesterone are some of the most powerful hormones. Their quality and amount directly interact with the cellular DNA program. Different types of estrogen substitutes compound the problems created by synthetic progesterone by creating poor message content. Health consequences occur when DNA programs receive poor directional information. The abnormal monthly cycle of a female describes the effects that occur when DNA receives poor message content.

Steroids, like estrogen and progesterone, are relatively simple molecules within the domain of the larger hormone molecules like insulin. The smaller the hormone (message carrier), the more exact the shape that the hormone needs to have in order to preserve message content.

In the size class of the steroids, changing a single angle in one chemical bond between carbon and hydrogen can change the message content and/or strength.

It has been known for almost fifty years that changing the angle between one carbon and hydrogen in estradiol changes the potency of the message content by a factor of thirty. Chemists denote this change as alpha to beta angle rotation.

The most powerful estrogen type in humans is Beta-estradiol. However, common estrogen replacement prescriptions contain, Alpha-estradiol that is thirty times more powerful than the naturally occurring human form, Beta-estradiol. In addition to the alpha type estrogen that horses make, they also make horse estrogen message content. Horse specific estrogen message content is contained in both equilin and equlinin. Many women are taking these powerful and altered message type estrogens in the prescriptions given to them for hormone replacement. These altered hormones are collected from the urine of pregnant horses or made synthetically from soy or yams.

The Monthly Cycle and Imbalance

Estrogen stimulates cell growth in estrogen sensitive tissues (breast, uterus, fat, and liver) for the first half of the female menstrual cycle. If left unopposed, the stimulant effects of estrogen lead to common ailments such as fibrocystic breast disease, uterine fibroids, breast cancer, uterine cancer, and unnatural growth of other estrogen responsive tissues.[8]

In the second half of the menstrual cycle, in a healthy state, progesterone counter-regulates much of estrogens' message content. Progesterone directs influence over DNA programs in the same cells that estrogen influences. Progesterone deficiency is a common problem.

The first of four reasons for this deficiency is the multitude of pervasive 'estrogen' mimics within the environment. This increases the total estrogen message for many women when compared to their ability to manufacture progesterone (adrenal chapter).

Second, the synthetic progesterone part of hormone replacement therapy intensifies the problem by using unnatural progesterone substitutes. Unnatural progesterone substitutes can inhibit natural progesterone production that is needed for the counter-regulation of estrogen and other youth preserving processes.

Third, progesterone deficiency relates to a nutritionally poor diet. Certain nutritional elements are necessary for adequate progesterone production. Each of these factors that contribute to estrogen dominance will be explained shortly.

This forth factor relates how female hormones become unbalanced and eventually produce disease. This common situation results when female owners are prescribed the wrong types of estrogen (in contrast to factor two above, which is caused by the prescribing of synthetic progesterone).

Many different natural and unnatural estrogens are prescribed to women by mainstream medicine. When the estrogen message content is out of balance, the wrong cellular message occurs chronically.

Four Factors Leading to Estrogen Dominance Relative to Progesterone

1. Estrogen mimics in the environment (hormone mimics).
2. Unnatural progesterone in hormone replacement therapies decreases real progesterone levels.
3. Nutritional deficiencies exacerbate the progesterone and estrogen imbalance (discussed within the six links in the ovarian chain of health, link three).
4. Hormone prescriptions commonly contain abnormal estrogen message content

In order to understand how prescriptions commonly disrupt the natural message in a woman's body, the natural state needs to be defined. When treatment strategies facilitate a recreation of the natural state, healing becomes possible. There is wisdom in the power of the female body to heal.

Three natural estrogens produced in the human body allow health. Each natural human estrogen type has an optimal percentage of the total estrogen message content within the body. When these are balanced, a coherent cellular message is realized. A deviation from the optimal relative percentages leads to an imbalanced hormone message with cellular consequences. For example, estriol has weak cell division stimulation tendencies, but it is the major natural form of human estrogen initially released from the ovary.

There are good reasons that the weakest estrogen is initially released within the pelvic cavity in the highest concentration. Estriol is very powerful in the maintenance and health of the vulva and vaginal tissues. It doesn't need conversion to the more powerful estrogen types.

This contrasts to B-estradiol and estrone, which contain powerful cell division message content directed at estrogen responsive tissues. This fact helps one begin see the advantage of their minority position.

Unfortunately, the patentable pharmaceutical estrogens are from the powerful cell division message type. This situation is completely avoidable if the patient obtains a prescription for the compounding pharmacist. Delivering natural estrogen via a patch, cream, capsule, sublingual drops, or vaginal gel can customize these prescriptions. A natural ratio and type between these three is individualized and determined by the twenty-four hour urine test results. This leads to a natural cellular message in the estrogen responsive tissues. The restoration of the natural estrogen message is the first step in healing from estrogen dominance.

Symptom control medicine ignores the natural estrogen message content found in the human owner. The typical prescriptions contain either synthetic versions or altered estrogens from horse urine concentrate. Relatively speaking, steroids, like estrogen and progesterone, are simple molecules in the domain of larger hormone molecules like insulin. The smaller the hormone (message carrier) the more exact the hormone needs to be in its shape to preserve the message content. The change of a single angle in one chemical bond between carbon and hydrogen can alter the message content and/or strength.

An example in futility is attempting to make even a slight change to natural estrogen by changing in the angle between one carbon and hydrogen in estradiol. This very small alteration in one bond changes the potency of the message content by a factor of thirty. Chemists denote this change as alpha to beta angle rotation. In addition to the most powerful estrogen type in the human, Beta-estradiol, these prescriptions contain, Alpha-estradiol, which is thirty times more powerful than the natural human form, Beta-estradiol.

Horses make the more powerful alpha type along with some beta types and in addition, they also make horse estrogen message content, equilin and equlinin. Many women are taking these powerful, altered message type estrogens in the prescriptions given to them for hormone replacement. These altered hormones are collected from pregnant horses urine or are made synthetically from soy or yams.

In the natural condition, humans make small amounts of the much weaker beta estradiol. This alone is a very powerful estrogen in the scheme of things. Imagine the potential consequences when the message content is multiplied by a factor of thirty. Yet, this is happening to millions of women who are taking unnatural mixtures of estrogen or synthetic versions. This fact leads to estrogen imbalances (number four factor). The fourth factor is the topic of this subsection. Physicians may be unaware of this chemical fact because they receive medical information through sources that are 'friendly' to the interests of drug companies.

If women are healthier with natural estrogen, why aren't more pharmaceutical companies manufacturing this? Natural prescriptions are not patentable and hence, not profitable. In order to obtain a patent, the natural estrogen or progesterone shape needs to be changed in some way. Small changes in molecules of this size are not possible without changing the message content that is inherent to the precise shape.

In the various birth control pill formulations, the shapes change even more radically compared to the natural shape of estrogen and progesterone. This example sites the estrogen molecule alterations that deviate from the natural human shapes. What about the consequences of altering progesterone, the counter-hormone of estrogen?

Synthetic Progesterone Substitutes as a Factor in Real Progesterone Deficiency for Its Message Content

Synthetic alteration of progesterone profoundly affects a woman's health for two reasons (factor two above). First, it is the building block molecule for many other steroids. Without adequate progesterone building blocks, other steroid levels suffer.

Second, like other natural hormones, the exact inherent shape of progesterone carries an exact message that is needed in the second half of a female's monthly cycle. It counters many of the effects started by estrogen in the first part of the menstrual cycle. The progesterone content, which rises in the second half of the female cycle, counters the cell division and fluid retaining effects of estrogen. Without adequate progesterone, females will tend towards estrogen dominance based disease such as fibrocystic breast disease, breast cancer, uterine cancer, premenstrual bloating, uterine fibroids, and migraine headaches. With the shape alteration of synthetic progesterone the message content changes and these tasks cannot be performed effectively. Hormonal balance occurs when the balance-counter-balance mechanisms are functioning properly. This includes proper timing and an adequate amount of real progesterone and estrogen.

Progesterone serves as a building block molecule for other important steroids manufactured in the adrenals and ovaries. The molecular building block, progesterone, is the source for testosterone, cortisol, and some estrogen. When owners have synthetic progesterone prescriptions in their body, the likelihood increases for creating an imbalance in the synthesis of other steroids. This concequence arrises because synthetic progesterone cannot serve as a building block for other steroids.

The message content of molecules the size of steroids, like estrogen and progesterone, is inherent in the precise shape. When the shape changes minutely so does the message delivered to the DNA. Healthy people have real hormones that carry accurate message content. Unhealthy people are the consequence of unnatural message content being delivered to their DNA.

Estrogen Dominance

Conspicuous clinical signs of estrogen dominance:

1. Pre-menstrual breast pain
2. Poor sleep quality
3. Fluid retention more than twenty four hours before the onset of the menses
4. Increased tendency toward premenstrual tension (increased irritability and combativeness) up to fourteen days prior to the onset of menses.

When an estrogen dominant imbalance persists, there is an increased likelihood for the development of diseases such as: fibro-cystic breast disease, uterine fibroids, breast cancer, shortened menstrual cycle, endometrial cancer, menstrual cycle migraines, osteoporosis, and weight gain. Being mindful of what the female body is saying will create awareness about estrogen dominance.

Clinical signs deserve attention into the 'why' and the 'how' of estrogen dominance. A brief review of the six links in the 'chain' of the estrogen and progesterone system will follow the ovary system. Within this discussion there is an explanation for how estrogen dominance accelerates the changes of middle age. Attention to these six links will increase the odds of a female owner having the best hormones that are consistent with good health.

Six Links in the 'Chain' - Good Health of the Ovarian System

Six links in the health of the ovarian system include:

1. Hypothalamus
2. Pituitary
3. Ovary
4. Blood stream transport system
5. Nuclear receptor at the DNA level within the ovarian hormone responsive tissues
6. Receptors manufactured as a result of ovarian hormones activation of certain DNA programs causing direction for the manufacture of new receptors (other steroid receptors and the 'lesser' hormones).

Different female owners suffer from different points of break down in the six links of the 'chain' within their ovarian system. Menopause results from a broken link at level three, the ovary. Some systemic illnesses affect level one, the hypothalamus. Some hormone abnormalities at the pituitary (level two) inhibit the ovary. The broken link must be correctly identified to restore hormonal balance.

Link One - Hypothalamus

The hypothalamus controls all the other links within the ovary system. Under activity of the first link creates under activity of all successive links of the chain. The amount of information that the hypothalamus sends is determined largely by the amount of estrogen it senses. Too much estrogen reaching this level weakens the link at this first level. When the hypothalamus turns down its informational direction of the ovarian system, other important hormones are affected. As long as the female ovarian system is in balance turning down the volume is appropriate. When certain estrogen prescriptions are taken, the hypothalamus gets fooled and doesn't direct the manufacture of other important hormones.

Sometimes various estrogens are prescribed without consideration for how this practice will decrease testosterone like steroids. The ovary, while releasing progesterone and estrogen, is also releasing testosterone (an important androgen) like steroids as well. Testosterone message is needed for rejuvenation. In this way, female owners who take too much estrogen can short circuit a powerful androgen message. The androgen message decreases because, link one, has been fooled by artificially high estrogens in certain female bodies.

In the example of estrogen replacement, the androgen deficiency results because hormonal replacements usually do not contain androgens. The hypothalamus assumes that when estrogen is elevated, testosterone is elevated as well. In the subsection on 'steroid tone,' there will be an explaination of the central role of testosterone-like androgens play in rejuvenation.

The amount of stimulatory information, which the hypothalamus sends into the ovary chain of health, is determined by the amount of estrogen it senses. When the ovary is healthy, it produces progesterone, estrogen, and testosterone. Estrogen replacement strategies usually do not contain the androgen. The elevated estrogen levels that these pills provide fool the hypothalamus, which further decreases testosterone.

Link Two - Pituitary

The master gland, the pituitary, regulates the other hormone glands. It manufactures many competing hormonal messages for release. The hypothalamus is the main director of the messages released by the pituitary. The pituitary then releases specific hormones directing the ovary. Hormones contain message content. The importance lies in which hormone messages are released from the pituitary. The quality of the mixture this gland secretes tells the ovary how to expend energy. This then becomes the dominant message. Adequate and rhythmic release of leuteinizing hormone (LH) and follicle stimulating hormone (FSH) released from the pituitary, nourish the ovary by giving specific direction to continue its natural cycle.

Conversely, in the master gland (the pituitary) is a powerful hormone, prolactin. The ovary becomes inhibited when prolactin is released beyond low levels. Even though many physicians have been groomed into the 'knee jerk' summary that prolactin stimulates milk production, the evidence clearly implicates prolactin as a powerful inhibitor of ovarian function. The confusion arises because they know that when women are pregnant steroid production becomes very high and the prolactin level also elevates. This false discrepancy is solved, when later in the pregnancy, the ovaries are powerfully inhibited by prolactin. It is the placenta, which cranks out huge amounts of steroids that are increased with the pregnant state. There are four common clinical states where prolactin, produced within the pituitary, induces ovary inhibition. There is no placenta to make up the difference in the lost steroids produced by the ovary in these cases.

The four states that stimulate pituitary release of prolactin include low thyroid function, birth control pill usage, chronic stress, and high serotonin. In these cases, the production of the ovarian component of steroids diminishes because these situations lead to increased prolactin. Steroids are so powerful if any one diminishes, the DNA content will go either dormant or hyper. Most people have a good feeling that when the DNA is not behaving, a danger to over all health exists. With an appropriate prolactin level, healing transpires.

Mechanisms for increased pituitary release of prolactin:

1. Birth control pill usage
2. High serotonin levels
3. Chronic stress
4. Low thyroid gland function

Increased prolactin levels are caused by increased estrogen used in birth control pills. Prolactin inhibits ovarian hormone steroid formations and release. The second hormone-induced mechanism associated with obesity is generally not in operation with pregnancy. This physiologic state has the growing placenta that generates needed steroids. The placenta manufactures androgens even though the ovary becomes relatively dormant by the fifth month of pregnancy. When female owners take birth control pills the body thinks it is pregnant and prolactin levels rise. Prolactin levels rise when estrogen levels approach pregnancy levels.

Potential obesity occurs because like pregnancy, the birth control pills increase prolactin levels. Unlike pregnancy there is no placental hormone factory to correct the inhibition of the ovaries for steroid production. Additional potential problems exist. Birth control pills do not contain androgens, only estrogen and progestins (synthetic progesterone substitutes). Androgen production can fall and some adrenals fail in the challenge to increase androgen production and obesity ensues.

High serotonin levels raise prolactin levels. This situation can occur when SSRI types anti-depressants are taken (section six).

Chronic stress tends to raise prolactin levels. Prolactin levels elevate when increased cortisol release stimulates prolactin release as part of the stress response.

Low thyroid gland function will stimulate the hypothalamus initially to release thyroid-releasing globulin (TRH). TRH is a very powerful secretogogue for prolactin release from the pituitary.

Link Three - Ovary

When the female owner is healthy her ovaries make appropriate amounts of androgens. In addition, the healthful state is typified by proper levels of estrogens, which are cycled with proper levels of progesterone. Each month a new cycle begins and cells receive the right amount of message content directing them to invest in rejuvenation activities. Rejuvenation activities keep the body young.

Around menopause the ovaries begin to fail and give up their steroid production role to the middle aged adrenal. Many years prior to this, steroid production begins to diminish within the ovaries. When clinicians miss this or treat with synthetic hormones, a female owner is on a accelerated path to an old body.

Nutritional deficiencies play a major role in ovarian disease. Common factors include a chronic tendency for the consumption of a 'processed food' diet versus 'real food' diet. Ovarian steroid production provides an example of how nutrition affects ovarian health. One central facet of ovarian function is determined by the rate at which cholesterol is converted to pregnenolone. The conversion rate is determined by how much aldosterone is present. This fact about the steroid manufacture rate is true for the adrenals, testicles and ovaries. In the ovary, testicle and adrenal DNA programs, adequate aldosterone is needed to start production of cholesterol Demolase. This initial enzyme involved in steroid manufacture is also known as a side chain cleavage enzyme.

A high potassium diet ('real food') stimulates aldosterone release. Processed food diets are deficient in potassium and pave the road for dysfunctional ovaries. This is an example of steroid interdependence for ovary health to be possible. Along with aldosterone, the healthy ovary needs vitamin C, plus A and B complex for adequate steroid production capabilities. The mineral zinc allows steroid synthesis to occur at high levels.

The mineral content between the two types of diets shows drastic differences. Real food contains natural minerals in the proportions required for health. Processed foods have drastically altered mineral content. The minerals, magnesium and potassium, become depleted in the act of processing natural foods. Unhealthy amounts of sodium, calcium, hydrogenated fats, and sugar are added to extend shelf life. This equals profits for the food industry. Processed food doesn't contain the proper ratio of the four minerals - magnesium, calcium, potassium, and sodium. Ovaries need the correct mineral ratio than other tissues in order to maintain aldosterone message content (adrenal chapter). The amount of aldosterone message content determines the rate of all steroids synthesis within the adrenals and ovaries. Natural food diets facilitate an increased aldosterone level.

Owners who eat dead food diets are potassium and magnesium depleted about the onset of middle age. A deficiency of potassium creates the need for increased insulin to process the same amount of sugar. In addition, potassium and magnesium deficiencies lead to high blood pressure; irregular heart rate; diminished adrenal and ovary steroid production; diminished red blood cell flexibility and decreased cell voltages (a weakened cell force field). The 'why' and 'how' of these facts are discussed throughout this manual. Proper mineral intake equates a better ovary and adrenal gland function.

Fourth Link - Bondage Fraction versus the Free Level of Ovarian Hormones within the Blood Stream

Transport of ovarian steroids is the fourth link in the ovarian system of health chain. There are three different ways ovarian steroids are transported within the blood stream.
1. In the red blood cell membrane (major fraction)
2. Trapped on bondage proteins, Western owners are often misled because of an incomplete inquiry into the level of ovarian hormones released and trapped in this compartment.
3. Small amounts travel freely in the blood stream.

The ovarian steroids, estrogen, progesterone, testosterone, and androstenedione, are usually transported within the red blood cells. Estrogen, while in transport within the red blood cell, can be acted upon by enzymatic machines and transformed into more powerful types of estrogens. By this mechanism, the initially released estrogen type changes in the periphery. The initial types of estrogen relative percentages, which are secreted from the ovaries, can be altered while in route to the distant target cell.

The liquid component of blood, plasma, also transports some ovarian hormones (testosterone, androstenedione, estrogens, and progesterone). Higher thyroid and estrogen hormone levels equal higher transporter 'bondage' protein levels. These hormones, when they occur at high levels, instruct the liver to make bondage proteins for all steroids within the blood stream. Some physicians are misled into thinking a blood drawn laboratory test looks good.

However, a higher bondage protein level means that a hormone measured in the blood may be misleading if the transport (bondage) protein level is either higher or lower than normal. The name of the transport protein for testosterone and estrogen is referred to as sex hormone binding globulin (SHBG).

The blood stream must contain this important protein for proper sex steriod function. Deviations from normal levels do two things to steroid message content. First, they alter the rate at which the liver can inactivate steroid levels. The higher the levels, the less readily the liver inactivates them. Conversely, the higher the level, the less readily the body cells access their informational content. When levels are high, they slow the ability of steroids to get into target cells (DNA programs). Only a fraction of steroids contained in blood cells and a fraction of the various steroids have the ability to get in the 'target' cells. Only when the steroids make it into the target cells can they activate the various DNA programs. When the DNA programs receive message content, they direct the cell's energy expenditure. Conversely, 'bondage' protein (SHBG) level determines the amount of steroid that can't escape from the blood stream. Steroids, trapped onto bondage proteins, are unable to deliver message content into cells until another hormone event changes their equilibrium. This last detail is beyond the scope of this book. These are variables to consider concerning steroids when interpreting blood test results.

Looking at only steroid levels in the blood can be misleading. A modest improvement in accuracy can be achieved with a SHBG level. When this protein level is high, large amounts of steroids could be circulating without a destination. A twenty-four hour urine test for steroid hormone excretion would be more accurate.

The effective level of a steroid's ability to bind and activate its DNA associated receptor (link five) is also a concern. Failure to consider the links that make up the ovary system chain has led many clinicians to falsely conclude that all is well.

Link Five - Integrity and Amount of Functional DNA Associated Nuclear Receptors in the Target Cell

Once an ovarian steroid successfully travels within the blood stream and enters the target cell, it needs to activate its DNA binding receptor. Without binding its receptor it cannot activate or repress a cells DNA program. When something is wrong with the receptor link, the message content of a steroid cannot be heard. A simple example of level five-associated receptor formation is the interdependence between progesterone and estrogen to manufacture each other's DNA associated receptors.

It takes a brave physician to prescribe the powerful steroid hormones without a lab test to back up the need. That is exactly what happens when post-menopausal females are given unnatural and synthetic hormones without checking to see what this will do to other hormone systems. Inferior scientific thinking is acceptable where `contrary' thinkers, who dare to think about the different links in the chain of ovarian dysfunction, are not. There is a legal medical 'witch hunt' that occurs when any physician thinks differently from the `herd'.

Physicians resist sticking their neck out medically or legally even though scientific revelations tend to back up the practice. This is one more way the complex effectively controls its best interest. This stranglehold will change if patients make a moral commitment (not) to litigate for the unforeseen consequences of what is (not) known about hormones.

Natural hormones are safer than their synthetic counterparts. When dealing with level five problems, safe dosages for patients are not known. One in nine female owners will get breast cancer. If her physician uses a natural approach and breast cancer develops, it constitutes an excuse for the licensing board to prosecute. However, if the physician uses synthetic hormones and does only a superficial hormone inquiry, the medical legal standard has been upheld even if a patient develops cancer. This reoccurring theme demonstrates how sound science is suppressed. The concern of the complex is to expose that a contrary physician's patient has breast cancer. The physician that suspectsthat he has a level five problem operating within a patient is caught between medical legal concerns and a patient who shows clinical signs of accelerated aging.

A dysfunction in the fifth link can mislead clinicians because patients often have normal blood and urine tests for different ovarian steroids. The prematurely aged female body will warn an astute physician that there is a level five problem in operation.

Whenever hormonal dysfunction happens at this level, the preceding four levels operate effectively. However, diagnosis is difficult. Even the best, most thorough tests available are not sophisticated enough to measure dysfunction in the message content the DNA is receiving.

Adequate zinc plays an important role in proper steroid receptor activation once the steroids arrive at the DNA associated receptor. The DNA associated receptor contains Zinc. Zinc is to steroid receptor activation as oxygen is to burning fuel within the mitochondria. Just as oxygen deficiency diminishes the power plant flame, zinc deficiencies prevent steroids from activating the different DNA associated receptors.

DNA associated receptors refers to the types of receptors for all steroids, vitamin A, and thyroid hormone. If the owner experiences a level five problem they should ask their physician about their zinc status.

A properly functioning fifth link is a prerequisite for the sixth link to function. The sixth link concerns protein receptors that are manufactured or repressed, on additional DNA segments, when the DNA is activated or repressed by a specific ovarian steroid. These activated or repressed DNA segments result in the increase or decreased amounts of receptors for the lesser hormones. In contrast, the fifth level concerns hormone receptors manufacture levels determined for the most powerful hormones only.

Link Six - Receptor Manufacture is Dependent on the Success of Ovarian Steroids for Activation of the DNA Program in the Steriod Target Cell

The sixth link concerns the receptor formation amounts for the lesser hormones. These lesser hormone receptors only occur as a result of successful activation of the DNA associated nuclear receptor. As the result of DNA activation by a specific steroid, the cell is directed to manufacture specific proteins. The instructions for the manufacture of specific proteins are contained within the genetic code - the DNA segment activated. Specific proteins directed to be synthesized lead to new receptors being made from these proteins. These specific receptors are manufactured for other steroids and other 'lesser' hormones. Hormones cannot deliver without their specific receptors being present on the target cell.

Most of the discussion at this level is beyond the scope of this book but a basic appreciation is warranted. At the sixth level interdependence of the different steroids, vitamin A, and thyroid hormone takes place. However, the final hormone receptors created at level six are constructed to receive the messages contained within the lesser hormones. An example of the lesser hormones receptor being decreased by estrogen's influence on the DNA program occurs within the liver. High estrogen states influence the liver DNA to suppress growth hormone receptors associated with IGF-1 release. When there are less receptors, which trigger the release of IGF-1, then growth hormone will tend to raise the blood sugar without compensation by increasing IGF-1 levels. This increased estrogen-caused defect leads to an increased insulin release. This is necessary for the growth hormone-caused blood sugar elevations to return to normal. The increased insulin then turns on the fat making machinery. This is an example of a level six problem, which leads the female owner to get fatter until someone helps her to normalize her IGF-1 again.

To eliminate confusion of the ovarian system, visualize six links in a chain. If one of the links is broken, the ovarian system failure profile appears. Common examples of this dysfunction include: hot flashes, irritability for up to two weeks prior to the onset of menses, insomnia, forgetfulness, breast tenderness, cyclical migraine headaches, fibrocystic breast disease, uterine fibroids, some breast cancers, some uterine cancers and some cases of obesity. These occur clinically regardless of which link fails. Even a well-run battery of ovarian steroid tests including urine and blood laboratory can be deceptively normal. In these cases, listen to the body and find a doctor who will look carefully for clinical clues.

The content of this section should alert the owner to the complexity of inquiry necessary to establish the level of ovarian function. Superficial inquiries, that have side effects and little to do with healing, lead to symptom control medicine. With opportunities for healing in mind, the time has come to discuss how various hormones interact as informational substances.

Chapter 7

Informational Substances

The amount of communication that occurs between different cells via the informational hormones is critical to health. These substances are secreted at numerous sites within the body and exert distant cellular communication. Informational substances are carried in the blood stream toward the target cell and are created to connect with a specific group of receptors. The shape that results from this combination generates a specific message within the target cell. The blood functions as a stream of information molecules.

Informational substances are of two types, rapid response and delayed response. The term delayed denotes the ability to affect the activity level of a cell's DNA program. Activated DNA programs make new cell proteins possible. One of the proteins made possible by DNA activation is the manufacture of certain receptors for the rapid response hormones (lessor hormones). They depend on proper amounts of the delayed type of informational substances activating enough DNA programs so there will be receptors when these hormones are released.

The term 'rapid' denotes informational substance types that only affect existing receptors and cellular machineries activity levels. These types of informational substances are rapid in their message delivery since they have no ability to directly instruct the DNA programs. When DNA programs are active or in states of silence, the protein levels are affected only after a delay within the target cell. Rapid response informational substance side steps this and stop short by having a message effect on what already exists in a cell.

Common examples of the rapid response type of informational substances are adrenaline and insulin. In general, rapid acting informational substances affect existing cellular machinery. Adrenaline and insulin only have effects on the activity level of preexisting cellular machines (enzymes).

In contrast, delayed informational substances have an effect on determining the types of cellular machinery and receptors created. Cellular machinery types and amounts are created when the delayed informational substances instruct the DNA programs. Only when DNA programs receive instruction are new cellular machines and new cellular structural components manufactured. These delayed types of informational substances act by binding directly to cellular DNA and turning off or on different genes. Examples of delayed informational substances are thyroid hormone, vitamin A, and all steroid hormones.

The rapid response informational substances are generally made from amino acid metabolites, amino acid combinations, or hormonal fat precursors. The final shape carries message and is created from these variously arranged molecular building blocks. Molecular building blocks, when processed into the manufactured hormone, carry information by virtue of their final shape. There are several sites of manufacture for each of the different types of rapid response hormones. Once released, the closest target cell receives the highest message content and the farthest the least. In this way the site of release sometimes controls the response. Without proper activation by enough types and amounts of delayed response type of informational substance, to the DNA programs, the rapid response hormones have a diminished ability to deliver message content. Rapid response informational substances are dependent on the delayed informational substances for receptor formation. Without a receptor they are unable to deliver their message content. The rapid response informational substances can only affect the activity level of existing cellular machinery and structural cell components. One of the structural cell components is the receptor it contains. In general, only the delayed informational substances determine the manufacture rate of cell repair, cell structures, and new cellular machinery.

Basic medical physiology texts are full of molecular and metabolic pathway descriptions of the individual rapid response type of informational substances. These descriptions detail the rapid response informational substances. It is more practical to simplify things down to the overall big picture. In this case, the big picture of the rapid response type of hormones means they only affect existing cellular infrastructure and machinery. All rapid response hormones are carried in the blood stream. The blood stream provides transport for release informational substances. In the nerves, these same substances are called neurotransmitters and the blood stream is not involved.

Communication occurs amongst the cells via numerous informational substances that flow in the blood stream. Factors that improve the quality of tone in this informational highway are reflected in improved owner health. Conversely, factors that decrease the quality of the informational tone in the blood stream predictably decrease health.

Traditional scientific dogma states that the central nervous system is the center of communication.[9] This dogma is being eroded by new data. Contemporary biochemical studies have revealed that information from numerous cells can direct the central nervous system. The classical notion of the central nervous system still has some truth in the control of its command of conscious thought processes, body movement, and tissue tone (as far as the nerve part of the central nervous system goes). Examples of nervous system movement include voluntary and involuntary types. Voluntary movements include ambulating, the mechanics of talking, and conscious urination. Involuntary movements directed by the classical nervous system are the hearts beating, most unconscious breathing, and digestion. Some of the blood vessel tension, airway tension (bronchial tone), and intestinal tone evidence tissue tone that is orchestrated by the central nervous system.

Not all cells have a nervous system connection. All cells have an informational substance connection. All cells depend on the quality of informational substances. Informational substances direct the cells in their energy expenditure. Whether or not cells are receiving quality information is central to longevity.

Quality informational substance content is a prerequisite to health. Healthy owners have optimal types and amounts of informational content flowing through their bloodstreams. This occurs at appropriate times and intervals and allows maximal cellular efficiency and harmony. Conversely, unhealthy owners have reflective poor qualities of types and amounts of informational content within their blood streams.

Their informational tone is out of sync with the needs of their cells that need proper informational direction on how to expend available energy. Energy usage is determined by the quality of the informational substances within the blood stream.

Good health cannot occur if the informational substances circulating in the blood stream are not the types and amounts that promote maximum cellular efficiency and vigor. Stressed owners carry and secrete informational substances that communicate stress messages to every cell. Common negative emotional energies such as fear, anger, guilt, and sadness are communicated to cells. Unhappy owners communicate 'unhappiness' messages to their cells via informational substances. Chronically sad owners secrete informational substances that decrease readiness to immune system cells. This decreases the ability to defend against rogue cancer cells, foreign invasion from yeast, bacteria, or virus' and from toxins.

Conversely, happiness, love, thankfulness, forgiveness, and hope stimulate the immune system to increase effectiveness that communicates through informational substances.

Science labels the informational substances hormones. Some of these same substances are called neurotransmitters when secreted by nerves. Numerous cell types secrete hormones. Each hormone conveys a specific message. The message content depends on the shape of the hormone plus the cell receptor type that it interacts with. Informational substance can convey varied content depending on the receptor it is designed to interact with. The combinations of shapes between the hormone and receptor creates message content. There are many different receptor that a hormone type can interact with. The resulting message depends on the hormone / receptor combination.

For example, cortisol (a steroid) molecule conveys different types of message content depending on which type of receptor it interacts with. When cortisol binds to the DNA program of the gonads, the message to direct energy away from androgen production and reproduction is conveyed. When CORTISOL binds to the DNA of a blood vessel smooth muscle cells, the message increases responsiveness to the adrenaline hormone. In other cells it instructs DNA programs in the conservation of energy. Directing these cells to stop their cellular infrastructure investment and rejuvenation activities conserves energy. This maximizes energy for survival.

All hormone's message content centers around how the body is directed to spend available energy. The energy expenditure is determined by which enzymes are active and which ones are quiescent. The hormones released determine which enzymes are active or dormant.

The numerous, different enzymes contained within the body are analogous to molecular machinery. Different types of machines are contained in specific work areas. These different work areas can be thought of as cell factories.

The different cell factories are called organelles. Mitochondria, endoplasmic reticulum, golgi apparatus, and nucleolus are organelles.

Different types of cells contain different types of enzymes (cellular machines). There are additional enzyme machines within the blood stream, in the area around cells, and on cell membranes. The enzyme types within a cell depend on the products and functions of each cell type. Each cell type generates specific products.

The integrity of the following two components are crucial determinants of the aging process: cell support structures (cell membrane and organelles), the integrity of enzymes (cell machines). It is the overall hormone mixture that determines whether energy is directed toward repair and rejuvenation or into chronic survival mode.

Hormones direct energy expenditure. The hormones present, direct this process and reflect how wise a body is at directing energy expenditures. The quality of the hormone message is one of seven main determinants of aging quickly versus aging gracefully. If the informational content contained in the blood stream is optimal, youth is maintained. Youth can only be maintained when the cells receive proper direction on the wise use of energy.

Wise use of energy involves adequate energy appropriation towards cellular maintenance, repair, toxin removal, and adequate cellular product formation. All of these processes depend on cells receiving appropriate informational direction. Cells direct energy toward rejuvenation and cellular infrastructure investment when they are given the appropriate informational substance message. Only the correct informational message will direct them to do so. The types and amounts of informational substances determine how the body spends energy. Hormone quality has a significant effect on healing and in slowing the aging process. The science exists to assess and improve the body's hormone profile.

How Delayed Informational Substances Affect Energy Management

Testosterone is of the steroid hormone class. Its excess or deficiency serves as an example of appropriate versus inappropriate hormone directions by an informational substance. The steroid hormone class is part the delayed onset type of informational message content. Testosterone because it is a delayed type of informational substance alters, the types and amounts of cellular energy available by its influence over a cells DNA program. The DNA program activated or silenced determines the maintenance and rejuvenation activities within the cell. When testosterone is present, it directs anabolic activities. Scientists denote the cellular buildup message content as informational substances that are anabolic. Anabolic means to build up. In contrast, catabolic processes means to use up. Before one can understand where the message of testosterone fits, an overall picture of steroid message content is helpful.

In the steroid class there are three basic types of metabolic activities controlled at the level of the DNA.
1. Water and salt content of the body
2. Cell survival (deferred cellular maintenance)
3. Cellular infrastructure investment and rejuvenation activities

The steroid testosterone activates rejuvenation and infrastructure investment. Cortisol is an example of the steroid class that directs body energy into maximizing the survival response. Part of the survival response makes fuel available by release for survival needs. Stress, whether real or imagined, is a catabolic process because fuel is made available by dismantling body cell structures where fuel is stored. With the help of cortisol, aldosterone controls salt and water balance (kidney chapter). Additionally, aldosterone controls the rate at which steroid producing glands manufacture other steroids like testosterone. Steroids are some of the central 'players' in how the DNA programs of cells are directed to expend energy. Thyroid hormones and vitamin A complex also work in this capacity.

The testosterone cellular message is one of cellular buildup and restorative integrity activities in male and female owners. To avoid confusion testosterone will be discussed as representative of anabolic steroids. The anabolic class of steroids is known as the androgen class collectively and includes testosterone, dihydrotestosterone, DHEA, androstenedione, and progesterone. Many of these can be peripherally converted to the others to varying degrees (ovary chapter). This allows for an increase in initially secreted potency without the masculine message in women.

Testosterone-like steroids direct buildup of the integrity of cellular components, in male and female owners by directly switching off or on DNA programs (genes). Testosterone gives the cell the message that cellular infrastructure investment and rejuvenation are important. This message results in strong bones, increased organ size and function, increased red blood cell production, increased immune cell production and function, increased bulk to muscles, and increased mental functioning abilities.

Certain energetic and lifestyle qualities promote testosterone production and secretion. Certain other energetic and lifestyle qualities decrease its secretion and production. Good information coursing through the blood stream is important. Testosterone is one of many necessary informational substances that help revitalize cells.

The intent of this subsection was to introduce the reader to the importance of containing sufficient anabolic message content. Without anabolic message content the cells lack direction to invest cellular energy in rejuvenation activities. Rejuvenation activities lead to healing. Healing requires an understanding of the three roles that steroid messages serve. The quality of representation of these three roles of steroids determines the steroid tone.

Chapter 8

Steroid Tone

Steroid tone is a useful construct to help predict the youthfulness of an owner's cells. Optimal steroid combinations and relationships promote cellular youth. Unhealthy steroid mixtures diminish cellular function. Cellular dysfunction accelerates the aging process. Cellular health improves as steroid tone improves. The appropriate amounts of steroids in the proper proportions create steroid tone. Optimal steroid mixtures direct cells to perform at maximum energy efficiency. Precise, proportional combinations of testosterone, DHEA, progesterone, cortisol, and aldosterone direct energy efficiently.

Maximum function and efficiency at the cellular level equals healthy owners through correct steroid mixtures. These appropriate steroid mixtures direct cells towards the efficient use of resources. Wise use of body energy equates cellular efficiency. Only when cellular efficiency occurs is youthfulness possible.

Highest Quality of Steroid Types and Proportions Instructing DNA Programs Equals Optimal Steroid Tone

Optimal steroid tone is only possible when the catabolic message content is balanced by the anabolic message content.

Steroids are powerful hormones because they turn the DNA program on and off. The cells are dependant on the quality of informational directions (hormone types and amounts) they receive. All other hormone types (immediate response type), if they act at all, act indirectly on cellular DNA activity. Immediate response hormones, in general, direct what already exists in a cell. Delayed hormone types determine what exist within a cell and they do this by their influence on DNA programs. When DNA programs are turned on, certain proteins, coded for activated DNA programs, are manufactured. Barriers limit the immediate response hormones as to where they can deliver message content. In contrast, the delayed-type hormones can go anywhere. It is only the steroid class, vitamin A and thyroid hormones that can go anywhere.

A youthful, physically fit owner operates in optimal hormone balance. Some owners are youthful physically at age 80 while others are prematurely aged at age 30. The choice is made by the sum of daily decisions and lifestyle behaviors that either promote wellness or accelerate the rate of the aging process.

Enhancement of steroid tone is a major principle, if youthful vigor is desired. Healthy owners have optimal steroid tone without exception. Optimal steroid tone is a question of balance between the steroid forces that oppose one another (catabolic versus anabolic forces). High quality steroid mixtures direct cells to spend energy wisely between cellular maintenance, rejuvenation, product formation (unique to each cell type) and appropriate rest.

Steroid tone is affected by stress. Stress increases the release of certain survival steroids in the stress response. Under stress the body perceives a survival threat and directs energy in to survival activities. These same steroids direct body energy away from cellular maintenance and repair activities. Chronically stressed owners are in a chronic survival pathway. These pathways predictably decrease steroid tone. When steroid tone decreases health as well decreases. Health decreases because stress hormones direct energy away from cellular maintenance, build up, waste removal, and repair activities needed to maintain the youthful state. The youthful state is gradually lost when stress steroid proportions increase above normal because the quality of steroid message content has deteriorated.

One of the stress response steroid hormones is cortisol. Cortisol is necessary in small amounts for proper cell function. In normal amounts, cortisol has a direct influence on many cell processes such as: immune regulation (turning down tone), maintenance of blood pressure (especially in moving from sitting to standing), limiting the inflammatory response from the mechanical strains of muscles, ligaments, and joints, and in the counter-regulation of insulin's message. In these situations the cortisol proportion of steroid tone is normal.

When chronic survival messages (stress) occur cortisol's production rate increases. The chronic increase of cortisol secretion creates an imbalance of steroid content within the blood stream. This leads to more survival message content (cortisol) and less rejuvenation message content (testosterone). The higher cortisol content lowers the proportional contribution of other steroids in the direction of energy.

When the body is in survival mode, energy is directed away from rejuvenation activities and into mounting a stress response by lowering the steroid tone. By definition, steroid tone is high when rejuvenation activity is high. Steroid tone becomes low when rejuvenation activity is low. Steroid tone is a construct to help conceptualize the adequacy of the body steroid mixture for maintaining youthfulness.

When steroid mixtures deviate from optimum, there are consequences to the message content. Without optimum types and amounts of steroid mixtures cellular injury and breakdown occurs. Developing one's knowledge for how breakdown occurs and ways to promote healing is imperative.

Cells need the correct informational message to heal. The function of cells depends on the hormone instructions they receive. Steroids turn on and off DNA programs within the cells and therefore are a primary consideration to maintain youthfulness. Steroid tone attempts to quantify the importance of the quality of instructions that cells receive from steroids.

Six Determinants of Steroid Tone

1. Health of the adrenal glands and gonads
2. Genetic inheritance
3. Environmental adrenal and gonad toxin exposure history
4. Nutritional adequacy for manufacture of the right steroids
5. Emotional lifestyle quality
6. Secretogogue influence on the adrenals and gonads. Amount of anabolic enhancement from the secretogogues

Five of the six determinants of steroid tone are under the influence of the owner and are responsive to healing strategies. The remainder of this chapter describes how to improve steroid tone. Section four describes the concept of steroid pressure. Section five explains how to improve steroid tone and pressures.

These six determinants can be manipulated to create healing. Female owners need more information about how the modern medical complex depresses their steroid tone. After this the discussion will apply to the steroid tone of both sexes.

Health of Adrenals and Ovaries Influence the Steroid Tone of Female's

As a female ages, her steroid tone depends more on functional adrenals. Females make less androgen in their ovaries than males make in their testes. Their ovarian derived androgens fall off more quickly than a man of the same age.

Healthy ovaries manufacture estrogens cycled with progesterone in a balanced and cyclical fashion. Significant amounts of androgen (androstenedione and testosterone) are also manufactured. Different female owners have different rates of decline in ovary-produced steroids.

The adrenals are the backup system for androgen steroid production in females. The female, like the male, needs adequate androgen production to maintain steroid tone. Only by maintaining steroid tone can the youthful human form be realized. When adrenals are healthy, they are capable producers of androgen-like steroids. DHEA (an androgen steroid) is only produced in adrenal glands. There is significant androstenedione production in the adrenal gland as well. Cortisol, the stress steroid, production takes place in the adrenal glands. Adrenals produce aldosterone that is vital for mineral and water balance (adrenal chapter). In addition, aldosterone determines the rate of production for all other steroids produced within the adrenals and the gonads (ovaries and testes). A low aldosterone production will diminish all other steroids production rates.

With these facts in mind the next level of steroid tone understanding is:

Steroid tone = adrenal (androgen steroids + stress steroids - excess stress steroids + aldosterone steroids) + ovary or testicle (androgens + progesterone + estrogens).

Very few physicians are trained in assessing steroid urine output. Fewer practicing physicians attempt to replace lost androgen production that results from the post-operative state of a hysterectomy. A progressive decline in muscle mass, increased tendency for weight gain, decreased libido, decreased mental acuity, and premature osteoporosis all result from this omission in the treatment plan. These consequences are produced from a decline in steroid tone.

Synthetic types of estrogens and progesterone substitutes make the androgen deficiency worse (ovary chapter). These substitutes are commonly given as the standard for hormone replacement therapy. Most of these estrogen prescriptions are made from the urine of pregnant horses. Alternatively, some prescriptions are made synthetically from yams or soy by a chemical process and the same chemical mixture results. These synthetic mixtures or horse urine derived estrogens are not healthy. Nor are they adequate substitutes for the human estrogen message content.

The optimal estrogen message is created by healthy ratios of three different estrogens (estriol, estradiol, and estrone). Optimal estrogen ratios occur within healthy females. Common prescriptions of estrogen substitutes contain an overabundance of alpha estradiol that amplifies the message of cell division by a factor of thirty within estrogen responsive tissues. The estrogen responsive tissues include the breast, uterus, cervix, vulva, vagina, ovaries, and fat cells (located within the hips and thighs).

These prescriptions also contain horse estrogens (equiline and equilinin). Horse estrogen sends out horse estrogen messages. The estrogen responsive tissues within the human female receive the unnatural horse estrogen message. The human females body was not designed to receive horse specific estrogen message content. Uzzi Reis, M.D., OB/GYN, author of *Natural Hormone Balance for Women*, says it very well. He asks, "Are you a horse? Do you eat hay? Then why take horse estrogen?"[10]

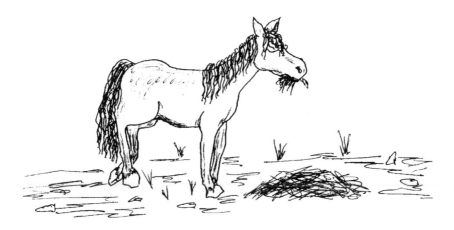

Part of the female steroid tone is from estrogen. Each estrogen has a different shape that determines the message content. When this natural shape is altered, the message contents change. There are over twenty different types of natural estrogen found in plants and animals. There are also unnatural environmental contaminants - the estrogen mimics. The estrogen mimics pummel most owners with inappropriate message content (adrenal chapter). An imbalanced message content caused by the wrong types and amounts of estrogen delivers a confused message to estrogen dependent tissues. The precise shape of natural estrogen has been altered which diminishes health. Properly proportioned amounts of human estrogens convey a precise message to the target cells that are necessary to maintain health.

Hormone replacement strategies that contain progesterone substitutes further compromise steroid tone. Only one real progesterone molecule occurs naturally. The precise shape of the real progesterone molecule contains the message content needed for true health. Altered or synthetic progesterone lowers steroid tone further by interfering with the biosynthesis of other steroid hormones. Other steroids require progesterone as building blocks. Progesterone substitutes retard this process. The process becomes retarded when progesterone substitutes fool enzyme machines that need real progesterone to build other steroids. The altered shape of synthetic progesterone cannot serve as a building block for other needed body steroids.

Natural progesterone is not patentable and therefore not profitable for manufacture by pharmaceutical companies. Complications occur with the use of progesterone substitutes. They always have side effects (a different shape changes message content). This fact alone leads to imbalances in steroid tone. Progesterone is necessary for building many other steroid hormones that are needed within the body. Real and properly proportioned steroids elevate steroid tone and a healthy body manifests.

An analogy given by the progesterone expert, John Lee M.D., states that progesterone is the basic 'chassis' for many other steroid designs. Dr. Lee points out that the progesterone substitute situation is like auto manufactures that use a common chassis for multiple car types. If the chassis is not properly constructed, the assembly process for the remainder of the automobile is halted at different points along the assembly line. Where this occurs depends on where the defective chassis lesion occurs. This leads to a marked slowing in finishing out different automobile types at the auto factory.

Similar to automobile assembly, synthetic progesterone substitutes can jam the steroid assembly process in female ovaries and adrenals. The 'assembly lines' are jammed within the enzymatic machinery of the cells because synthetic progesterone has an altered shape. The altered shape is close enough to get into the assembly line (enzyme machine) but not close enough to build from. No new steroids can be built because the substitute steroid is not the correct shape to be processed into other urgently needed steroids. However, it is close enough in shape to natural progesterone to get into the enzymatic machinery. Once these substitutes are engaged in the enzymatic machines, they compete with the process of natural progesterone converting to other needed steroids.

Steroid mismatch, quantified in severity by a diminished steroid tone, leads to a poor quality of life. This is the first part of a complex problem. Part of the solution is in obtaining an accurate steroid hormone profile. The twenty-four hour urine test quantitative and qualitative is a start for addressing where one stands in steroid tone.

The unfortunate female that continues to take synthetic, imbalanced hormone messengers often feels lousy while on an accelerated path to old age, as well. One of the central problems with altered mixtures of steroids (prescription estrogens and progesterone substitutes) is that they interfere with and diminish the androgen component of steroid tone. The lower steroid tone that results puts the female in androgen steroid deficiency. The androgen message content needed to rejuvenate cells isn't available. A deficiency in the androgen message content allows DNA programs to respond inappropriately in regard to cellular maintenance and rejuvenation activities.

The adrenals and gonads perform independent tasks to maintain steroid tone. Adrenals have unique hormone products that will be discussed in detail here. This will be followed by a discussion of the adrenal contribution to the androgen class of steroids (build up and maintenance) by the synthesis of DHEA. The adrenal contribution to steroid tone depends on the health of these glands. This is the first determinant of steroid tone and the adrenal component of this will be reviewed first.

Manufacture sites for the different components of Steroid Tone

Adrenal component:	Gonad:
DHEA	Estrogens
Cortisol (normal levels)	Progesterone
Diminished with excess cortisol levels	Testosterone
Androstenedione	Androstenedione
Aldosterone	Progesterone
Estrogens	

Each of the above steroids has precise message content needed by cells in order to expend energy efficiently. When correctly proportioned, the cells receive the message to spend energy wisely, which allows for youthfulness.

There are six determinants of steroid tone. Five of the six the owner has control over. This subsection is divided into six parts for each of these determinants.

First Determinant - Health of Adrenals and Gonads

The adrenals and gonads contribute to steroid tone by their unique contributions and overlapped contributions. This subsection will explain:

1. How chronic stress lowers adrenal contribution to steroid tone
2. Steroid tone created from adrenals and gonads depends on adrenal manufacture of aldosterone.
3. Types of adrenal androgens manufacture compared to the gonads
4. Overlap between estrogen and progesterone produced in the adrenals and gonads.
1. Introductory remarks about powerful androgens manufactured in the ovaries and testes.

The contribution of the adrenal gland to steroid tone will be the first consideration in this subsection. The adrenals part of the first determinant of steroid tone is a good place to start the discussion. It concerns the effect of chronic stress on steroid output of the adrenals.

Chronic Stress, Adrenals, and Steroid Tone

Survival is the primary role of the adrenal glands. Survival of chronic stress comes with a high price on steroid tone. Physiologically, standing up is stressful. The change in gravitational force is tremendous when going from sitting to standing. Without a concerted interplay between cortisol and adrenaline, this would not be possible. Cortisol, secreted by the adrenal cortex, puts blood vessels in a responsive state each morning before waking up. Adrenaline, made by the inner part of the adrenal, also increases when one is upright or stressed. The body is designed for a certain average level of cortisol manufacture. The body design can handle occasional stress, as well, without detrimental effects.

The human body needs minimal amounts of cortisol for the maintenance of high steroid tone. A cortisol deficiency results in a fall in blood pressure following then on into unconsciousness. Sufficient adrenal output of cortisol facilitates correction of falling blood sugar, as well. The more insulin that is available, the higher the amount of cortisol needed to counteract insulin's requirement to take sugar molecules out of the blood stream. Cortisol also serves to tone down hyper-vigilance of the immune system. In health, this results in the prevention of inappropriate activation against body tissues manifesting as autoimmune disease and allergies.

When the secretion of cortisol is higher than normal, the body directs energy away from cellular maintenance to accommodate the stress reaction whether real or imagined. Deferred maintenance occurs when the body temporally lowers steroid tone to survive a perceived threat. The human body can handle occasional deferred maintenance. Survival of a perceived threat by the body redirects body energy into fuel release (catabolic) and out of rejuvenation pathways (anabolic).

The job of steroid hormones is to reroute body energy as the situation merits. When there is a survival situation, more cortisol (catabolic) and less androgen (anabolic) are released and steroid tone therefore decreases.

This is similar to the situation of deferred maintenance in a car. An owner can get away without an oil change once in awhile. When the body perceives one stress after another, the aging process begins. There must be adequate time for continual repair and cellular maintenance activities.

The stress response can become complicated with the discussion of the numerous physiological particulars and associated hormone cascades and feedback loops. Summarize mentally, when the body perceives a survival threat, time is essential to maximize physical energy. The body is smart enough to know that an oil change, cellular garbage removal, spark plugs changes, etc. are poor uses of energy when survival is the issue. If this threat becomes chronic, then deferred maintenance has consequences to the physical body.

Hormones carry the messages that direct energy expenditure. For this reason, cortisol production increases drastically when stress occurs. High cortisol production directs energy away from rejuvenation activities and into maximum energy for physical strength and alertness so the body can survive the perceived stress. Beyond the stress response, there is an additional adrenal steroid hormone, aldosterone. Aldosterone is important to the overall strength of certain cell types. In many ways, the aldosterone level is the supreme determiner of steroid tone.

Aldosterone – Maintenance of Steroid Tone

The adrenal glands respond to a narrow control range of salt and water balance that is largely controlled by the amount of aldosterone message content. The adrenal cortex secretes aldosterone within the glomerulosa layer. Potassium level, stress, and angiotensin type two are the three determiners for the amount of aldosterone that the adrenal gland releases.

The secretion of aldosterone directs three main events directed by its instruction of various cell's DNA:

1. Increased sodium retention relative to potassium removal from the body.
2. Increased cellular charge (increased power to the cell force field) of cardiac and brain cells
3. Increased steroid biosynthesis in the adrenals and gonads.

All steroids manufacture rate are dependent on adequate aldosterone levels. There are shared roles that the adrenals and gonads have in relation to steroid production. Steroid production rates within both of these glands will determine steroid tone. Conversely, they are different in the unique steroid products they each produce. Aldosterone manufacture takes place in the adrenal glands. The amount of aldosterone produced determines how much of the other body steroids are manufactured. When aldosterone production goes well there is the benefit of increased steroid tone. When aldosterone production goes poorly, there is liability of decreased steroid tone (adrenal chapter).

Androgens – Contribution to Steroid Tone

The adrenals and gonads share in the manufacture of androgen steroids (the builders and maintenance stimulators). By far the major androgen manufactured within the adrenal is DHEA. This overlap of androgen production between the adrenals and gonads is a backup system for the maintenance of steroid tone. Health wise, it's advantageous to have both glands helping in the production of steroid tone. High steroid tone promotes these activities in an efficient and youthful manner. However, in a culture that takes female ovaries on a regular basis, the backup system is better than nothing.

The contribution of DHEA to steroid tone begins to rise at age 7 and peaks around age 25. This level then proceeds to decline throughout life and reachs about 10% of peak levels in the last year of life. DHEA levels decline more quickly in people with high insulin states. High insulin requires an increased cortisol message to counteract the message of insulin to lower the blood sugar too far. The adrenal then needs to direct the manufacture of more cortisol preferentially. High stress seems to cause DHEA levels to fall in order to accommodate increased cortisol biosynthesis. Cortisol and DHEA are manufactured from cholesterol stores within the adrenal.

There are many different types of androgens made in the body. DHEA is only one of many. Each body tissue has its own preferred androgen that maximizes its anabolic response. When cells receive their preferred androgen, they invest appropriately in repair and rejuvenation. When directions come from the preferred androgen, the body will remain vigorous and vital.

Lung tissue seems to prefer DHEA (anabolic message) that is balanced with the right amount of cortisol (catabolic message). Blood vessels seem to respond in rejuvenation with a preference for DHEA and only small amounts of cortisol as the counter balance message. Muscle cells seem to prefer testosterone for maximal activation in rejuvenation and growth. Skin benefits maximally from dihydrotestosterone. The heart needs balanced input from testosterone, thyroid, cortisol, and DHEA for continued vitality. The brain, while healthy, concentrates DHEA at five to six times the plasma level of this anabolic steroid. This fact has led some researchers to declare DHEA the youth hormone. It would be more accurate to say DHEA is one of the youth hormones and qualify it within the concept of balance. Owners can only have steroid balance when their steroid tone is high.

Progesterone and Estrogen – Contributions in Men and Women to Steroid Tone

Adrenal glands make progesterone and estrogen. Adrenal production of these hormones can become very important in the menopausal years of a woman. Menopause creates a drastic reduction of ovary activity for steroid production. This source for these hormones is important throughout life for men. Men need the message content of these hormones for their steroid tone, just like women, but in lesser amounts. Healthy adrenals supply men and women with adequate amounts of these steroids.

Gonads - Steroid Tone

Optimal steroid tone is realized when adrenal glands and gonads are healthy. Alternatively, health can be regained if these glands have been damaged with an accurate real hormone replacement program. A real hormone replacement program requires an accurate 'hormone report card' before the physician can advise an owner in the continuum from health to diminished function. Part of the hormone report card is an assessment of steroid tone. This is best ascertained by a well-run twenty-four hour urine test.

Both the six links in the ovary system and the adrenal system need to be intact for healthful steroid tone to come from the gonads and adrenals. The adrenals can help failing gonads. Function of either system needs to be determined by an accurate assessment of steroid tone. Sometimes supplementation is necessary for the owner with failing glands for their rejuvenation program. This program will help these owners heal from the effects of low steroid tone (ovary chapter and adrenal chapter).

This subsection is leading up to all six determinants of steroid tone. Five of six of these determinants are additional considerations, which can allow healing to occur without chronically prescribing hormone replacement. Low steroid tone often requires the help of a knowledgeable physician. It helps to separate the contributions of the adrenals and gonads (ovaries or testes) to overall steroid tone.

Adrenal component of steroid tone:
DHEA
Cortisol (normal amounts only)
Cortisol diminishes tone in excess
Androstenedione
Progesterone
Estrogen
Aldosterone

Gonad component:
Estrogens
Progesterone
Testosterone
Androstenedione

A health assessment of the adrenals and ovaries is the first determinant of steroid tone. The other determinants have a moderating influence on initial steroid tone. The testes work with adrenal glands promoting steroid tone. The only difference between ovaries and testes, as far as steroid production is concerned, is in the relative proportions of the different gonad derived steroids.

The proportions of estrogen and progesterone are higher and testosterone and androstenedione are lower in women. The opposite proportions exist in men. When testes cells are healthy, these glands will activate (secretogogues below). Injured testes generate lower steroid tone. These cases need to have the six links in the testes system chain of health assessed (testes chapter). Sometimes the assessment leads the physician to recommend real hormone replacement therapy. In other cases the four other determinants of steroid tone, that an owner controls, can be corrected. Nutrition of the glands is one factor that powerfully influences steroid tone and is under owner control.

Nutritional Adequacy and Steroid Tone

Physical signs occur in people who eat processed foods. Puffy, bloated faces, sagging skin, and loss of muscular definition exemplify the nutritional deficiencies processed food causes. Fast food restaurants are an excellent place to make these clinical observations.

Before the owners' manual, unless you were an Asian who imbibed in good quality ginseng, less androgen would be manufactured with each passing year. Less androgen manufacture leads to lower steroid tone and the ungraceful decent into old age.

Poor nutrition causes gonad and adrenal cells to have decreased ability to free up cholesterol and move it inside the mitochondria. The mitochondrion is the site within the gonads or adrenal glands cells where cholesterol is converted into early steroid precursors. Cholesterol needs to move into the mitochondria for the first step of steroid manufacture to occur. Once cholesterol moves inside the mitochondria it is converted into the various steroid hormones. The end product within the mitochondria is pregnenolone, a necessary starting molecule from which to build all other steroids. After pregnenolone is formed inside the mitochondria from cholesterol, it undergoes conversion to other steroids outside the mitochondria. This internal conversion from cholesterol to pregnenolone is more difficult as the owner ages.

There are four reasons the conversion of cholesterol to pregnenolone becomes a roadblock with age:

1. Aldosterone content within becomes diminished secondary to a processed food diet.
2. Necessary vitamins and cofactors for biosynthetic reactions of these conversions are diminished.
3. Cholesterol is deficient within the adrenals and gonads
4. The common method of taking pregnenolone supplements has possible detrimental side effects.

This fourth additional point needs emphasis before proceeding with the remedies for the other three causes of diminished steroid biosynthesis. This additional factor exposes many short sighted and half thought out approaches to steroid replacement. Pregnenolone supplementation can partially bypass the need for these mitochondria first step reactions. The side effect of taking pregnenolone as a supplement for waning steroid production is that it contains cortisol-like message content of its own. Increased cortisol message content is warranted in certain clinical situations. In most situations, when it is within one's blood stream after oral ingestion, it will contribute to decreased overall steroid tone. Steroid tone is negatively influenced when cortisol message content rises above a very low threshold. In the normal state, pregnenolone never enters the blood stream in increased amounts. It converts within the adrenals and gonads into other steroids.

To counter act these problems, pay attention to the first three nutritional factors of adrenal and gonad support. The first of the three nutritional factors affecting the health of these glands is the owner's history of diet preference. This determines the aldosterone level of most owners. Aldosterone levels are affected with either a 'real food' diet or a 'processed food' diet. As aging proceeds, eating processed foods leads to an eventual depletion of one's mineral balance. Around middle age owner's bodies become deficient in mineral balance through the chronic ingestion of processed foods. Processed foods have the wrong mineral proportions. The right mineral proportions are necessary for high steroid tone. Real foods (unprocessed and natural) will have a much higher proportion of potassium and magnesium content. Real food sodium content is lower than processed food. The opposite situation of mineral balance exists in owners who arrive at middle age with a history of a preference for processed foods (dead food). This food type is diminished in its potassium and magnesium content from food processing. Processed foods usually have high amounts of sodium added. Many middle-aged owners, who eat processed foods, prematurely suffer the consequences of a decline in steroid tone.

The central steroid defect from a chronic 'dead food' diet is diminished aldosterone production required for normal blood pressure. Some bodies still try to produce appropriate aldosterone in this chronic situation of a dead food diet, but high blood pressure predictably results. The dead food diet is high in sodium and low in potassium. The human body was designed to ingest the reverse mineral content, which the processed food diet provides. Sodium retention beyond healthful amounts causes fluid retention, which causes elevated blood pressure. The other group senses inappropriate sodium content and therefore reduced aldosterone levels. The price paid by these owners' is a diminished steroid synthesis resulting from diminished aldosterone levels.

The owner who takes an active role in the procurement of a real food diet (section three) has an advantage. The 'dead food' (processed) diet accelerates the path to an old body in two major ways. First, diminished aldosterone or elevated blood pressures are the choices given to the body that is fed dead food. When a body chooses the lower aldosterone route, steroid tone suffers and the owner ages faster. Conversely, when a body chooses to maintain steroid tone by keeping aldosterone elevated in the presence of a processed food diet, the blood pressure elevates. When the blood pressure elevates the owner again gets older by a failure to honor the second principle of health, avoiding hardening processes.

The second reason steroid production rate begins to fall with advancing age is the deficiency in vitamins and cofactors. Vitamins and cofactors are necessary for the manufacture of many different steroids. These are additional nutritional dependent factors that effect steroid tone. Enzymatic machinery must be in good working order to allow efficient steroid biosynthesis. Individual enzymes (cellular machines) need specific trace minerals and cofactors in order to perform in the creation of the different steroids. Only when steroids are manufactured at appropriate rates can steroid tone be high.

An analogy is the automobile that has a full tank of gas, but all the oil is drained out. In addition, the spark plugs and carburetor are missing. Missing components are like the cofactors and vitamins which steroid producing enzymes (machines) need, to make the necessary steroids. When there is a cofactor deficiency, steroid production diminishes. When steroid production diminishes steroid tone falls.

A partial list of vitamins required for the manufacture of steroids is vitamin A, pantothenic acid, folate, most of the B vitamins, and vitamin C. The adrenal gland has the highest tissue concentration of vitamin C in the body under healthful conditions. This fact might provide a clue as to why vitamin C is so important in the owners continued survival from the prevention and stress of illness. The stress of surviving an illness requires an increase in steroid production. The need for vitamin C goes up with stress and illness.

The accessories, in the car engine analogy, lends itself to understanding the reason that dietary attention and discretion become so important as owners navigate their search for health and happiness. Youth can survive for a while without the critical nutrients needed by cellular machinery. Youthfulness that endures cannot. 'Father time' is there to observe old cellular parts struggling to work their normal life span without molecular replacement parts. The body can only acquire new molecular parts through dietary intake of the molecules needed (section three).

Food processing destroys important nutrients required for the production of enzymes. There are at least five B vitamins contained in whole grains that decrease by half within one week of grinding it into flour (half life = time for half to be gone-). Oxidation of these unstable and bulky molecules occurs after the grinding process. Vitamins are positioned precisely within the seeds molecular architecture to confer stability. When grains or seeds are ground into flour this process destroys the protection provided by the architectural framework. The grinding process exposes these unstable molecules to the oxidative forces diminishing their nutritional value.

Oxidation takes place in vitamin-fortified foods exposed to heat, air and sunlight for the same reasons. Just because manufactures add vitamins to the box or can doesn't mean they are still intact when the owner ingests it. This is in contrast to real food that still contains vitamins and minerals that the creator intended.

Vitamin supplements are more stable, but absorption characteristics differ widely from brand to brand. Vitamins preparations and vitamin-fortified foods are deficient in some of the vitamins and are removed when food is processed. Folate, panothenic acid, and lipoic acid are especially susceptible during food processing. Compounding the deficiency problem is the fact that many vitamin fortified foods and supplements are deficient in these three vitamins. When one of these is missing it is as if there is a malicious conspiracy within the food industry to make owners weak and old. The weakest link in a chemical reaction sequence will stop a body process. In a pantothenic acid deficiency, carbohydrate and fat combustion is greatly curtailed. With a lipoic acid deficiency, carbohydrate can only be converted to lactic acid that builds up in the tissues and is evidenced as sore and achy muscles. Adrenal and gonad tissues need tremendous amounts of fuel for energy. Therefore, when these vitamins are deficient steroid tone diminishes.

Additional trace minerals are needed within the adrenals and gonads for maintenance of steroid tone. Minerals like zinc and magnesium need adequate stomach acid for absorption. Many western owners are prescribed medicines that block acid production. These owners could therefore become deficient in many of these critically needed minerals despite a healthy diet.

A diet containing sufficient organic and unprocessed whole grains, vegetables, eggs, fish, meats, nuts and fruit promote steroid tone. A real food diet promotes steroid tone by the fact that it contains the proper proportions of minerals and vitamins to promote the health of steroid producing glands (other body tissues as well).

Many plants also contain antioxidant (anti-rust) molecules that confer particular benefits to specific tissues. Examples include lycopines found in tomatoes for prostate health, bioflavonoids found in berries for blood vessel health, acanthocyanins found in 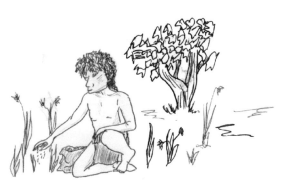 bilberry for retina health, silymarin found in the milk thistle for liver health. Carelessness in how these foods are processed can destroy much of the anti-oxidant content and their potential benefits. The lower the anti-oxidants in the diet, the more needs for anabolic steroids to direct increased repair. Increased repair is necessary when there is diminished protection from the oxidants. When oxidant damage occurs, there is more need to elevate steroid tone to compensate for increased injury rate. Increased steroid tone compensates for the increased injury rate because when steroid tone is high, anabolism is high. In order to derive the intended benefits of sufficient steroid tone, purchase only quality supplements or real foods that comes from fresh organic sources.

When certain tribes throughout the world are studied, it is observed that they enjoy remarkably good health and greater freedom from the ravages of chronic disease. These tribes share a common denominator of a diet high in plants that have high progesterone or progesterone precursors. Some of the plants known to contain relatively high amounts of progesterone or progesterone precursors are: pomegranates, European mistletoe berries, panax ginseng, Mexican wild yams, halotorrhea floribunda, and possibly soy products.

Environmental Toxins and Steroid Tone

Many toxins exert their effect on adrenal and gonad health. Environmental affects on steroid tone (hormone mimics subsection) increase the estrogen-like message content in an owner's body. Increased estrogen message content creates problems in anabolic balance and in estrogen responsive tissues that include men's prostates. Many of these mimics and toxins are far reaching in their ability to disrupt the ideal natural hormone message content. When this natural hormone message content is imbalanced so is steroid tone. There are effective measures that limit exposure to environmental toxins that diminish steroid tone. Limiting exposure to these toxins can restore the message content provided by anabolic steroids.

There are several lifestyle practices that limit toxin exposure to steroid producing glands. First, limit exposure to hormone mimics. Consume organically grown food whenever possible. The food supply is where most of the hormone mimics invade an owner's body. Clean water consumption avoids many of the hormone mimics. Stay away from golf courses because of the heavy use of hormone mimic-like molecules. Education about toxins in the home is important. Avoid the counter-productive stress of being paranoid; just try to reduce chemical exposure within reason. Ideally, with public awareness of the consequences of continued industrial, agricultural, and food distributors practices that allow this problem to perpetuate, things will change for the better.

Genetic Inheritance and Steroid Tone

Genetic predisposition toward weakness or strength is a component of steroid tone. Some owners have strong adrenals and gonads that increase their advantage for creating steroids. If the increased steroids are of sufficient quality then a longevity advantage follows through an increase in steroid tone. Some owners are born with weak adrenals and/or gonads. The weakened glands do not supply steroids sufficiently. Following the advice of the other five determinants of this subsection will help make things right.

The cornerstone to coaching a borderline functional owner, inregards to adrenal and gonad health, is an accurate steroid report card. Only with an accurate assessment will there be any hope of correctly replacing steroids that begin to wane around middle age. An accurate assessment contains a blood analysis and a twenty-four hour urine test for steroids. These values are the baseline for later treatment and inquiry.

Genetic inheritance knowledge is useful in that it helps the owner understand potential weakness. Genetic weakness predisposes owners for disease. Awareness about personal genetics allows ways to pay special attention to weak links that are carried on DNA programs. Family history falls into the realm of consideration. Hormone assessment increases accuracy of the current situation.

Steroid tone has a genetic component, although the genetic component is a mind twist to understand. There are two different angles to consider in regards to genetics and steroid tone. First, and the most common, is the genetic consequences that result from diminished steroids instructing the DNA. Without sufficient steroid message content instructing the DNA programs the genes do not operate properly. Second, genetic variability results from poor quality in regard to the proportions of steroids produced. Both of these genetic variability's are worsened by the other five-lifestyle redeemable habits discussed in this subsection.

Some family lines produce extremely strong bodies because they produce a superior steroid tone. Other genetic lines produce less vital strength in the adrenals and gonads. Vitality wanes when gonads and adrenals begin to fail in their production of a rhythmical and adequate steroid message to cells. This is falling steroid tone.

The role genetics plays in many common degenerative diseases often is sensationalized in the effort to market what is for sale within the complex. Much genetic vulnerability can be overcome by lifestyle modification. With careful assessment, many genetically predisposed owners with low steroid tone can be helped by supplementations of real steroids in the correct physiological doses. The science that empowers owner's to actively improve their genetic vulnerabilities collides with the more lucrative approaches of the complex. Improvement in steroid tone empowers owners to avoid genetic weakness from manifesting.

Emotional Energies and Steroid Tone

The overall emotional quality has a powerful effect on steroid tone. Positive emotional experience communicates to steroid producing glands to increase the steroid tone mixture output (section six). Negative emotions influence steroid glands to believe survival is the issue. When the body perceives a survival threat, either real or imagined, stress steroids increase and rejuvenation steroids decrease. When chronic negative emotions occur, this mechanism lowers steroid tone.

America is a stressful place to live in many respects. Deadlines, job insecurities, modern life complexities, noise pollution, environmental pollution, and electromagnetic pollution take their toll on the human body. The body experiences these emotional stresses energetically by the informational substances it secretes. The stress response informational substances include cortisol. When cortisol levels increase the relative proportion of this message content among other steroids increases as well. This proportional change will lower steroid tone.

There are specific dynamics in the way cortisol opposes androgens and the energies that direct this process. The dominant emotional energy determines how the body spends available energy. The hormone messages that get secreted result from, in part, from the different emotional energies. In this way the different types of emotions have a profound effect on energy usage patterns.

Studies have shown that teammates testosterone increases immediately before a competition and remains elevated during the event. Studies also show that the teammates testosterone will remain elevated when the game is over, only if they win. This is the contrast between the negative emotions of losing and the positive emotions of winning. The outcome of the event not only affects the quality of emotions, but the quality of steroid tone. Studies have also shown chronically depressed owners have lower DHEA levels than the aged matched controls that are not depressed.

The quality of emotions affects on overall steroid tone can be understood in a general way. The adrenals have the choice of making more DHEA or more cortisol. Positive emotional experiences usually allow DHEA levels to remain adequate. Positive emotions translate into the body as a low stress situation. When the body perceives a low stress situation, more energy is available for rejuvenation activities. However, when the body perceives the survival threat of negative emotions, more cortisol is needed. The body has limited energy. Hormones are the directors of energy expenditure. The stress response channels energy expenditure by the types of hormones that are summoned.

When negative emotions cause stress hormones to increase, the energy is directed into catabolic pathways. Catabolic pathways consume body structure. The survival response involves the inhibition of rejuvenation activities and increased fuel availability within the blood stream. Increased fuel availability brought on by stress is a primitive design feature. Modern stress differs from primitive stress, which usually involved a physical challenge. Physical challenges need extra fuel to maximize strength. Modern mental stress requires no physical response. The result of this design feature, in a setting of chronic negative emotions, is increased catabolic direction of energy and decreased anabolic direction of energy. The cortisol message content is increased and the androgen message content is decreased.

DHEA is one of the body's main androgens. All androgens convey a general cellular message that says to invest adequate cellular energy into rejuvenation and infrastructure investment. Cortisol, because it is catabolic, directs cells to put a on hold cellular rejuvenation and infrastructure investment. Negative emotions direct a powerful message channeling energy into catabolism by increasing cortisol predominance. Only low cortisol conveys a harmonious and less dramatic message. When the body perceives a survival threat, high cortisol secretions direct energy toward survival pathways. Survival pathways are necessary in mounting a strong physical response at the expense of cellular maintenance and rejuvenation. Emotional energy has a powerful effect on steroid tone.

Excess cortisol has the ability to direct energy away from youth maintenance activities. The message content from high cortisol levels directs energy toward survival. Some scientific circles have called the chronic elevation of cortisol the 'death hormone'. This title refers to its message contnent to deference of cellular maintenance activities when cortisol is chronically elevated. This accelerates wear and tear changes because there is less anabolic message content. One of the seven deterrents to wear and tear changes (old age) is having adequate message content to rejuvenate. Message content to rejuvenate comes from the anabolic steroids. When anabolic steroids are in balance with the catabolic steroids, steroid tone is maintained and health is more likely.

As a general rule, the faster the metabolic rate in body tissue, the more vulnerable it becomes to deferred maintenance activities. High metabolic rate tissues, like brain and heart tissue, consequently become more vulnerable with decreased steroid tone. The overall quality of the mixture determines high or low steroid tone. High steroid tone quantifies the tendency for percentages of different steroids in the blood stream to approach optimal.

High steroid tone directs the body to invest appropriate energy in repair of the wear and tear associated with changes inherent in life activities. High steroid tone directs appropriate rest intervals and is synonymous with the balance of message content between anabolic and catabolic steroid hormones. Optimal steroid tone needs to occur if youthfulness and healing are to occur. The quality of emotions has a powerful effect on the consequent steroid tone.

That emotions effect steroid tone is an essential concept to combat the ravages of life and emerge as an owner who ages gracefully and lives life fully. The fact that positive emotions promote high steroid tone means there is an increase of appropriate levels of testosterone, DHEA, androstenedione, and progesterone relative to the total amounts of cortisol-like substances within the blood stream. The balance between opposing steroids makes the difference.

The human body needs re-building activities followed by rest periods. All building and the owner become the stiff body builder and/or the aggressive personality types. When energy is directed to the extremes of a body builder physique or the aggressive personality type, too much unhealthy anabolism takes place. Cortisol induces appropriated cellular rest periods in the healthy state. Balance needs to occur between rest and adequate periods of androgen secretion. Emotional energy either facilitates or upsets this balance.

The physical stress of vigorous exercise causes a temporary elevation of cortisol that directs energy toward maximal strength activities. This means cellular maintenance decreases. The difference between exercise stress and emotional stress is that physical exercise increases testosterone as well as cortisol when emotions allow it. When the emotions allow it, testosterone remains elevated after exercising and cortisol levels decrease. During the stress of physical exercise there is no need for extra insulin because the increased blood sugar, directed by cortisol, is appropriately consumed by physical exercise.

In marked contrast, with emotional stress, only cortisol is secreted. The message of cortisol is completely different in the absence of the testosterone message. The message difference results more from the increased insulin required and the lack of testosterone when mental stress occurs.

Part of the stress response is the soaring cortisol secretion relative to other steroids. Chronic stressful emotions raise cortisol levels relative to other androgens. This accelerates wear and tear within cells because cortisol directs cellular energy to emergency situations. The body response to an emergency situation is always the same. The body directs energy out of rejuvenation and increased fuel availability from body structures (protein, fat, and carbohydrate).

The more metabolically active the body tissue, the more vulnerable it becomes to deferred maintenance activities. The brain has one of the fastest metabolic rates within the body. Therefore, chronic emotional stress has the potential to contribute to the rate of brain aging quickly. The brain ages more quickly because the chronically directed energy goes into survival pathways. When survival pathways are active, rejuvenation (repair and maintenance) activities are inactive. These changes become physically manifested in diminished cell membrane integrity, aging intracellular factories, and enzymatic machinery. There is also a tendency for oxidized fats and proteins to build up inside cells. As oxidized fats accumulate, they condense into waste known as lipofuscin. Clinically, the aging brain manifests in a slower reaction time and progressive memory impairment for new events and concepts. (a red neck).

The dominant hormone message is often a reflection of dominant emotional energy. Positive emotions of love, forgiveness, joy, hope, and contentment convey to the body that all is well. The body naturally produces steroids consistent with that emotional state. Conversely, negative emotions of hate, anger, fear, and sadness direct an increase in the production of stress hormones. Beyond the effects of emotions on steroid tone are factors that increase rejuvenation-type steroids. Scientists call such factors secretogogues.

Secretogogues and Steroid Tone

Secretogogues enhance the output of the rejuvenation message content contained within the steroid class called androgens. Androgen message content increases when secretogogues increase. Examples of secretogogues are regular exercise and certain plants like panax ginseng.

Counterbalances to stress are the practices that promote secretion of strength and rejuvenation steroid hormones (DHEA, testosterone, and progesterone). Secretogogues promote secretion. Given adequate nutritional support and adequate adrenal and gonad health, certain practices promote optimal secretion of body building steroids and promote elevated steroid tone. Without some of the three criteria of adequate nutritional support, adrenal and gonad health being present there cannot be an adequate response to a secretogogue. Secretogogues can't pull strength hormones out of a dying gland. The shriveling gland affects other functions.

An analogy for this involves the similarities between factories and cells. Old gonads and adrenals are like an order to a factory and the condition of the factory is in disrepair. The disrepair is evidenced by aged factory support structures (organelles) and aged machinery (enzymes) that is worn out and falling apart. Very little, if anything, can be done to fill the order (hormone creation). Before the factory can respond to the order, it needs to be remodeled and upgraded in its infrastructure and machinery. The adrenal and gonad 'factories' are similar in that they need the proper infrastructure investment provided by adequate molecular replacement parts and the right hormones (message content) for direction. Sedentary owners send the wrong message content (hormones) and their 'factories' tend toward disrepair. This is the root of the saying, 'use it or lose it'. Exercise is a secretogogue directing cells to improved message content and invest in rejuvenation.

Owners with poor steroid tone hate to exercise. This is from long standing habits that produced an attitude. Part of the problem lies in the fact that sedentary owners have a diminished secretogogue influence in their lives. There is also a significant biochemical component for this aversion. Poor steroid tone is predictable when physical condition deteriorates. Out of shape owners have steroid mixtures that reflect poor physical exercise habits. Conversely, a well-trained athlete possesses sufficient types and amounts of steroids that reflect high steroid tone. Highly trained and physically fit cells of an athlete invest maximum cellular energy in maintenance and rejuvenation. Their cells receive the proper message to invest in rejuvenation. To the highly trained athlete, regular exercise acts as the secretogogue stimulant for anabolic steroid production.

Chronic stress of modern life makes matters worse by encouraging cells to invest energy foolishly, which accelerates wear and tear on the body. Stress reroutes life-sustaining energy into survival mode. When poor exercise habits are added to the daily routine, deterioration becomes more aggressive in assaulting the body form. The higher the stress in life, the more need to counter balance with secretogogue. Exercise is a reliable secretogogue. Owners in the middle of modern life stress need to exercise.

Unhealthy owners need to know that the body wants to heal. The body needs the correct informational message to do so. Higher steroid tone carries the information needed to heal the body. Optimal steroid tone doesn't return over night. It is a gradual process just like getting unhealthy is a gradual process. Understanding that with the passage of time, vigor and vitality will increase as the owner persists in improving the quality of informational messages that her/his cells receive. The secretogogues like exercise help owners begin healing. Their cells begin to receive improved information from higher steroid tone that exercise provides. The secretogogues increase the amount of energy available for cellular rejuvenation and infrastructure redevelopment. These restorative activities increase because steroid tone increases. Owners committed to their recovery program notice positive changes every time they look in the mirror and in the improvement in the way that they begin to feel as the months go by. Recovery doesn't have to be expensive or complicated. Recovery can start today with a commitment to understanding the nutritional needs and the emotional environment that gives and takes energy from the owners life. The body begins to heal with improved nutritional quality and through a daily walk, stretch and breath exercises.

The ability of exercise to increase steroid tone crosses over into its effect on emotional energy as well. Positive emotions confer an energetic rhythm to cells by facilitating improved quality of informational substances that course through the blood stream (section six). The emotional energy of happiness, joy, laughter, self-love, and forgiveness are all ways to increase the rate of healing. Exercise adds positive emotional energy to an owner's life. This is effective beyond it's secretogogue influence.

An owner is asked to remember the last time they felt happiness and what it felt like. This is instructive as far as remembering what the cells felt via the informational substances. Happiness energy directs a reflective release of the appropriate informational substances that communicate to the cells that all is well. This message allows the cell to harmoniously interact with maximum efficiency and aliveness.

Chapter 9

Four Misunderstood Steroids

The four misunderstood steroids are thyroid hormone, vitamin A, vitamin D, and aldosterone. Many in the scientific community will now protest. First, they will protest this point because in a peripheral way, aldosterone and vitamin D are already considered steroids. Their inclusion here is because they have steroid-like power to regulate the DNA program of cells. Second, thyroid hormone and vitamin A are generally not classified as steroids. However, thyroid and vitamin A are among the most powerful hormones, which include the steroids, in that they determine the activity of the genetic program. Like steroids, thyroid and vitamin A directly bind DNA and carry message content by virtue of their precise shape. All of the misunderstood steroid-like hormones regulate cell DNA by the amount of their presence or absence. The fate of the body is so dependent on how well these four hormones are released; they will be briefly described.

Steroid-like Properties of Aldosterone

Aldosterone is the first misunderstood steroid hormone to be considered. There is currently a narrowness of thought that regards the impact of aldosterone on certain cells. Many physicians think in terms of water and salt balance only when considering aldosterone. Aldosterone influences certain cell types in their ability to increase cell membrane charge. Maintenance of an optimal cell charge only takes place when there is adequate instruction from aldosterone and thyroid hormones. These two hormones instruct certain DNA genes of cells to activate and increase the force field (cell membrane charge). In the maximal function of cardiac cells and nerve cells this is particularly important. The stronger the force field created by a cell type, the more work it is capable of performing (section 3 and 5). A more powerful electrical charge gives added protection from inappropriate penetration of harmful ions (excess calcium). This is important for the continued operation of a nerve cell (section 6).

One of the seven indicators of aging within is diminished cellular charge. Lastly, aldosterone has a fundamental role in the instructional activation of gonad and adrenal DNA. When the DNA programs of these glands are activated in this way, the steroid manufacture rate increases.

Certain medications, called angiotensin converting enzyme (ACE) inhibitors, lower blood pressure by poisoning the ability of the adrenal gland to release aldosterone. There is currently a debate concerning the exact mechanism of how these prescription drugs work. Aldosterone diminished release is the mechanism physicians are given.

Blood pressure is lowered through several other but under reported mechanisms (sections one, the adrenal and kidney chapters). For the purpose of the current discussion, only the aldosterone lowering mechanism is pertinent because of the secret side effect.

Very few doctors are educated about the importance of aldosterone in stimulating the adrenals and gonads in steroid production. A lower aldosterone message content to the heart and nerve cells diminishes the ability of these cells to increase their force fields to the strength required for maximum function (section five). Diminished force fields within nerve and heart cells lead to an inability for these cells to perform.

There are circumstances where aldosterone production must be suppressed. When physicians become aware of the importance of aldosterone, they will understand the appropriate times and methods for accomplishing this. They will also avoid reducing aldosterone production when suppression is inappropriate.

This narrowness of learning that occurs in medical educations is one example of how well informed patients can help curious physicians understand what science has revealed. Alternative methods for natural ways to heal high blood pressure are more fully discussed in section one. The current medical system controls the behavior of physicians through a mixture of three things. Acceleration in busy work takes away from a doctor's time and desire for new learning. Second, people that become 'certified experts' are the ones who learn early on to keep their mouth shut when they stumble upon scientific inconsistencies while being indoctrinated with the official view of medical treatment strategies. Third, the medical legal rule of the 'standard of care' must not be violated. Any deviation from the sanctified approach will alienate a physician into a legal battle with the complex. The medical industrial's viewpoint has profit to consider.

This being said, never under estimate the power contained in even one man's life when he lives it properly. Like ripples in a pond spreading forever outward, so it is when at the grass roots, people begin to create ways for their physicians to again practice and learn different ways that lead to healing.

Steroid-like Properties of Thyroid Hormone

The thyroid hormone, like the steroids and vitamin A, shares the unique ability to penetrate through many body chambers and barriers. It also shares the powerful ability to reach and direct the DNA programs of cells. This powerful ability instructs which genes, under its influence, get turned on and off. The only other hormones that are this powerful are the steroids and vitamin A.

Fragmenting this small group of hormones, which instruct the DNA programs, leads to their interdependent roles to be misunderstood. Alternatively, it would be more scientifically consistent to group thyroid, vitamin A, and the steroids together in a umbrella class which denotes their special powers to instruct genetic programs. Hormones that instruct DNA programs are conceptually 'steroid like' even though molecularly they are of a different class.

This grouping would then lend itself to a definition of steroid-like tone. Steroid-like tone is a complete assessment of the message content which reaches the DNA of cells. Deficiencies of vitamin A and thyroid message content lead to receptor problems with the mainstream steroids. The important role that thyroid message content plays within cells will be explained in the thyroid chapter. The role of the thyroid is disconnected from other steroids and vitamin A within the clinical setting. This unfortunate mindset causes the larger group, of which thyroid is a hormone member, to be misunderstood.

Vitamin D and Steroid-like Properties

Vitamin D is misunderstood as a steroid because its role of instructing the DNA of the cell is downplayed. A more complete assessment of steroid tone would include this in the evaluation. This steroid's measurement is not commonly available in the 24 four-hour urine test. Vitamin D precursor is made within the skin from cholesterol when sunlight strikes it. At the level of the kidney, the final decision is made about activating the precursor or degrading it for removal in urine. The kidney makes this decision based on how much calcium is available within the blood stream.

Vitamin D instructs different DNA programs of the cells in how to interact with calcium. When too much vitamin D is available within the cells, they take in more calcium. Too much calcium has consequences such as brittle bones, soft tissue calcification, kidney stones, and mineral imbalance. In addition, magnesium deficiencies exacerbate calcium imbalance. On the opposite extreme, too little vitamin D causes loss of calcium.

Vitamin A and Steroid-like Properties

By its name, vitamin A is immediately misunderstood. Unlike all other vitamins, vitamin A contains message content by virtue of its molecular shape. In addition, vitamin A has the ability to go anywhere within the body and deliver message content to the DNA program of a cell. This is in contrast to other vitamins that work by facilitating chemical reactions within the cells. Vitamin A behaves more consistently as a hormone. In contrast, by calling it a vitamin, there is a tendency to hit an intellectual roadblock that needs to be crossed in order to appreciate the consequences of this molecule's deficiency or excess. A real food diet (section three) would supply ample vitamin A and little tendency to develop deficiency of this important substance.

Vitamin A must be obtained in the diet and can become toxic, at high levels, because it amplifies its instructional content of cellular DNA beyond healthful parameters. The only way to overdose on vitamin A is to take high dosage supplements (above 50,000 IU a day) for over three months. Too much vitamin A causes thinning hair, dry and scaly skin, bone spur formation, and brittle bones.

Too little vitamin A leads to diminished functional abilities of cells that coat the body (skin and cornea) and cells that line body cavities (the gastrointestinal tract and lungs). Conditions like ichthyosis vulgaris are caused by a vitamin A deficiency. Skin cancers are promoted by this deficiency as well. There is little encouragement from physicians for decreasing cancer risks by taking adequate vitamin A. Adequate adrenal function depends on vitamin A to instruct adrenal cell DNA activation programs. In the healthful state, the liver is filled with vitamin A and able to release it as needed.

Vitamin A is a complex of similar vitamins that promote cell maturity. Immature cells are a central property of cancer cells. Adequate vitamin A complex intake is a cornerstone for the prevention of cancer. Almost all cells contain DNA programs that are responsive to the message content of vitamin A complex. Some vitamin A derivatives occur in plant seeds. These prevent cell division until they are removed when the right conditions occur. For example the right conditions occur when the planting technique is correct. Likewise, within the body, Vitamin A's message content seems to be involved in keeping the cells from undergoing rampant cell division. This fact is almost entirely ignored by mainstream cancer specialist in attempting to stop cancer cell division (tumor growth).

This section was to help science become more consistent for the four misunderstood steroids. In the chapters that follow insight will develop about these four misunderstood steroids. In the next chapter, the message content of the thyroid hormone and the reasons malfunction of this gland often missed in the clinical setting will be explained. In addition, methods of healing from this problem will be addressed.

Chapter 10

The Thyroid

The amount of thyroid message content determines how hot the power plants (mitochondria) flame will burn within the cells. For healing purposes terms like metabolism and respiratory quotient will be side stepped in favor of understanding why a hot burning cellular 'power plant flame' becomes desirable. Standard thyroid tests used today are often falsely reassuring. Understanding and considering the many variables is pertinent to thyroid functions at the cellular level. The idea here is to avoid being misled into a prescription for anti-depressants when the true culprit is low thyroid function.

The first part of this chapter reviews some of the general variables of thyroid function. Later in the chapter these variables will be organized into the seven links of health chain for thyroid health. All seven links need to be discussed along with the confounding variables if the medical inquiry is to be trusted as accurate.

Many variables are not routinely considered in today's office setting. Hence, many owners are on an accelerated path to an old body because one or more scientifically valid variables interfered with the accuracy of their test.

Envision a wimpy, feeble furnace that heats a home with worn out components and blocked air filters. No matter how much the fuel mixture increases or air is added to the room, until someone repairs the worn out parts and cleans the air intake the furnace will always burn poorly. When the furnace burns inefficiently, the home is cold.

This is what owners with low thyroid function have within their many trillions of cellular power plants. Their cells have adequate fuel, usually to excess, but their power plant flame is so weak it can't burn any hotter. Thyroid hormone gives informational direction at the cell level to the DNA programs. With adequate thyroid hormone, comes instructions that direct the DNA program to spend energy on the repair of the mitochondria (power plant components). Without continuous repair and rejuvenation within the mitochondria, the ability to combust fuel and create energy packets are compromised. The energy packets are needed by the cell to perform useful work and to charge cell membranes to maximum voltage.

Almost all cell types depend on an adequate thyroid message. Thyroid message content allows for energy generation used for cell work and heat maintenance (except in the brain, lymphatics, spleen, and testes). The thyroid message instructs the DNA of the cells to make appropriate power plant (mitochondria) investments. This includes new structural rejuvenation in the form of new mitochondrial structural proteins and enzyme machines.

There is the need for constant synthesis of the specialized structural power plant fats, cardiolipin. Power plant fats are an integral part of the mitochondria structural architecture. Some cell types have up to 2000 mitochondria (power plants) in each cell. All the mitochondria in the body combust a common fuel derived from carbohydrates, protein, or fat, which is acetate. Fuel will combust in the presence of adequate oxygen. In order to burn protein, the liver must change it into carbohydrate (a process known as gluconeogenesis). In turn, all carbohydrate before it can be combusted within the power plant must be converted into acetate. In the end the power plants can only burn one type of fuel, acetate. Acetate is derived from all three-food groups when the proper vitamins and cofactors are present (chapter one) to convert them to acetate.

Even though the brain does not need thyroid hormone message content to stoke its furnace to capacity, it does need the help of thyroid hormone for generation of an adequate cellular force field and waste removal. The ability of thyroid hormone to improve the cellular 'force field ' is enhanced by adequate aldosterone. Both of these hormones are from the steroid-like class in that they penetrate deep into the cell and provide their message directly to the DNA. When thyroid hormone message content delivery is accomplished, the activated DNA leads to protein synthesis. The protein synthesis which thyroid message content directs increases the number of enzyme machines that generate the electrical charge within the cell membrane (section 3). This is in addition to DNA activated protein synthesis of improved mitochondria structural components for most other cells.

In summary, the thyroid hormone tells the DNA of the cell to switch on synthesis of programs that maximize the mitochondria performance and integrity. This is not true within the brain. In nerve and cardiac cells adequate thyroid along with aldosterone, are fundamental in powering up the cell membrane charge (section five) to maximal potential. The thyroid has steroid-like powers. It sets the stage for the capability of the cells in regards to the generation of energy for work and heat. Like the steroids and vitamin A, thyroid directly determines which DNA programs are activated or silenced within a cell. Within the whole group, each of these hormones specific shape conveys different message content to the DNA. The proportions between each hormone type within this powerful group determine what the genetic program is doing.

Inefficient cellular furnaces are also inferior at the incineration of the ever-generated cellular trash. This is probably how the condition of myxedema accumulates within the skin of untreated hypothyroid patients. Myxedema denotes puffy bloating of the skin and occurs in severe cases of low thyroid function. Just below the front part of the knee is one common area of accumulation. These cells clog with accumulating cellular trash that normally burns within the cellular furnace.

Owners that have too much thyroid are similar to a furnace that burns too hot. When the cell power plant burns too hot, the cell has to throw in the 'furniture and house structural components' (doors and flooring). These structural components become necessary because the needs of the furnace cannot be met by usual amounts of fuel delivery alone. Untreated high thyroid leads to marked weakness and body wasting. Too much thyroid depletes the structural integrity of the cell in order to keep the cellular power plants stoked.

The thyroid gland itself is dependent on message content from the pituitary gland, which instructs it to produce its product, thyroid hormone. The thyroid gland also needs the pituitary derived message content to maintain proper size. Nutritionally, the thyroid needs quantities of the amino acid tyrosine and a continuous supply of iodine. The thyroid then needs the ability to release adequate thyroid hormone daily. Once the thyroid hormone is released, in order for it to be fully activated, it needs a precise removal of one of its specific iodines out of a total of 4 on a single thyroid molecule. Unless the right iodine is removed, the thyroid message is lost. Certain mineral deficiencies lead to inactive enzyme machines whose task is to remove the correct iodine. Many owners run into trouble here. They have defective activation mechanisms in operation.

Iodine deficiency and iodine excess inhibit thyroid gland function. Various drugs hamper the ability of the body to take the right iodine off. When certain medications do this they make the owner functionally hypothyroid. Instead of removing the precise iodine that confers the most active form of thyroid hormone, a different iodine is removed and it becomes worthless.

Almost all thyroid released from the gland has 4 iodines per hormone molecule. The most active form only occurs when specific iodine is removed. This conversion creates, what doctors like to call T3. If any other iodine is removed off of the 4 iodines contained on each thyroid hormone molecule, then the rubble becomes worthless. When rubble is produced instead of the active form of thyroid hormone, cells lack appropriate direction within the thyroid dependent DNA programs.

Selenium deficiency decreases the ability for activation of thyroid to T3 within the brain and placenta. When these organs are unable to activate thyroid to its more active form, T3, they each receive decreased message content. Decreased message content in the brain of T3 will lead to diminished ability of the nerve cells to charge their membranes. This has two consequences. First, the nerve will have diminished ability to perform work (easy fatigue and mental slowness). Second, the nerve will have diminished ability to protect itself from harmful ions that are waiting to get inside and bind to the nerve cell's delicate contents. Western trained physician don't counseled owners about these facts?

Acute illness, trauma, cancer, kidney failure, and myocardial infarction can lead to faulty iodine removal. Scientists like to call this inactive form, reverse T3. When the wrong iodine is removed, reverse T3 is created. Reverse T3 has no biological activity (no message content). Measurement of a 24-hour urine test for T4, T3, and reverse T3 is the most accurate way to assess thyroid adequacy at the tissue level.

Stress decreases thyroid responsiveness to the pituitary message content to activate it. The doctor can measure a normal pituitary hormone message, TSH, directed at the thyroid gland, but when stress is present thyroid function diminishes. When thyroid function diminishes, the cells receive decreased thyroid message. Unfortunately, the measurement of a TSH only is the standard of care for thyroid inquiry. When stress increases this value is misleading.

There are many additional perturbations on the effectiveness of thyroid message content at multiple levels from stress. Stress also increases secretion of acute phase reactant proteins into the blood stream. The acute phase reactant proteins include complement, C-reactive protein, fibrinogen, and interferon. Interferon further suppresses thyroid activity during times of stress. Normal TSH levels can be misleading when increased interferon is released during stress. The anxiety of the blood draw can temporarily increase free values of thyroid hormone. Lastly, cortisol levels that increase during stress also suppress thyroid gland activity by suppressing the master gland, the pituitary.

This all makes sense when one thinks about repairing the power plants when the body perceives an emergency (stress). Repair activity is a low priority when survival is the message that the body receives. The body cannot discern the difference between real or imagined stress. The physiological response to mental and physical stress is initially the same. Stressed owners, by nature of body design, tend to be hypothyroid even though their lab tests come back normal.

Some common clinical signs of low thyroid function are:

1. Hair is coarse, prematurely gray, and sparse.
2. Skin is dry and yellowish
3. Voice is husky and low
4. Thinking is slow
5. Memory is poor
6. Cholesterol is increased in the blood stream
7. Armpit temperature before getting out of bed is less than 97.6 degrees
8. Bowel movements tend towards constipation
9. Lateral edges of the eyebrows are missing.
10. EKG voltage tends to be diminished
11. Cold intolerance compared to the normal population.

Other symptoms surface as the consequences of turning down the power plant flame within the cells. Consistently low body temperature is a good clinical marker of those owners who have tissue level thyroid resistance, but possibly normal thyroid levels of T4, T3, and reverse T3.

Some people have normal levels of thyroid parameters measured by even the best testing methods available. They may still have a thyroid problem. There has been an association of attention deficit and hyperactivity disorder with this type of thyroid resistance. Thyroid resistance means that thyroid levels are normal, but the receptors for receiving thyroid message content are diminished. One of the consequences of diminished thyroid message content within a developing brain is attention deficit disorder. This evidence suggests that the thyroid plays a role in normal brain development.

Lastly, the thyroid can be inhibited by the food ingested. Certain foods contain thyroid-inhibiting substances that are found in foods from the Brassicacae family of vegetables - rutabagas, cabbage, and turnips. All of them have been documented to inhibit thyroid function. Lony elucidates the importance of this. She is a 25-year old who developed swelling in her thyroid area. Standard testing showed that her thyroid function diminished. The specialist involved with her care was unaware that certain foods consumed in excess can produce this swelling. This particular patient loved large helpings of rutabagas, cabbage, and turnips. When this patient discontinued this practice, her neck swelling subsided. Despite this, her specialist is still found to be advocating her need for continued medical therapy. The world of certified experts and the near extinction of the generalist have consequences.

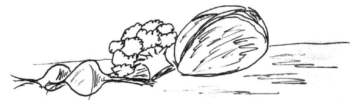

This subsection was about general considerations for what the thyroid does and needs. In the next section the general considerations are organized into the seven levels of where the thyroid system can fail. The seven levels are best conceptualized in their interdependence by seven links in a chain. When the weakest link fails the system fails. Science is present to do a better job of inquiry as to the true status of thyroid message content reaching cellular DNA programs.

Seven links in the Thyroid Chain of Health

First Link - Hypothalamus

The hypothalamus releases TRH (thyroid releasing hormone) when stimulated by three different mechanisms - lowered amounts of T4 and T3 (active thyroid hormones) in the circulation, cold weather, and adrenaline. One of the jobs of the thyroid is to provide the mechanism for warmth. Cold weather increases the need for heat production. Adrenaline is released when body temperature begins to fall. Adrenaline also helps raises body temperature by stimulating fat to enter the blood stream. The fat liberated heads for the trillions of cellular power plants. When adrenaline reaches the hypothalamus it begins the first step of raising the body temperature. Adrenaline within the hypothalamus stimulates the first link in the thyroid chain, the release of TRH. The TRH released will then go directly to the pituitary. When TRH is in the pituitary, its message stimulates this gland to release TSH (thyroid stimulating hormone). This is the second link of the thyroid chain. Before discussing the second link of the thyroid chain it is worth mentioning the processes that inhibit the first link.

The natural inhibitory factors of the first link (TRH release) are high circulating levels of T4 and T3. There is a certain class of blood pressure and prostate shrinking medications called alpha-blockers that inhibit this first link. When this medication is prescribed, the clinical signs for the hypothyroid state should be rigorously followed. When the first link is inhibited, these owners will tend to have diminished thyroid message content instructing their DNA program. This is in contrast to the natural control of the hypothalamus in that both increased T3 and T4 will decrease first link activity. There is no need to stimulate the chain with seven links into activation if there is already enough active thyroid message content within the body. In the case of the alpha-blocker medications, the first link is fooled by the medicine itself. If this medication is necessary, then thyroid supplementation should be considered at the first sign of inadequacy.

Second Link - Pituitary

Link two in the thyroid chain of health is the pituitary gland. The pituitary gland is often called the master hormone gland. It has some control over how the many endocrine glands grow and perform their task of making specific hormones. The glands that the pituitary has some control over are the gonads, the thyroid, the adrenals, the parathyroid, and the endocrine aspect of the liver, the pancreas, and the kidneys. The general theme of the how much the pituitary is stimulating a hormone-producing gland is a controlled process.

The first general control is by how much of one or more of the hormones manufactured in that gland are sensed within the blood stream reaching the pituitary. The second general control, at the level of the pituitary, is through other modifying molecules that augment or inhibit pituitary secretion. Conceptually, secretion modification is either helping the pituitary 'listen' or 'ignore' what the hypothalamus (first link) is directing by TRH release.

When the pituitary receives the message from the first link, it is in the form of TRH. The pituitary response to TRH may vary. There are some powerful competing forces within the pituitary gland itself. The summation of these competing messages will determine whether or not the pituitary 'listens' to what the TRH released by the hypothalamus is instructing. The competing messages must be summarized at the level of the pituitary, which either enhances or inhibits the pituitary response (listening ability or deafening ability). It is the summation of these competing messages at link two, which determines whether the pituitary listens to the message or ignores it.

Factors that increase the pituitary's ability to listen are high estrogen states and the diminished activity of link five, the de-iodinases. The enhancement of the link two response in the presence of estrogen demonstrates how ovary status and thyroid are interrelated. Hot flashes during early menopause are caused by the wide fluctuation of estrogen levels. The hot flashes are either lessened or intensified by the thyroid and estrogen interdependence.

Inhibitors of pituitary responsiveness to TRH message content are the hormone somatostatin, dopamine, and other dopamine agonist like bromocriptine. High cortisol levels caused by stress will also lower the pituitary response to TRH. All of these molecules inhibit the pituitary from releasing TSH when normal levels of TRH are instructing it to do so.

Part of the stress response inhibits link two in the thyroid function chain. This makes more sense when one understands the simultaneous stimulation of link four. Link four is discussed below but it is the level (link) where thyroid is transported within the blood stream. When cortisol levels increase in the blood stream, thyroid hormone is displaced from its carrier protein. The freed thyroid hormone content in the blood stream can rapidly exit into the numerous cells. When thyroid hormone levels increase inside cells, the effect is that the cells immediately begin stoking the power plant flame for energy production. This seems like a contradictory action of cortisol message content to different levels within the thyroid function chain. It is resolved when remembering that the body was designed to survive physical stresses.

Stress affects multiple levels of the thyroid system chain of health. The first level that stress interferes with is the pituitary gland (second link). The creator did not design the body to be mentally stressed day in and day out from modern life. The body was designed to handle short burst of stress - like running from death. The design of the body, when stress occurs, is for maximizing an increase in physical energy quickly. This is accomplished by the quick displacement of thyroid hormone off its carrier protein within the blood stream. This displacement allows a burst of thyroid hormone to enter the cells. This surge of thyroid hormone stimulates the mitochondria in the cells (through DNA program activation) to produce more energy. The ability to do this comes with a price. The body has turned off the pituitary (link two). This means the other links, below level two, are depleted quickly. When physical stress is the issue, the body is smart enough to know that the manufacture of more thyroid hormone is a waste of energy in the short run. However modern stress is different in that the time course can become chronic. This situation explains how chronic stress inhibits the level of thyroid hormone within the blood stream. Eventually the thyroid hormone becomes depleted from cortisol inhibiting effects on the pituitary. When the pituitary link is inhibited by stress hormone, the successive other links eventually run out of thyroid hormone.

In order to understand how the common testing of the second link, the TSH level, can fool the doctor when stress is involved the fourth link needs to be mentioned out of turn. The fourth link depends on all prior links. In the short run, the stress reaction triggers the carrier protein, the fourth link, to dump massive amounts of thyroid. However, cortisol inhibits the prior links, including the pituitary. The higher links inhibition diminishes the release of more thyroid hormone for further body use. Chronic stress therefore eventually depletes what was available within the blood steam before stress occurred.

Chronic stress is therefore one clinical situation where the physician can be fooled with a normal TSH result. The TSH result may be normal, but the successive links are not. When lower links are not functioning properly, numerous cells lack adequate thyroid message content within their DNA programs. When the DNA programs fail to get these important messages, cells fail to spend energy on thyroid directed rejuvenation. Adequate rejuvenation, at the cell level, is partly the responsibility of thyroid message content. The best assessment for this is the armpit temperature and a twenty-four hour urine test for thyroid hormone.

Third Link - Thyroid

The thyroid gland is the third link in the chain in regard to power plant function and cell membrane charge within the trillions of body cells.   Ideally, the thyroid manufactures adequate thyroid hormone when directed by the pituitary. Like the pituitary, there are many competing messages within the thyroid that either interfere or enhance the thyroid gland's ability to 'listen' to the pituitary message. When the thyroid listens to a healthy pituitary, adequate amounts of thyroid hormone are released into the blood stream. Stress will diminish the pituitary directed TSH amount released even when the thyroid is becoming 'deaf' to its message (link two).

Many physicians are unaware that excess iodine in the diet poisons thyroid gland function. Thyroid function will decrease with too much iodized salt in the diet. This is an effective and simple treatment for an overactive thyroid gland. Other thyroid gland inhibitory substances that can be found in food are nitrates, thiocyanates, perchlorate, lithium, and possibly fluoride.

At the level of the thyroid, there is the potential that an owner's antibodies will attack their own thyroid tissue when the adrenals are weak and unable to retain normal immune function. Weakened adrenal status is an early indicator in the disease process that can potentially save the thyroid from total destruction. William McKenzie Jefferies, M.D., in his book *Safe Uses of Cortisol*, explains the 'how to' parameters very well. This education is about adrenal dysfunction and its role in this type of thyroid gland disease.

The thyroid gland link affects the ability to have healthy cellular power plant flames and maximally charged cells. Certain edible plants poison the gland's ability to perform these tasks. The Brassicae family that includes broccoli, cabbage, turnips, and cauliflower are some of them. Only large and frequent amounts produce a wounded thyroid gland (goiter) but it does happen.

Fourth Link – Blood Stream

All blood stream transport parameters are the fourth link in the chain of thyroid health. The blood stream transport system delivers thyroid hormone to the body cells. Body cells require adequate amounts of thyroid hormone transported in the blood stream at all times.

The major thyroid transport parameters are:

1. The amount of thyroid carrier protein within the transport system.
2. The blood stream, the amount of substances within the transport system that desires to displace thyroid off its carrier protein.
3. The rate of thyroid release into the transport system.
4. The rate of thyroid hormone destruction by the liver that constantly removes thyroid from the transport system.
5. The ability of the cells to suck thyroid out of the transport system.
6. The proportion of 'dead thyroid' hormone within the transport system.

The thyroid gland is like a faucet dumping more thyroid hormone into the blood stream and the cells are constantly removing it. This sucking action promotes the idea that the cells act like a drain removing thyroid hormone that is dumped into the blood stream by the thyroid gland. The ability of the cells to suck out thyroid hormone is retarded by the amount of thyroid hormone in the blood stream that binds to its carrier protein (thyroid binding globulin or TBG). The amount of thyroid hormone in the blood stream is where modern medicine stops looking. It usually ignores links five through seven.

The amount of thyroid in the blood stream is an estimated value when a laboratory measures it. The blood sample measurement of thyroid hormone contained in the blood stream is estimated before drain-off mechanisms deliver it to the cellular DNA programs. The carrier proteins are large enough to escape the ability of the drains to suck various hormones out of the blood stream.

Thyroid hormone can bind to its carrier protein and resist the drain sucking it out of the system.

The liver is the first big drain that sucks thyroid hormone out of the blood stream. Healthy livers have more power to suck the small amount of free thyroid hormone out of the blood stream. Only free thyroid hormone, not bound to a carrier protein, can enter the cells. The rate, at which the liver sucks out thyroid, forms a powerful drain off from available thyroid hormone to the other cells. Only the free level of thyroid hormone can be sucked out of the blood stream by the liver.

A healthy liver deactivates many hormones more quickly, including thyroid. In the case of thyroid hormone, when it is freely circulating it has little ability to prevent the liver sucking action so it can deliver its message content to other cells. The creator countered this problem by designing various carrier proteins that bind their hormones tightly while in transit within the blood stream. 99.9% of thyroid hormone binds to its carrier protein.

Certain factors will raise or lower the amount of free thyroid in transit in the blood stream. When the blood stream fails to have adequate carrier proteins, for thyroid, in order to keep the same level of hormone in the blood stream, the thyroid has to increase its production rate. When the drain (liver) is more effective at the removal rate, there has to be a greater faucet flow (the gland secretion rate) to keep the transport system levels the same. In these situations the thyroid gland has to work harder to keep blood levels adequate.

Certain drugs induce a larger liver drain (faster liver metabolic rate) for hormones like thyroid. Some of them are Phenytoin for seizure disorders, rifampin an antibiotic for tuberculosis, carbamazepine a psychiatric medicine. A larger liver drain is synonymous with a faster removal rate. These medications increase certain enzymatic machinery within liver cells.

The amount of carrier protein in the blood stream is another competing force to thyroid drain off by the liver and other cells. The higher the carrier protein levels, the better the prevention of various drains sucking out thyroid hormone. By avoiding the liver enzymatic machinery, the cells are also limited by their ability to remove thyroid. Chronically high levels of cortisol and estrogen promote an increase in carrier protein levels. This is a double edge sword in that these high levels help keep the liver drain at bay, but also prevent the drain leading into the tissues (cellular DNA level). In other words, an amount of thyroid hormone in the blood stream is less available to the cells. Despite the cells having no access to normal amounts of thyroid, the blood test will look deceptively good.

Women who take birth control pills can have signs of low thyroid function despite normal blood tests. This side effect results from high estrogen content stimulating an increased production rate of the carrier proteins. The blood test will measure a normal value of thyroid, but does not routinely measure the level of carrier protein in the blood stream. The amount of carrier protein for thyroid directly competes with the ability of cells to access thyroid hormone for their DNA programs. When increased cortisol or estrogen levels persist, the levels of thyroid binding protein increase. When binding of thyroid hormone increases, the hormone has trouble releasing into the tissues because it is trapped within the blood stream. In this situation thyroid is bound to high levels of carrier protein that trap it in the blood stream. Unless thyroid hormone can deliver message content to the level of the DNA program, in the trillions of cells, a normal level in the blood stream does little good.

Certain factors lead to a decreased level of thyroid carrier protein levels. When these factors exist, the opposite situation results. The liver can drain off the thyroid hormone produced more quickly making the thyroid work harder. The cells can access the thyroid hormone more easily while a higher level is free. The thyroid gland needs to make more thyroid hormone per day to keep blood levels in the normal range. Carrier protein levels decrease when there are increased androgen steroid hormones, chronic illness, and starvation conditions.

Certain agents within the blood stream (fourth link) are able to displace thyroid hormone off of its carrier protein. There are certain acute physical situations that occur in life where the body suddenly needs massive amounts of thyroid in the tissues. Mental stress and certain medications can inappropriately elevate thyroid dumping off its carrier protein. Regardless of how thyroid gets displaced, these situations can make blood test measurements appear normal when they are not. The inappropriate displacement of thyroid hormone off its carrier protein will reverberate all the way down to the cells DNA program.

Situations, in addition to stress, which displace thyroid off its carrier protein are aspirin, phenytoin, phenylbutazone, diazepam, and increased blood heparin. These situations make thyroid hormone more available to the liver drain as well as the tissue DNA program drain. Heparin increases the amount of free fatty acids secondary to activating lipoprotein lipase. When lipoprotein lipase is activated, there is an increase of fatty acids in the blood stream. Increased cortisol and epinephrine levels, occurring with related stress, also cause the increased fatty acid. This leads to thyroid hormone displacement, as well. Stress hormones cause a sudden increase in free fatty acid levels in the blood stream. Heparin and stress both displace thyroid off its carrier protein. Once thyroid hormone is displaced it becomes more available to the drains.

The amount of 'dead' thyroid versus active thyroid hormone in the blood stream must be considered. Illness can rapidly raise the amount of dead thyroid hormone in the blood stream. Scientist call the dead thyroid hormone, reverse T3. Clinically, the thyroid can be making its hormone properly, but some other process can kill off message content by deactivating it. Unless physicians routinely check this in chronically ill patients, they will miss opportunities for healing a problem caused by a low thyroid hormone level.

Link Five – Enzyme Machines & Selenium

There are enzyme machines that amplify the message content of the thyroid hormone. These machines, the de-iodinases, are link five in thyroid chain of healthy cellular power plants and maximal cell charge abilities. The presence of adequate selenium is necessary for these machines to function. Selenium deficiency will prevent the important body enzyme machine, de-iodinase, from activating thyroid hormone to its full power. Scientists denote this activation as conversion of T4 to T3. T3 is eight times more powerful for telling DNA programs what to do. For any amount of thyroid, this conversion amplifies the message content by a factor of eight.

Link Six – DNA Receptor

The DNA receptor that the T4 and T3 binds to around the DNA are link six in the chain of healthy cellular power plants and maximally charged cells within the body. Like other steroid-like hormones, thyroid hormone is interdependent on other steroid-like hormones for the completeness and integrity of its receptors. Steroid-like hormones and thyroid cannot activate DNA programs without adequate functional receptors at the level of the target cell. There needs to be adequate vitamin A and cortisol message content or the thyroid hormone won't have completed receptors. When the thyroid receptors at the DNA level are incomplete, the thyroid hormone's message content delivery becomes impossible. This is known as peripheral thyroid resistance. When peripheral thyroid resistance occurs, blood tests can be within normal for thyroid parameters, but these people are far from well. They have all or many clinical signs of diminished thyroid function.

In this situation an astute physician who notices the clinical signs of hypothyroidism, but normal blood values will cautiously try supplementation strategies. These strategies are worthwhile when armpit temperatures are consistently low. He will also make an inquiry into the levels of vitamin A and cortisol.

All prior links in the system can function perfectly, but if link six is defective, these owners will present like any low thyroid function owner. Their blood values can all be normal. At the level of the cell DNA program, where it matters, the ability to receive message content is impaired because the receptor is incomplete. Often the culprit is that there are insufficient vitamin A or cortisol levels. These two hormones are needed in order to direct the DNA to finish the manufacture of the thyroid DNA associated receptor. These patients are best diagnosed by a twenty-four hour urine test for steroids and thyroid hormones. The vitamin A status can be surmised by a lab test or by physical signs (unhealthy skin for age).

Link Seven – Receptor Formation

The receptor formation that thyroids message content directs as a result of DNA program activation is vulnerable to an inappropriate attack by the immune system. This is link seven in the chain of thyroid health. The hierarchy of hormones subsection will make the seventh link in the system of thyroid health more comprehensible.

Steroid-like hormones are the only hormones that directly activate cellular DNA programs. Thyroid hormone is a member of this group. The consequence of DNA program activation is that the segment of the genetic code activated leads to the manufacture of specific types of proteins.

Some of the DNA programs activated by thyroid involve proteins that become receptors for other 'lesser' hormones. These other hormones depend on adequate thyroid message content for the manufacture of their receptors. Without their receptors presence, it does little good to have these other hormones arrive. Hormones cannot deliver message content without their receptors being present. Many diseases arise because of receptor formation deficiency or receptor destruction. Asthma is sometimes caused by this defect in the receptors needed by epinephrine to keep the airways open.

Some thyroid message content is directed at the manufacture of cell membrane receptors for the recognition of adrenalin (epinephrine) in the lungs. In some owners, their adrenals fail to keep their immune system from attacking these types of receptors. In some types of asthmatic patients, adrenaline receptors in their lung airways are inappropriately destroyed by their immune system. This is an example of a level seven problem with thyroid function. This level does not involve the part of thyroid message devoted to power plant flame improvement in the cells. It involves other parts of the thyroid message that direct different DNA programs to manufacture adrenaline receptors. High blood eosinophils, or a reversed ratio between lymohocytes and nuetrophils (right shift), are a good sign that this is occurring (adrenal chapter).

The discussion about the seven links in the chain of thyroid system health is useful for understanding how the common thyroid clinical inquiry is often incomplete. Some of the popular blood tests can be inaccurate. Sometimes the twenty-four hour urine test can be deceptively normal. It is valuable to consider the stress level operating in a owner's life. Lastly, the medications and foods that are ingested can have dramatic effects on thyroid message content. The clinical signs of low thyroid function are often the most accurate.

Chapter 11

The Testes

An ailing physician almost one hundred years ago stumbled on the central role that the testicles play in the maintenance of health. He had been suffering from progressive deterioration of his musculoskeletal structures and depression. Out of desperation, he acted on a scientific inkling that the testes were somehow related to youth. He received the world's first testicle transplant from a cadaver. Anti-rejection techniques were not understood back then, but while the transplanted testicle was still functional, he noted dramatic improvements of his mental outlook and physical abilities. He also noted a dramatic improvement in his muscle contours and size. In addition, his arthritic symptoms lessened considerably. Lastly, he noticed both an increased zest for life and a heightened vitality in his physical stamina.

About the same time, across the Atlantic Ocean, one of the first endocrinologists, Albert Lamond, M.D. was conducting autopsies on the testicles of extremely long-lived men. He also researched male prowess and abilities of his living subjects. He noted consistently that testicular health was a predictor of the health of the man. In addition, to his research on testicles, he was one of the first physicians who prescribed extracts from the different endocrine glands. These extracts included the thyroid, pancreas, ovary, testes, adrenals, and occasionally the pituitary. He became world famous for his success at reversing some of the effects of aging.

Eugene Shippen, M.D., in his book *Testosterone Syndrome*, writes "I have never seen an older male patient in excellent mental and physical health whose testosterone levels were not well within the normal levels."[11] Most of men's testosterone is made in their testicles.

What the complex sells often skirts around central hormonal considerations that predictably begin to decline at the onset of middle age. Testosterone decline often manifests in men as decreased libido, loss of skeletal mass, loss of muscle mass that produces sagging and less taut skin (especially on the face and arms), loss of liver function, loss of kidney function, joint and diffuse body aches, loss of confidence, decreased concentration ability, memory deficiencies, hot flashes, and progressive fatigue. In addition to these symptoms, there is also the tendency for increased body fat. As testosterone falls the fat synthesis message of insulin becomes more powerful.

None of these symptoms are surprising when one understands testosterones importance to health. The powerful role that steroid-like hormones play centers on their ability to switch off or on the DNA programs. Testosterone is a steroid hormone. Its shape is such that when it binds to DNA, its message directs cellular energy toward infrastructure investment and rejuvenation. A lowered testosterone level creates a deficiency in cellular rejuvenation message content. When there is less rejuvenation message content, the DNA programs fail to activate at the youthful level. Without rejuvenation activities occurring, the wear and tear of aging begins. On average aging begins in middle-aged men and continues for the remainder of their lives. Eventually the man begins to have a 'worn down by life look'.

Science is all there, but it is often disorganized and disjointed in the presentation. Without an organized presentation, many physicians are unaware of the relationship of the degenerative processes and the relationship to decline in the male hormone, testosterone. The emphasis and presentation in medical schools often fail to educate physicians in these congruous facts.

The holism of these facts relates a strong correlation with physical and mental decline to the fall in testosterone. A fall in testosterone is often remedied by simple replacement therapies or lifestyle changes. These programs can be used to prevent and/or reverse the decline into an old body physique (low steroid tone).

In order to decide where one stands between normal and deficient testicle function, there needs to be a competent, thorough inquiry into one's steroid hormone status. The common standard of care is often superficial and misses opportunities for healing. The testes evaluation is similar to the adrenals and ovaries so far as the links in the chain to consider before ruling out testicle dysfunction.

Six Links in the Chain of Testicle Health Care

There are six links in the chain that need to be intact or testicle dysfunction will occur.

1. Hypothalamus
2. Pituitary
3. Testes
4. Blood stream transport parameters
5. Peripheral conversion to estrogen before it delivers the testosterone message
6. DNA receptor completeness - Very little known about this in the mainstream textbooks and therefore beyond the scope of this manual

The reason these are all mentioned together is that many well-meaning physicians miss one or more of these levels in their workup considerations and will therefore miss opportunities to heal. There is a popular tendency to prescribe synthetic testosterone substitutes in lieu of the real hormone. Similar to hormone replacement for women, these patentable substances have altered message content because their shape has been changed. The message content of steroids is inherent in their exact shape. A change in the shape changes the message content that the DNA receives. Clinically, these shape changes manifest as side effects.

One common example results from the chronic ingestion of the synthetic hormone replacement, methyl-testosterone, which is given to men and women. The side effect is increased tendency develop bloody cysts in their liver (peliosis hepatis). This is not known to occur with natural testosterone. One other caution, some testosterone injection preparations contain a deliberate contaminant, mercury. The mercury contaminant is under the hidden code name, thimurosil, in the inert ingredients. This is a known liver and neuron toxin.

Before a discussion of the six ways to break the links in the chain of the testosterone message occurs, these pit falls need to be addressed. Awareness of the side effects of contamination and substitution will help to prevent another problem from developing. Be cautious about taking prescribed hormones.

First Link – Hypothalamus

The first link in the testicle system of health is the hypothalamus at the center of the brain. The decisions of the hypothalamus facilitate or inhibit all other links in the testicular chain of health. When the first link is activated it secretes GRH (gonadotrophic releasing hormone). The amount of GRH released in men and women is determined by estrogen content. The amount of body estrogen inversely determines the activity level of the hypothalamus (first link).

Trouble lies in the fact that there are many environmental estrogens in the food supply (estrogen mimics). Increased estrogen from the food supply can fool the hypothalamus to believe the body has all the sex hormones it needs. For this reason the sperm count of men has fallen worldwide.

The increased environmental estrogen makes its way inside the body. The increased estrogen message content that results, tells the hypothalamus there is enough testicle steroid production. The estrogen content in men and women determines the hypothalamus activity for stimulating the gonads to increase steroid production. Steroid production rates are determined by body estrogen content as body design assumes when estrogen reaches a certain level, the other steroids are at a certain level as well. This is erroneous with environmental estrogens. They increase estrogen without increasing the other gonad steroids. For men, a diminished first link activity reverberates all the way down the testicle chain of health. Testicles need informational direction from the previous links. When this direction diminishes the testosterone dependent sperm production rate falls off. Like the other endocrine glands, without information the testicles begin to shrivel. The precautions listed earlier in the adrenal chapter are applicable.

Second Link - Pituitary

The second link in the chain to testicle health is the pituitary gland that hangs off the underside of the brain. There are several competing hormone messages in the pituitary that either facilitate or harm the ability of the pituitary to activate the next link in the chain, the testicles. Like the second link (thyroid), these hormonal factors either facilitate the pituitary's ability to listen or turn a deaf ear to the message content of the hypothalamus when it releases GRH.

When stress levels increase, the release of the hormones in the pituitary cause testicle activity to be suppressed. Normally, when unstressed, the hormones that stimulate the testes are suppressed by the elevation of cortisol. Cortisol elevation at the level of the pituitary suppresses the release of follicle stimulating hormone (FSH) and leuteinizing hormone (LH). The testicles need these two hormones that the pituitary manufactures and releases for growth and production of their testicle products.

Simultaneously, with cortisol, an additional hormone is released in the stress response, prolactin. Prolactin is also manufactured in the pituitary. When prolactin exceeds normal levels, the gonads (ovaries or testicles) are inhibited. In the case of the male, their testicles are inhibited when prolactin levels increase from chronic stress. Chronic stress diminishes the size of the testicles. The size of the testicles decreases with theconsequent decreased production of steroid at the direction of the prolactin message content.

When steroid production decreases the rate of sperm production decreases. If this is the suspected problem, a serum prolactin level is in order. A twenty-four hour urine test for cortisol is also helpful in establishing the cause of diminished testicle function. Other causes of prolactin elevation that have the same side effects are serotonin re-uptake inhibitors prescription medications (or anything that raises brain serotonin levels) and decreased thyroid function because thyroid-releasing hormone (TRH) is also a powerful stimulator of prolactin release from the pituitary. High blood estrogen levels that commonly occur in women taking birth control pills and excessive exposure to hormone mimics will also elevate prolactin levels. Conversely, lower estrogen levels stimulate the pituitary to release LH and FSH because the hypothalamus and pituitary are sensitive to estrogen levels.

Link Three – The Testes Level of Function and Directions

The informational directions received determine testes level of function. If testes receive both growth factors (LH and FSH) and nutritional molecular building parts (section three) the production of sperm and steroid hormones tend to be adequate. If however, it receives primarily prolactin message content there tends to be inhibition of testicle function.

At the testicle level, there is an additional powerful hormone, aldosterone that determines the ability of the testicles to make steroids. Aldosterone is manufactured in the adrenal glands. Steroid production is stimulated and enhanced by aldosterone levels. It is the steroid hormone responsible for beginning the manufacture of steroids from the raw material, cholesterol. Without sufficient aldosterone message content the testicle has difficulty in starting the steroid manufacture process. Factors that increase aldosterone levels will also lead to increased steroid production in the testicles. Increased steroid production in the testes leads to increased message content reaching the cells to invest available energy in rejuvenation. Conversely, factors that diminish aldosterone levels will cripple the testicles ability to manufacture steroids. The third link of testicle health, the testicles themselves, depends on proper message content from the adrenals and pituitary.

Some owners that arrive at middle age after eating a processed food diet can no longer handle normal aldosterone levels without a simultaneous increase in blood pressure. The crux of the blood pressure problem is not aldosterone, but the chronic ingestion of reversed ratio minerals content which deviate from body design. When the mineral content of food is reversed, the body will eventually develop health problems around middle age.

Middle age is often accompanied by a breakdown of the body's ability to deal with years of ingesting a reversed mineral content diet. In the case of the testicles these owners, if they are going to continue to have adequate testosterone, will tend to have high blood pressure. If the body decreases aldosterone production to help keep blood pressure normal, the testosterone level will fall. Certain medications prescribed to treat blood pressure have the potential to lower testosterone. They also lower aldosterone production rates (chapter three).

Blood pressure problems with aldosterone are avoidable when the owner consumes a diet with proper mineral proportions. Real food has proper mineral proportions. Processed food (dead food) has the wrong mineral proportions. The potassium and magnesium content are generally depleted when food is processed. Processed food tends to have large amounts of sodium added to prolong shelf life. This combination can poison the testicles around middle age. They are not receiving enough aldosterone, which decreases to lower the blood pressure. The body was designed for at least three times the intake of potassium compared to sodium. When mineral consumption occurs in these designed proportions there is no problem when aldosterone levels are elevated. Blood pressure elevates on the reversed mineral proportions diet (processed food) with the side effect of fluid retention. This occurs because of the incompatible reversed mineral ratios contained in the processed food diet. Rather than just educate physicians and owners about this simple consequence of a processed food diet, owners are given blood pressure prescription medication.

Around middle age some testicles turn down the production rate of testosterone because aldosterone elevation, while on a processed food diet, will elevate blood pressure. Alternatively, some men are prescribed blood pressure lowering medications, the ACE inhibitors, which lower steroid production rates. The steroid production rates in both cases decreases from the consequence of testicles receiving diminished aldosterone message content. On the other extreme are male owners who continue to make adequate testosterone while consuming a dead food diet. These individuals experience increased blood pressure around middle age. The blood pressure elevates with increased aldosterone on a processed food diet due to the altered mineral content. The altered mineral content contains increased sodium and diminished potassium and magnesium. These reversed mineral proportions are in direct conflict with general body design. Chronically altered mineral intake will cause sodium to be conserved as well as water. This combination elevates blood pressure.

There is an important but uncommon exception to this general pattern. Some owners manufacture the hormone atrial natruretic peptide (ANP) at high levels. ANP is a powerful peptide hormone made within the heart. When this hormone is manufactured at a high rate and it is not destroyed before it reaches the kidney, it can override the desire of aldosterone to conserve sodium and water and blood pressure remains normal. Although these owners have an override system that allows for increased aldosterone despite a processed food diet, they will be unhealthy in other ways. This lack of health is explained in section five.

Both the testicle and high blood pressure problem are completely avoidable when an owner adheres to a real food diet (section three). A real food diet is naturally high in potassium and magnesium and low in sodium. A real food diet is consistent with the way the human body was designed to interact with mineral proportions. The mineral proportions in food affect powerful hormone systems. Altered mineral proportions disrupt the testicle system.

Link Four – Blood Stream Transport

The blood stream transport level of testosterone is often the only link in the chain that ever gets any inquiry. European studies have shown that the majority of steroids are carried in the red blood cells. There are other ways that steroids are transported. One is on carrier proteins. There is also a very small amount of steroids free within the liquid phase of blood. The higher the amount of carrier protein, for a particular steroid, the lower the free amount within the serum. This is a similar concept that occurs with thyroid in that it is a double-edged sword. On one edge a higher carrier protein level impedes the rate of the liver sucking the various steroids out of the blood stream. On the other edge, it impedes the cells ability to suck them out, as well.

The new fact is that the steroids are transported in the red blood cells themselves. The amount of steroids transported in the red blood cells is the larger proportion of the total amount in transport in the blood stream. The amount of steroids and carrier protein in the red blood cells is not routinely measured. This means a blood value from different owners could mean different things entirely. The higher the estrogen or thyroid levels, then the higher the carrier protein's level will be. These two hormones direct the liver to increase production of carrier proteins. For the same total serum levels that occur in two different patients there could be an entirely different risk for deficiency of testosterone. An owner with a very high carrier protein levels could be extremely deficient at the DNA level in the cells. If he is unfortunate enough to receive only a total serum level and not have the carrier protein level included, he will be misdiagnosed if the protein level is higher than normal.

Until an accurate and routine laboratory test becomes available for the red blood cell contribution of steroid transport, physicians and owners will have to wait. It is likely that the flexibility of red blood cells powerfully determines how readily a steroid, like testosterone, can enter cells at the capillary level (chapter 2). Similarly, the mechanical squeezing (flexibility) of all red blood cells is largely ignored as far as this factors' contribution in determining the rate of oxygen delivery to the cells. The same red cell flexibility factor is ignored for steroid delivery (chapter two) rates at the capillary level into the cells themselves. These problems with the accuracy of blood measurements of steroids lends further credence to the value of a twenty-four hour urine test for steroids and thyroid output. Someday there will be additional measurements in the blood stream that includes a more accurate assessment of these variables.

Link Five – Peripheral Conversion of Testosterone to Estrogen

The prevention of the peripheral conversion of testosterone to estrogen is the fifth link. When the male owner is healthy, there is very little testosterone that converts to estrogen within the male body. The testicles make the majority of testosterone, which does little good for the cells if it is converted to estrogen before it can deliver its message content to the DNA programs in the cells.

When testosterone converts to estrogen before it can deliver message content, a powerful unraveling of the male form begins. The male form can only be maintained when the proper proportion between estrogen and testosterone is maintained. Certain factors alter the optimal ratio around middle age. Until these factors are effectively mitigated, supplementation of the manufacture of testosterone in the testicles will do little good. In these cases it is preferentially converted to estrogen. The higher estrogen within the male body has powerful repercussions on not only the male form, but also the testicles themselves (first link).

Three common factors that increase the conversion rate of testosterone to estrogen are increased body fat, zinc deficiency, and methyl donor deficiency. Minimizing each of these three will allow testosterone to increase. When testosterone increases, the cells receive the message to increase rejuvenation. When rejuvenation increases, cells increase their infrastructure development activities. Adequate infrastructure redevelopment is reflected in the mirror as an improved physique.

Increased body fat creates a vicious cycle of increased estrogen. Fat cells contain an enzyme called aromatase that converts testosterone to estrogen. The more fat, then the more aromatase present to convert testosterone to estrogen. Increased estrogen perpetuates an increased body fat in the male in the same way as a female. Some well-meaning physicians prescribe testosterone for middle-aged patients and get poor results. Until aromatase activity diminishes, testosterone supplementation is counter productive. Often these males get cranky and irritable and begin to develop breast tissue. An estrogen level from a blood sample or a twenty-four hour urine test should be included in the hormone evaluation for men.

There are two possible methods for side stepping aromatase activity. The first is in sticking to a low carbohydrate diet that will decrease insulin and reduce fat production. Once fat levels have decreased, testosterone supplementation may be effective. The second method to consider is prescribing of dihydrotestosterone (DHT), which cannot be converted to estrogen as readily and is ten times more powerful than regular testosterone. Keep DHT away from the male scalp. This is the form of testosterone creates male pattern baldness when it reaches high levels in the scalp tissue. A cream is best for this reason and can be applied to the abdomen and breast areas. DHT will tend to support prostate growth. In the estrogen dominant male, DHT will probably shrink an enlarged prostate. Increased estrogen has more of a growth promoting effect on the prostate than DHT does. It is important to follow serial PSA's when there is any doubt. In the case of the middle aged male, there is always doubt.

There are two methods for decreasing the activity of the aromatase enzyme. First, normal amounts of zinc inhibit aromatase activity. The highest concentration of zinc is found in oysters. This may explain why oysters have long been associated with aphrodisiac activity. Second, keep the methyl donor system healthy. The methyl donor system is healthy when there are sufficient methyl groups for the DNA stabilizing, hormone creating, and hormone deactivating system (section three).

The body needs a methyl group at the rate of one billion times a second. When owners continue to eat processed food, they will eventually become methyl deficient. It will take a methyl off of testosterone with the help of the enzyme aromatase. When this happens testosterone is converted into estrogen.

Nutritional deficiencies can disable the hormone system by multiple mechanisms (section three). Before discussing nutritional building blocks that make up the body form, a hormone pecking order needs to be established. By understanding the hierarchy of hormones in the body, owners become less gullible to the agenda of the complex.

Chapter 12

Hierarchy of Hormones - Informational Substances

Before proceeding with this book, it helps to have a concise grouping of how the different hormones can be separated into a successive hierarchy. The hierarchy between the different hormones concerns their degree of influence and length of action when compared to one another. There are four basic groups of successive levels of influence on how the body spends energy. Hormones direct cell energy usage. The more powerful the hormone group, the more central it is in the energy direction determination.

It helps to elucidate the common error of how mainstream medicine often focuses on the 'lesser' hormones. The lesser hormones get the press coverage while the more powerful hormones are only peripherally addressed. By taking this approach to chronic disease treatment strategies, symptom control is all that is possible. Symptom control medicine always has side effects and has nothing to do with healing. When the hormonal hierarchy is added back into the discussion the error is easy to expose.

Grouping the different informational substances (hormones) into four groups will help in understanding the relationship of the many various hormones. Also, many chronic degenerative diseases will begin to have healing solutions.

Common degenerative diseases amenable to healing once the hormone hierarchy is addressed are: adrenal gland caused asthma, rheumatoid arthritis, systemic lupus erythematosus, osteoarthritis, adult onset diabetes, obesity, some cases of heart disease, ulcerative colitis, Crohn's disease, some liver diseases, some kidney diseases, some cases of senility, and muscle wasting diseases.

All of these diseases have an increased likelihood of a solution when the clinician attends to these disease treatments in a logical progression from the most powerful hormone imbalances down to the weakest. When supplementation strategies are needed, real hormones are used because they contain accurate message content. The body was designed for real hormone message content. Whenever the altered shaped of the synthetic substitutes are given in place of real hormones, there will be side effects. When the shape is changed, to obtain a patent, the message content is changed.

The four groups in the hierarchy of hormones are:

Level 1 - the supreme commanders of body energy

This powerful group of hormones directly switches off and on different DNA programs. The DNA programs activated in a cell determine the activity of the cell and the degree of repair (rejuvenation). The activity and repair determine the usefulness of the cell. When cells are given good informational direction from the level one hormones, they will be productive and healthy. The quality of the mixture and amount of level one hormones reaching the over one hundred trillion cells is a central determinant of health. An owner's health is powerfully influenced because these hormones all contain message content that instructs the DNA genetic program.

The level one hormones are the only hormones powerful enough to directly interact and instruct cellular genetic material (the DNA). The quality of the proportional mixture between these hormones determines the highest level of energy expenditure possible and the direction that available energy will take. At this primary level it determines whether a cell is using available energy efficiently or not. This class of hormone has access to every body chamber (skin chapter).

Level 2 – the amino acid chain

All hormones message content is about directing cellular expendable energy, likewise with the level two hormones. Level two hormones deliver a message when they bind to a cell surface receptor (their own unique type) or they bind a receptor inside the target cell. The level two hormones are only able to influence cell energy expenditure on existing cell structures and enzymatic machinery activity. They are not able to directly interact with the DNA programs in the manufacture of new cell structures or new enzymatic machinery. Only level one hormones are powerful enough to do that

Insulin and glucagon are examples of level two hormones. Like other level two hormones, they are made up of a specific sequence of amino acids that are twisted around in three-dimensional space. The shape of these specific sequences and resulting twist contains precise message content. Insulin and glucagon are also an example of level two hormones that contain opposite message content. The message content difference between insulin and glucagon directs the target cell to spend energy in the opposite way. Consistent with level two hormones, each can only affect existing cellular enzymatic machines or structural content. Insulin turns off the enzyme machines that glucagon turns on. Likewise, the message content of glucagon turns off what insulin turns on. Each of these opposing hormones has enzyme machines that they activate. The direction of energy within a cell is determined by which enzymes are quiet or active.

The liver cells are instructive as an example of opposite energy direction between the message content of insulin and glucagon. Insulin directs liver cell energy into fuel storage. Fuel is stored in various locations, but insulin stimulates the liver in the manufacture glycogen, triglycerides, cholesterol, and LDL cholesterol. Insulin also inhibits the liver from turning amino acids into sugar and fat. The more insulin in the body, the more these activities are occurring within the liver. Glucagon directs the liver in the release of stored fuel and curtails new cholesterol and triglyceride manufacture. It also stimulates the liver contained enzymatic machines to make sugar from available amino acids.

Some level two hormones are further endowed with the ability to leave a 'last will and testament' before being chewed up into component parts by intracellular machinery. Intracellular machinery eventually dismantles the level two hormones. There is an intermediate step. The last will and directive of some level two hormones occurs between activating their receptor and being dismantled. The last will and directives are additional messages to the cell created by level two hormones. This directs the types of level four hormone precursors that are formed. These messages exist for a limited time. During that time, the level two hormones affect which level four hormone precursors a cell will receive message content from. Insulin and glucagon are good examples of how a hormone's presence determines which level four hormone precursors are formed. Also consistent is the fact that level four hormones precursors, stimulated by insulin, have the opposite effect on cell energy, when mature, as the direction that glucagon level four hormones impart.

Level 3 – the subservient hormones

The level three hormones are composed of single amino acids, which have been structurally modified or are from short chains of amino acids. These hormones depend on directives of the higher hormones 'stage setting'. The level one and two hormones set the stage for structural integrity and enzyme machinery contained in a cell. The level one hormones at the DNA level centrally determine the stage setting. In turn, the level two hormones determine the activity of the setting, the enzymes. The level three hormones channel blood and fuel to the cells. However, the level three hormones depend on level one hormones directing the manufacture of their receptors. Without enough level three-hormone receptors being made, many chronic diseases begin (asthma from epinephrine receptor deficiency).

Biogenic amines, cytokines, bradykinin and endothelin all belong to this class of hormones. Dietary deficiencies can effect development and manufacture of these hormones. Many different vitamins are important for the biogenic amines manufacture. In general, the level three hormones have an effect on the caliber of blood vessels and properties of the cells in these vessels in a certain area of the body.

The level three hormones (muscle chapter) delivering message content in a certain blood vessel determines much about the oxygen availability, nutrient delivery, waste removal, stickiness of the vessel wall, clotting tendency, and immune cell behavior.

Level 4 – local acting, subservient hormones

These hormones exist for seconds, only long enough to deliver message content to nearby cells. Within seconds of their release they are deactivated. These hormones only having an influence for both the duration and as far as the sound of their 'voice' will travel. This is in contrast to the other three levels of hormones that can travel more extensively in delivering their message content.

Some of the level four hormones, like nitric oxide gas, have powerful penetration abilities through body barriers. Although nitric oxide has powerful penetrating abilities, its message content delivery ability is limited due to its rapid deactivation. This short lifespan diminishes the distance of influence of nitric oxide message content.

Other level four hormones, like the ecosanoids (hormonal fats) that include prostaglandins, leukotrienes, and lipoxin are also limited by their short life spans. The ecosanoids come from essential fatty acids (hormonal fat precursors). These include Linoleic, linolenic, and arachidonic acid. All three of these essential fatty acids can only be obtained in the diet. The type of diet determines which level two hormones message content will predominate.[12]

An example of the opposing possibilities of level two hormones and how they determine what level four hormones are possible occurs between insulin and glucagon. The opposite message content contained between glucagon and insulin has a powerful influence on which level four precursor hormones are possible. High carbohydrate diets tend to promote the pro-inflammatory hormonal fat precursors to line many cells. Low carbohydrate and high protein diets promote anti-inflammatory hormonal fat precursors. The type of level two hormones limits the possibilities for which level four hormone precursors line numerous cells. Those hormonal fat precursors that line the surface of cells determine the likelihood of developing or preventing some malicious chronic degenerative diseases. Some diseases effected by the presence or the absences of hormonal fat precursors are cancer, heart disease, arthritis, depression, fatigue and immunodeficiency syndromes.

There are three principles about the ecosanoids (hormonal fats) that are important. First, only green plants can make two out of three of these hormonal fat precursors called the essential fatty acids. Animals like salmon that live in the wild eat plankton and therefore contain significant amounts of these two plant manufactured essential fatty acids. Farmed, grain-fed animals are raised without these essential fatty acids presence. The green plant manufactured essential fatty acids are linolenic and linoleic acid. Free-range chicken eggs are good sources for these plants derived essential fatty acids. Wild game such as elk and deer are also sources for these two essential fatty acids. These are good sources for essential fatty acids because of the high content of green plants in their diet. Green plants are the source of the anti-inflammatory fatty acids, linolenic and linoleic acids. Non-green roots and grains are more likely to contain the pro-inflammatory arachidonic acid. Store bought chicken, meat and eggs, because the animals are grain fed, will be higher in the arachidonic acid type.

Second, eating all the right essential fatty acids can still output the wrong hormonal fats. These hormonal fat precursors are subservient to the more powerful higher hormones. Level two hormones like insulin and glucagon determine which hormone fat precursors become created from essential fatty acids in the diet. The essential fatty acids in the diet are the raw material created for precursor hormonal fats. The balance of message content between insulin and glucagon predetermine which precursors are created.

Third, hormonal fat precursors are ideally contained on all the cell surfaces. When released, these hormones have a limited area of influence because of their short lifespan. Scientist denote this shortened hormone lifespan by the term paracrine. Paracrine hormones can only deliver message content in the immediate area of release. All level four hormones are paracrine in nature. The level four hormones are only released when triggered by higher hormones. Sub-optimal hormonal fat message content has a powerful influence on several chronic diseases.

The hormonal fats are so important that many powerful medications work by poisoning their ability to be produced. Some medications that work by poisoning hormonal fats are aspirin and related non-steroidal anti-inflammatory medications, cortisone derivatives, and the newer cox 2 inhibitors. These symptom control approaches have consequences to the balance of fine tuning abilities occurring in cells. All of these redirect body energy. With an understanding of hormonal fats and how to optimize their function, one can work with their body and begin healing.

Nitric oxide has a powerful ability to lower blood pressure and is also within this fourth class of hormones. It can only briefly increase blood delivery into its local area of release. This is how the medication Viagra works and why all the warnings about it lowering blood pressure are given. The medicine content of nitric oxide increases blood flow to the penis. The synthesis of this natural blood flow regulator requires the presence of the nutritional co-factors arginine, tetrahydrobiopterin, FMN, FAD,and thiols. These are contained in garlic, folate and riboflavin.

Be aware of the hierarchy of different hormone groups and what dietary factors are required for them to be produced. Owners who have optimal balance at each level are in good health. Conversely, a lowered quality of informational content occurring at any of the successive levels or dietary deficiencies leads to health consequences. The science exists to help owners receive better hormones and good nutrition.

In the next chapter the owner will begin to understand how the different molecular parts are assimilated and how deficiencies lead to breakdown processes.

SECTION III

YOU ARE WHAT YOU SUPPLY AND ABSORB

Principle 4

The fourth principle of health has two interconnecting parts. The first concerns the quality of function in the digestive organs. The prevention of body breakdown occurs because only functional digestive tracts can maximize the absorption of nutrients. The second part of the fourth principle is the need for quality molecular replacement parts in the digestive tract. The owner needs to make good nutritional decisions or there will be insufficient building blocks for the digestive tract to absorb. Reactions of life use up molecular parts quickly. There is a continual need for new sources of quality parts. Molecular replacement parts serve in making body structure, fuel, maintaining cellular electrical charge, hormones, and as part of enzyme machine activities.

Structures that are alive, cells and tissues, require a constant supply of quality molecular replacement parts. The process of life degrades molecules. This chapter concerns how these molecular replacement parts are obtained and assimilated. When replacement parts assimilate, the rejuvenation program continues.

Inadequate supply strategies for obtaining the needed molecular replacement parts are the fourth path that leads to an old body. The fourth principle of longevity concerns how to obtain and assimilate quality molecular replacement parts. Quality parts are necessary to prevent the old body manifestation that results from the accumulation of worn out parts. Many ownders fail to comprehend the obvious consequences of inadequate molecular replacement parts or a deficiency in quality. Often this disconnection results from scientific communication being explained in an abstract manner.

Each cell type needs a continuous supply of specific replacement molecular parts. These molecular replacement parts are needed in specific amounts and sufficient quality to maintain healthy cell function. The processed food diet is deficient in regenerative replacement parts. Deficiency, excess, or inferior quality interferes with health.

When the digestive tract fails from either mechanism, health consequences ensue:

1. Cellular trash accumulation
2. Loss of cellular integrity (old worn out molecular parts)
3. Deficient molecular parts needed to manufacture adequate informational substances (hormones and neurotransmitters)
4. Inadequate cellular charge (mineral imbalance)
5. A progressive deficiency in the ability to maintain cellular energy requirements (vitamin deficiencies, rust and poor quality fuel intake)

This section concerns processes two, three, and five. They are determined by the fourth principle of health. Processes of cell trash water removal and cell charge have other determinants.

Negative Digestive Mechanisms:

1. Cellular trash accumulation
2. Loss of cellular integrity from lack of molecular replacement parts
3. Deficient parts to manufacture new informational substances
4. Mineral deficiencies that cause a diminished cellular charge (decreased cellular force field)
5. Diminished fuel supply lines that make cells vulnerable to injury

Chapter 13

Digestion

The Body is Analogous to a Temple that is Alive

The ongoing assimilation of molecular replacement parts is similar to the non-living building world. There are fundamental building blocks, each with specific roles in creating the overall whole (wire, bricks, two by fours, windows, light sockets, trusses, etc.). These components have the potential, when assembled correctly and proportionally, to become an elaborate temple building. Multiply the architectural complexity of the ongoing body molecular parts replacement program. Throughout life this replacement program is necessary for healthy structure and function.

The body can be thought of as a dynamic, living temple that will, in time, wear out constituent molecular parts as it pulsates with the life energies. The wear and tear creates accumulation of defective molecular structural components and enzyme machines. The temple requires precise maintenance of internal structure and energy flow parameters. It is only able to obtain these from other temples (living things). These other temples must be precise in dismantling or rubbish instead of replacement parts is left. The precise dismantling of these temples is referred to as digestion.

Healthy owners have digestive systems that assimilate continuously needed replacement parts into the body. Availability of sufficient parts results from precise dismantling of other temples in the digestive tract. The absorption of these molecular building blocks and fuel sources (to power the 'intra-temple electronics') occurs in a rhythmic fashion. After absorption of these parts, they are reassembled into components (cell structure or enzymes) or consumed as fuel in the cellular power plants (mitochondria).

The reactions of life diminish when the digestive tract malfunctions in its ability to precisely dismantle a molecular building block. The lack of replacement parts leads to many chronic degenerative diseases.

Digestion fails because of:

1. Poor nutrition choices
2. Improper dismantling ability of critical structural components that are needed to replace worn cellular structural components, or cellular machines (enzymes)
3. Poor quality communication between digestive cells secondary to sub-optimal hormone tone
4. Injury to various digestive chambers and structures

Digestive Tracts and Molecular Supply Lines

All too often the nutritional integrity of cells is superficially addressed. Many owners age at an accelerated rate unnecessarily. The disassembly of protein, carbohydrate, and fats relies on numerous digestive juices. These juices must occur in a specific sequence and be of a sufficient amount. Protein disassembly is a prototypical example of the three different food groups that can facilitate comprehension of problems with the dismantling process - digestion.

Proteins are comprised of twenty different molecular shapes (amino acids linked end to end). Each amino acid type has a different shape and is endowed with unique chemical qualities. The order of sequence of amino acid connection and the proportions of different amino acids determine the resulting properties of a protein.

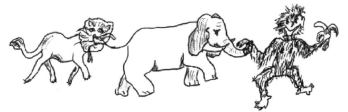

It helps to visualize twenty different miniature animals as analogous to the twenty different amino acids that make up protein. Different animals occur in various sequences and numbers as they line up. The average number of amino acids strung together in a protein equals five hundred. This allows a mental picture of the average protein molecule. This chain would have so many tigers, so many elephants, etc. The specific order of these shapes and the amount of each type confers a unique chain (20 different building block shapes, corresponding to 20 different amino acids that can link together to form a protein). In order to build this chain the body can only obtain the different lions, tigers, and bears from properly dismantled (digested) other chains (protein meals). In order to build new necklaces, a tiger separates as a whole tiger and not a half of a tiger and half of an elephant. If this occurs, the building block potential of the different shapes is reduced to rubbish.

The body can only produce twelve different amino acid types. It cannot manufacture the other eight. When the body manufactures its own amino acids, it depletes essential acids that must be obtained in the diet. The best situation occurs when an owner consumes proper proportions and amounts of all twenty amino acids.

The healthy digestive tract, when presented with these chains (proteins) starts methodically dismantling them. The proteins must be precisely disassembled or useful replacement parts are not absorbed. When amino acids are absorbed, they are used for building new proteins (chains). The unique order and amounts of different amino acids confer specific qualities and abilities for a protein. Some proteins contain many sulfurous amino acids. Other proteins have extra nitrogen. Still other proteins have extra acid content. The overall order and content determines protein function.

Some proteins are used for structural integrity (cell membrane, organelles, hair, bone, ligaments, etc.). Some serve as transport vehicles in the bloodstream for critical minerals, steroids, and gases (calcium, testosterone, and oxygen respectively as examples). Other proteins are used as cellular machines (enzymes). Still others are used as informational substances (insulin, glucagon, and IGF-1).

The body requires a continuous supply of quality building blocks (amino acids) in order to maintain availability of the different protein types. Amino acid building blocks need to be structurally intact when absorbed. The digestive process is worthless without precise dismantling of consumed protein meals into component amino acids.

Molecular Replacement Parts Require Precision Dismantling

The public is led to believe digestion is analogous to food that is grounded in a blender. The perpetrated story implies that this slurry is then sucked into the bloodstream and divided into the different body cells for use. The temple analogy can expose this gross simplification.

If a building were to explode into rubbish, there would be little salvage ability in the way of reusable structural components (intact doors, windows, trusses, flooring, appliances, etc.). In order to have any reusable structural components derived from a temple building that is dismantled, there needs to be a precision dismantling process. There can be reusable components with precision dismantling. This is similar to the human body digestive process that needs to be orderly and precise in its ability to dismantle the various food building blocks, nutrients, vitamins, and chemical reaction facilitators (cofactors).

Shrink down to the size of a molecular glass ship. In this glass ship take an imaginary trip through the digestive tube. The trip down the digestive tract from mouth to anus involves passage through multiple chambers. Each chamber concerns specific digestive process that needs to occur before movement to the next chamber becomes appropriate. These processes occur all along a healthy digestive tube.

The digestion that follows each meal is an orderly and precise process as it dismantles the food consumed into the building block molecular components. Next, these molecular components are absorbed at specific sites along the tube. Once these different molecular replacement parts are absorbed, they eventually are secreted into the blood stream. There they are distributed to different body cells and reassembled into new temple components or burned as fuel. Disease and old age results when the supply of these necessary replacement molecular parts becomes scarce.

Only when there are adequate molecular supply lines, adequate workforce, optimal workforce environment, integrated communication with the salvage ability team and sufficient enzymatic machines will there be sufficient cellular rejuvenation. This leads to new cellular structural repairs, new transport vehicles, new cellular factories, new informational substances, and adequate cellular trash removal.

Without adequate cellular rejuvenation all the cells are forced to make due with old cellular machines (enzymes). There is an accumulation in cellular trash. The cellular factory components are aged. An increased amount of degraded molecular parts that are forced to work long after their useful life spans is the end result.

The Task at Hand for the Digestive Tube

The accomplishments of a healthy system after a meal is best understood when the different components of that meal are isolated. These isolated components need to be discussed in regards to their unique contribution and their particular dilemma before body assimilation occurs. Once these basics are reviewed, a trip down the tube in the glass ship is in order.

How to Dismantle Carbohydrates

Carbohydrates break down into sugar and are the quickest food group to be absorbed. There is almost 100% absorption of sugar within a healthy owners digestive tract. Fat is the slowest and protein is only absorbed a little quicker than fat. Carbohydrate meals are followed by hunger because this fuel type is removed quickly from the digestive tube. An empty digestive tube leads to a strong desire to eat. Carbohydrate intake obligates the insulin hormone to be released. Insulin is necessary to process elevated blood sugar that results from carbohydrate intake. As insulin increases, there are grave consequences in the stimulation of eating behavior.

Eating behavior is stimulated when unnecessary carbohydrate intake occurs. This intake increases the insulin level beyond the nutritional needs of the body creating a vicious cycle between the insulin-induced obsession for food and the consumption of carbohydrates. As insulin levels rise, weight gain occurs. Insulin is the most powerful of all growth factors for fat. The failure to counsel trapped owners about this fact leads to unnecessary suffering in the western world today.

Carbohydrates, whether complex (bread, potatoes, pasta, or grains) or simple (fruit, sugar, corn syrup, honey), break down into one or more of the simple sugars (glucose, fructose or galactose). Intestinal absorption of sugar is independent of insulin level.

Insulin is needed only after the intestines absorb sugar and dump it into the blood stream. The amount of insulin needed becomes proportional to the sugar load absorbed. The other food groups, protein and fat, need very little insulin for cellular uptake of these fuel types. When enough insulin releases into the portal vein then the blood sugar returns to normal levels. The exception occurs with insulin resistance (liver chapter).

The insulin resistance problem compounds when carbohydrate consumption takes place without potassium. Processed food diets contain less potassium relative to carbohydrate consumption. Real food diets (natural and un-adulterated foods) will contain high potassium relative to carbohydrate content. When owners pay attention to this, tolerance for carbohydrates increases. When potassium is present less insulin is needed for the amount of carbohydrates. Potassium is crucial to take sugar out of the blood stream. Only real food contains sufficient potassium with carbohydrate. Processing food removes potassium (mineral table, Section 1)

Ignoring this simple fact about potassium-depleted foods will eventually cause insulin resistance. Insulin resistance means that more insulin needs to be secreted for the carbohydrate load in order to return the blood sugar to normal. The blood sugar returns to normal with less insulin with the availability of potassium. One potassium molecule is needed to move one sugar molecule out of the blood stream.

Potassium deficiencies are a big component of health issues that begin in middle age. The degenerative processes that begin with potassium deficiencies in middle age often cause obesity, abnormal cholesterol profile, decreased steroid tone, high blood pressure, nervous irritability, diabetes, and decreased energy levels. Middle age disease can sometimes be avoided when the digestive relationship between potassium intake and carbohydrate intake is realized.

How to Dismantle a Protein

There are 20 different amino acids that occur as building blocks for numerous proteins. The types, amounts, and order of amino acids confer unique properties on each of these proteins. These properties can be structural in nature (hair, connective tissue or surface dead skin layers), transport (carrier proteins for cholesterol, the sex hormones, fat, oxygen, and carbon dioxide in the bloodstream), or enzymatic machinery (Krebs cycle enzymes in the mitochondria that allow orderly, controlled combustion of fuel groups in the presence of molecular oxygen). Some proteins can be one category of an informational substance class (insulin, IGF-1, glucagon, etc. in group 2 of the hierarchy of hormones).

Each individual amino acid is unique in shape and electrical charge. Some are further endowed with additional sulfur or extra nitrogen atoms that confer important properties and abilities. For example, sulfur contained on methionine is the carrier of the methyl group donor system. Another example of special properties of individual amino acids occurs with the amino acid glutamine. Glutamine can donate its extra nitrogen group in the formation of amino acids from sugar. The various amino acids have different atomic make-up. Some behave like oil in water (hydrophobic), while others mix in water (hydrophilic).

The body can manufacture twelve of the twenty different amino acids that comprise the building blocks of all body protein. The eight amino acids the body cannot manufacture are called essential amino acids. Only one food source contains all eight essential amino acids, the egg. The egg is the only complete protein source. Nutritionists designate the egg as having a biological value of 1.00. All other protein sources (meat, beans, rice, chicken, fish, and nuts) have a fraction of this completeness of essential amino acids.

Each protein type is made up of various amounts and sequences (the chain) of twenty different amino acids. There is no nutritional value, for building block purposes, when the digestive tract fails to precisely dismantle protein molecules. This precision is a prerequisite for obtaining the continuous supply of amino acids needed for ongoing rejuvenation projects.

There are additional concerns if consumed proteins are only partially digested (fragments that contain three or more amino acids). The absorption of amino acid sequences three or more long has the potential to activate the immune system. This is the basis for starting food allergies in infants fed foreign proteins before their digestive tracts are developed. When the digestive tracts are not ready to digest protein completely, they will leak the partially digested protein fragments into the blood stream. Once these protein fragments are floating in the blood stream they will activate the immune system of an infant. When the immune system is activated an allergic response is possible. The immune system sees that same sequence from the ingestion of food and reacts on those proteins.

Partial digestion and absorption of protein fragments can be a powerful immune system activator resulting in autoimmunity. Autoimmunity means that the body's own immune system attacks its structure. One cause of autoimmune disease occurs when certain processes injure the integrity of the tube of the digestive system. When the tube integrity becomes compromised it will leak undigested fragments that normally do not penetrate until they are completely broken down. Examples of these diseases are rheumatoid arthritis, systemic lupus erythematosus, and some thyroid diseases. Some clinicians call this 'leaky gut syndrome'.

Normally, the digestion process disassembles larger molecules that would activate the immune system. The immune system is programmed to activate against foreign sequences of protein. Foreign proteins are found on viruses, bacteria, fungus, and partially digested proteins in food. The body circumvents protein meals containing foreign protein amino acid sequences by dismantling these proteins into their constituent amino acids. Individual amino acids are too small to activate the immune system. These small building block molecular parts, (amino acids) are transported in the blood stream where they are taken into different cells. Once inside the cells, the individual amino acids are recruited to synthesize new proteins. Once inside the cells, these amino acid molecular parts are used to create complex structures without the immune systems activation in the blood stream.

A Component of Old Age Results from Old Proteins

Old age or chronic disease occurs when the integrity of the individual proteins begin to breakdown. It helps to think of the animals that make up the imaginary chain. As they become deformed, acquire worn down edges, or attach to debris, they become less functional. The diminished ability to replace proteins as they break down and wear out defines a crucial process of aging. Poor nutritional absorption, that results from the lack of efficiency in the digestive tract or misguided protein choices, cause decline in protein dependent cellular rejuvenation.

The face of someone who is old and decrepit is the result, in part, of the lost protein integrity. At the molecular level this is nothing more than damaged individual amino acids, which alter the overall affected protein structure and function. The functions of protein encompass their role in cellular support. Support functions are compromised when the underlying protein shape becomes deranged. Deranged proteins have a diminished ability to perform other functions like work and trash removal. These old faces, at a molecular level, have accumulated cellular garbage, poor informational substance message content, decreased cellular electrical charge, and accumulated cell rust.

All owners will head this way more quickly without proper nutrition motivation. Better daily nutrition choices that impact cell regeneration and healing is a place to start. Optimal digestive juices and operative digestive structures are integral parts of healing.

Surprises About Where Protein Comes From

Approximately 50% of digested protein comes from meal content; 25% from proteins within the digestive juices that digest themselves after they perform their roles; and 25% comes from sloughed cells that line the intestinal tube that are also digested. The intestinal tube lining cells have a life span of only 3-5 days. They are sloughed into the tube and are degraded by digestive juices into their original building blocks and then these molecular parts are recycled into cell rejuvenation programs. The individual amino acids are interchangeable molecular building parts. As long as a building block (amino acid, fatty acid, vitamin or cofactor) is chemically intact it is free to be used or recycled into any cell synthesis or rejuvenation project.

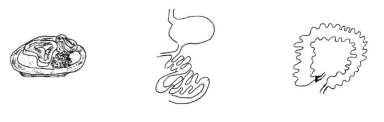

50% meals   **25% intestines**   **25% colon**

The ability of an amino acid to interchange is terminated when its structure is damaged. Replacement of a molecular part only becomes necessary once wear and tear weakens function. In healthy owners, cells constantly dismantle damaged proteins and efficiently replace them with new proteins.

Healthy bodies have adequate ability to supply the needed molecular replacement parts. Adequate replacement parts facilitate efficient cellular trash removal systems and adequate informational substance content. Fat is another molecular building part that the body requires for structural integrity.

Some Facts About Fat and the Reasons They Have Been Kept a Secret.

Four important roles of fat (lipids):

    1.   Cell structure and water retention (simple fats and cholesterol)
    2.   Hormone precursors
    3.   Fuel
    4.   Brain fats keep nerve cells happy

Lipids (fats), fatty acids, triglycerides, and cholesterol make up the basic structural fats of the body. These building parts are often used as a covering for trillions of cell membranes. These occur as part of the cell covering structure (plasma membrane) and organelles (cell factories). These structural fats are integrated between varying combinations of interspersed proteins. These membranes are composed of both the simple structural fats and the more complex, specialized structural fats. Lipids with extra molecular parts like phosphate or choline are in the complex group. Ultra-specialized fats have additional properties in body function by their role in specialized cells and organelles.

Beautiful skin demonstrates the importance of structural fat. It polishes the surface and prevents shriveling by retaining water. Prevention of cellular water loss is a major function of fat. Inadequate fat content, in type or amount, causes or accelerates water loss. Shriveling and cellular inefficiency occur when water content decreases. Second, certain lipids (fats) behave as informational substances. These can be thought of as hormonal fats and are derived from the essential fatty acids. The body cannot produce essential fatty acids. They must be acquired through dietary sources and absorbed by the digestive tract.

Essential fatty acids can be transformed into message carriers (hormones). Hormones have their own message content contained in hormonal fats that promote information exchange between neighboring cells. These messengers are the ecosanoids classified as the level four informational substances (section two). Availability of essential fatty acids plays a role in the prevention of heart disease, arthritis, and inappropriate immune activation.[13]

Ecosanoids are in three groups: prostaglandins, leukotrienes, and lipoxins. All of these ecosanoids are derived from arachidonic acid, linoleic acid, or linolenic acid. The three fatty acids are the only known essential fatty acids. Dietary choices and the higher level hormones circulating in the body determine what type of essential fatty acid eventually develop in cells. Consuming good fat leads to prevention of inflamamation, prevention of heart disease, and optimization of the immune system types of message content.

To have good message content, there needs to be the right higher hormones (section 2). When level two hormones are good, there will be direction for proper precursor hormonal fat to be manufactured from the dietary derived essential fatty acids.

Some owners consume diets that lead to the promotion of heart disease, inappropriate activation of the immune system, and inflammation producing fatty acids (informational substance precursors). These disease exacerbating hormonal fat precursors are produced on cell surfaces when insulin predominates. When precursor hormonal fatty acids are made from disease promoting types of fatty acids, some body processes will activate inappropriate message content. These messages are inappropriate because they promote diseases (immune and heart chapters).

The third role of fat in the body is to serve as fuel. Per gram of weight, fat provides triple the energy content of protein, and double the energy content of carbohydrates. Only optimal hormone message content permits accessibility of this excellent fuel source to the cells for caloric needs. This is largely determined by which hormones dominate the message content. If the wrong hormones dominate message content, the fat cell content is off limits as fuel. This condition, and all the complications to other body systems, traps the body in obesity (section two).

The fourth role of fat concerns the electrical circuitry of the central nervous system. These electrical insulator types of fats possess unique types of components that provide for maintenance of proper nerve conduction and health. The human brain has more fat weight than nerve cell weight illustrating this point.

Plant Leaves Provide the First Clue that Lipids are Cool

The ordinary plant leaf demonstrates the water conservation role of fat in the cells. The leaf endures hours of hot sunshine without crinkling or wilting under normal conditions. Leaves possess the right amount of molecular surface structure to retard moisture loss. The leaves are rich in lipid-derived wax. Wax is just slightly modified fat. The fat that lines the surface of the cells provides similar water conservation properties in the skin cells. Oils float on the surface of water and provide a vapor barrier against water loss.

The lipid lining of the cells serves to keep cells from shriveling up. A shriveled group of skin cells manifest to the naked eye as wrinkles. Inadequate cell membrane lipid in types and amounts provides one mechanism that leads to wrinkled cells.

The faces of owners who adhere to a low fat diet acquire deep creases between the inferior lateral margins of the nose extending downward towards the edge of the mouth. Later, more wrinkles crease these faces. Inadequate fat content accelerates water loss causing changes.

'Dietary Fat is Bad' - Misinformation Campaign is Successful

Lipid (fat) has been given a bad name by the medical industrial establishment. For many years, people have fallen victim to disjointed information. This happens when the dogma for sale and dispensed by the sanctioned scientific literature is sensationalism.

Availability of information has a profound influence on the practice patterns of medical practitioners today. Some have encountered the medical opinions of authorities like, Bernstein, Atkins, Schwarzbein, and others. Their unique viewpoints led to a curiosity about what scientific knowledge had been ignored. Scientific knowledge is often ignored in a profit driven health care system because it is less profitable.

There is a big difference between 'diet derived fat' versus 'liver synthesized fat'. Owners who acquire fat from too much diet derived healthy types of fat have a lower health risk than owners who absorb fat from liver manufactured sources. Fifty years ago, medical research documented that liver manufactured fat was solid (hard) compared to many dietary sources of fat.

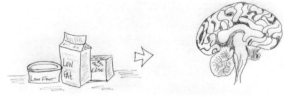

The liver will only manufacture fat if it is given the informational message to do so. The hormone that directs the liver to make carbohydrates into fat is insulin. Insulin can be thought of as the body's fuel nozzle and hose. When the nozzle is correctly inserted, the food groups can be taken up into the cellular fuel tanks. When all the cellular fuel tanks are full (this occurs in the well-fed, sedentary state) insulin directs the liver to manufacture fat from diet-derived carbohydrates. Insulin directs the liver to manufacture carbohydrates into fat only when it is spilling backwards into the blood stream. Carbohydrates spill backward into the blood stream when the cell fuel tanks are full. The higher the carbohydrate consumption, the more insulin needed to process the sugar load. The higher the insulin level, the more message content is directed at the liver to make carbohydrates into fat (triglycerides).

The higher the insulin contents in the bloodstream, the higher the 'volume' direction at the appetite center of the brain. The volume control of the appetite center is the amount of insulin message content that will stimulate the next feeding urge.

The higher the insulin content, the more "locks" that will be placed on access to fat cells for energy mobilization. The overall message content of insulin with in the body is concerned with the storage of fuels. The body can store fuel as fat or to a limited extent as glycogen. The amount of body fat possible is limited by the amount of insulin that the pancreas can produce. The greater the pancreas production rate of insulin, the more weight gain tendency when there is dietary indiscretion.

Good Reasons to Fear the Insulin Directed Manufacture of Fat

When insulin directs the liver to manufacture fat, it is called LDL cholesterol (the bad cholesterol). This type of cholesterol does damage by accumulating in the blood vessels. LDL cholesterol accumulates in the macrophages that line the arteries. The higher the manufacture rates of LDL cholesterol, then the more likely the accumulation of this type of fat and cholesterol within the arteries. This becomes a likely process in those owners who tend toward high blood insulin levels. These owners eat high carbohydrate diets or are stressed. Understand this is important if health is to be maintained.

Macrophage collection of LDL cholesterol problems can show up in laboratory tests as increased LDL cholesterol and/or elevated triglyceride level. This text will refer to LDL. In the next few subsections it will be explained why the macrophage cells, being stuffed full of LDL cholesterol, are a problem for blood vessels.

Macrophages Stuff Themselves on LDL Cholesterol

There are some owners who have a rapid exit rate of LDL cholesterol out of the blood stream, due to the size of their drains and into their fat cells. Their blood fats (LDL cholesterol) stay down even when they eat insulin-producing foods. Not all owners are insulin sensitive. Owners who can eat carbohydrates without retaining fat in the belly area (spare tire of middle age) demonstrate this. There are other owners who indulge in high carbohydrate diets. They have a genetically larger drain (fat cells) once LDL cholesterol is dumped from the liver into the blood stream. These owners will become fat, but their abdominal fat cells are so proficient at the removal of liver manufactured fat that the serum levels of LDL cholesterol stay normal.

Most owners are insulin sensitive and will follow the increased insulin message into two health problem areas. For most owners health problems occur in the form of progressive obesity and additional elevation of LDL cholesterol and triglycerides in the blood stream. An elevation of the LDL cholesterol and triglyceride collects in the macrophages that line the blood vessels. These owners do not have a sufficient sized 'drain' off in their fat cells. The drain is the exit rate of LDL out of the blood stream by fat cells compared to the rate of liver output of LDL production. Owners who are deficient in vitamin A and thyroid will have a slow down in the removal of blood fat.

In a certain proportion of these insulin sensitive owners, the chronic increased carbohydrate load, sedentary lifestyle, and their body size, combine to exhaust the ability of the pancreas to make enough insulin. At this point, the blood sugar starts to rise. Scientists call this situation adult onset diabetes (90% of all diabetic victims). Some manage to output all the insulin that is needed to keep their blood sugars normal. Both of these groups go on to develop heart disease and are unaware that high insulin levels fuel the problem (liver chapter).

Why the Body Needs Cholesterol Supplied Through the Diet

Cholesterol is just a type of fat. Each type of cell requires a certain amount of cholesterol for structural integrity. Cholesterol content in a cell is meticulously regulated to prevent destructive cellular health consequences. Liver manufactured fat is always packaged with cholesterol before being dumped into the blood stream. Once the cells have absorbed the maximum load of cholesterol there becomes little metabolic opportunity for liver secreted cholesterol. The amount of cholesterol secreted by the liver increases with rising insulin levels.

The Big Difference Between Liver Manufactured Fat and Dietary Fat is a Secret

Fat is always packaged with varying amounts of cholesterol, but technically cholesterol is a modified fat molecule. Fat and cholesterol need to associate with protein in order to float in the blood stream. The variable that makes a fat available to the metabolically hungry cells concerns the construction of carrier proteins.

There is a distinction in the difference between carrier proteins occurring between the liver manufactured fat and fat from the diet. Diet derived fat has less potential to accumulate in blood vessel walls. The carrier protein of dietary fat contains a protein package that has less potential to plug up a vessel. Where fat originates is the crucial difference between transport packages. When fat-cholesterol-protein complexes originate in the digestive tract following a meal, the metabolically hungry cells easily absorb them. When insulin directs the liver to make cholesterol-fat-protein complexes, they are designed for storage and not immediate fuel needs.

The insulin message content is concerned with fuel storage in the body. The majority of fuel storage occurs as fat. Normal amounts of diet derived fat form complexes that are rapidly assimilated by the metabolically hungry cells (skeletal muscle, cardiac muscle, kidney, etc.). Liver manufactured fat is designed to form complexes that are not readily cleared from the blood stream except by fat and macrophage cells. Insulin directed fat-cholesterol-protein complexes are less able to serve as fuel. They are designed by the direction of insulin, the fuel storage hormone. The body is smart and consistent. The consistent message of insulin causes greater amounts of stored fuel (fat). The insulin directed fat-cholesterol-protein complexes are designed with fuel storage in mind.

The Unique Way Fat is Absorbed from the Diet Illuminates the Fallacy of the 'Fat is Bad Campaign'

A physiologic fact clarifies the lack of stickiness of diet-derived fat on vessel walls. Dietary fat and cholesterol are absorbed via the lymphatics, which is different from all other nutrients. This exposes lymph vessels to the highest vessel concentration of cholesterol and fat. Atherosclerosis of lymphatic vessels is unheard of. Hemodynamically, lymph fluid moves in a sluggish manner compared to blood. If there were anything sticky about diet derived fat, it would be more pronounced in the sluggish lymph vessels.

There is a difference between the type of cholesterol-fat package that blood vessel walls are exposed to, and the cholesterol-fat-package that are in lymphatic vessels following a fatty meal. This difference explains the true cause for the majority of heart disease. The insulin directed liver manufactured cholesterol-fat packages coat blood vessel walls in the macrophages. Lymphatic vessels are not exposed to insulin manufactured cholesterol-fat packages. They are only exposed to diet derived cholesterol-fat packages that are not deposited along lymph vessel walls.

Even though lymph vessels are sluggish in flow characteristics and exposed to very high levels of diet-derived fat, they do not plug up. Anatomically the small intestine delivers fat and cholesterol following a meal via the lymphatics. The protective factor for lymphatic vessels involves the fact that they have no exposure to liver manufactured cholesterol-fat-protein complexes (LDL). Intestinal lymphatic vessels drain eventually into the left neck area, the thoracic duct. In this location the fatty parts of digestion are dumped into the blood stream.

In contrast, the other products of digestion such as protein, carbohydrates, minerals, and vitamins, etc., are dumped directly from the intestinal cells into the blood stream via the portal vein. The portal vein collects all blood and nutrition (except fat and cholesterol) from the digestive tract and takes it straight to the liver.

The blood vessels clog up whenever insulin levels rise to the point of directing excessive manufacture of the sticky type of cholesterol-fat packages or LDL cholesterol. This is sticky because it is taken up by the macrophages that line blood vessels. Macrophages are immune system scavenger cells that under well-fed circumstances bed down on blood vessel linings and stuff themselves with LDL cholesterol.

When liver derived fat-protein-cholesterol complexes (LDL cholesterol) are created beyond a healthful rate, they incorporate into macrophages in excessive amounts. Excessively stuffed macrophages with LDL cholesterol grow and grow. Year after year they continue to accumulate LDL cholesterol and eventually form giant cells called foam cells. Foam cells are the earliest lesions recognized by scientists as the beginning of heart disease.

Some of the places that macrophages bed down and become foam cells are in coronary arteries, hearing apparatus, kidney vessels, peripheral leg vessels, and retina. These tissues prefer fat for fuel. The LDL cholesterol accumulation trouble compounds in a sedentary owner.

High insulin levels in sedentary owners allow LDL cholesterol to collect in the macrophages continuously. These cells permit fat to collect due to lack of exercise. After many years, this vicious cycle allows fatty streaks to grow enough to block blood flow. Blood flow can suddenly worsen in these narrowed areas when other factors promote blood clot formation. When severe enough, the constriction causes cell death to cells that are down stream from the blockage.

The other common mechanism for the sudden loss of blood flow is vessel spasms in the narrow area. These two climaxes are the typical scenario for the number one killer of Americans past middle age. Earlier available information on this subject has been disjointed and fragmented.

High insulin producing bodies produce more fat. Insulin directed cholesterol-fat packages, which are designed for storage depots. These packages designed for the storage depots of the body are slow to drain off out of the blood stream. These individuals have an increased risk for heart disease when they are living sedentary lifestyles, have unmanaged stress (section two) and/or consuming high insulin promoting diets. All three of these risk factors increase insulin levels. Increased risk arises from increased tendency for macrophages to ingest more LDL cholesterol than is healthy.

The relationship between high insulin levels and sedentary lifestyles is the crux of the problem for over ninety percent of all heart disease victims. The other risk factors for heart disease development accelerate the primary disease producing mechanism in the blood vessels. Rather than focus on the hopeless mantra about some owners genetics, empowerment comes from focusing on how dietary and lifestyle changes prevent the problem.

Some owners have a greater tendency for heart disease based on primitive survival strategies. A survival advantage was obtained in prehistoric times when a body could store fat in times of plenty in order to survive periods of famine. Owners that made more insulin had a survival advantage. The food supply was never predictable so there was no accumulation of blood vessel fat.

The modern day food supply is uninterrupted to these same survival equipped insulin producing machines. Add to this the greatly increased insulin requirement that is necessary to handle a chronic ingestion of processed food that is secondary to diminished potassium content. These same owners are now fat producing machines.

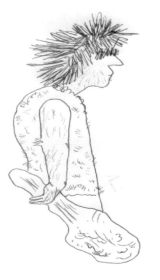

An owner still has the ability to turn off his fat making machine. This fat making machine in the liver, turns off by consistently choosing a low insulin diet, doing aerobic exercise, and stress management (sections one and two). Instead of helping owners understand this, they are sold on what is for sale by the complex.

Unfortunately for the average owner there is little incentive by the complex, to share (publish and sensationalize) this basic scientific understanding. The 'fat is bad campaign' is largely hype that allows the relationship between insulin and blood vessel disease to remain a secret. Knowledge about the insulin secret jeopardizes the more lucrative approaches for treatment of blood vessel disease.

The Weak Spot in the Campaign of the Complex Against Dietary Fat

The 'fat is bad' media campaign has a weak spot. Simply monitoring the cholesterol profile while on a high good fat/protein and low carbohydrate diet exposes the weak spot. This dietary approach is in direct contrast to the official campaign against fat, and in favor of a high carbohydrate diet.

The owners who try a high protein/fat and low carbohydrate diet for three months or more (while they defer judgment) will likely see several improved health benefits. At the end of this time period, each owner should assess the improved mental clarity that occurs because there is less 'brain fog'. Hypoglycemia induced by high carbohydrate diets has stopped. They will also notice a decreased appetite due to the fall of insulin levels. There is less brain appetite center stimulation for the next feeding event. There will be consistent weight loss because of lowered insulin levels that free the 'locks' on the bodys access to fat stores. Finally, there is a dramatic improvement in the cholesterol profile due to less insulin message content instructing the liver to make carbohydrates into LDL cholesterol.

Insulin excess is the cause of most cholesterol problems and the development of clogged blood vessels. Chronic increase in stress also raises insulin levels. Other hormone imbalances increase abnormal fats and other risk factors for vessel disease (section one, two, and the liver chapter). The imbalance between potassium and sodium increases the need for insulin. Increased insulin is required for large amounts of carbohydrate in the diet.

Attention to thyroid function, adequate androgen output from the adrenals and gonads (testis or ovary), optimal cortisol output, and IGF levels are important for normal fat parameters. Aerobic exercise should be optimized enough for muscles, skeleton, and cardiovascular system to be utilized to full capacity. When these are attended to, this contrary diet will put the owner on the path of longevity.

The high protein/good fat and low carbohydrate diet becomes less controversial when reviewing the epidemiological studies that have noted the absence of heart disease in cultures that consume a low carbohydrate, but high fat/protein diet. Eskimos exemplify this fact. Eskimos also exemplify the relative safety of obesity acquired through over indulgence in fat intake. Many Eskimos are obese because of the arctic climate. The type of fat Eskimos make is opposite to liver manufactured fat that arises from a high carbohydrate diet. When these same Eskimo people begin to adhere to a high carbohydrate diet, after about 20 years, they develop heart disease at rates similar to their western contemporaries.[14]

This correlates with the absence of heart disease in America until around 1900. Up until this time, the general population survived on a high fat and protein diet (chicken, meat, eggs, and beans). The carbohydrates that were available were unprocessed containing high potassium content. When the potassium content is high, the need for insulin diminishes. After the turn of the century, as processed sugar and cereals became available, the twenty year rule began to tick. This epidemiological tool measures the time between a change in cultural behavior and a public health effect. By the 1920's heart disease had become an epidemic in America.

Chemically Reactive Fats in the Diet Causes Heart Disease

The consumption of unhealthy fats are not allowed in high fat diets if one wishes to be free of blood vessel disease. The people of the world that are free of heart disease, while they indulge in a high fat and low carbohydrate diet, are not the ones that consume high amounts of chemically reactive fats. Chemically reactive fats are partially hydrogenated vegetable fats. This distinction about good fat and bad fat is often overlooked and leads to confusion in the minds of clinicians as well as owners in regard to the safety of high fat diets. Diets made up of real fats are safe while diets made up of large quantities of chemically reactive fats are not. Chemically reactive fats contribute to oxidation (rust) in the blood vessels.

The chemically reactive fat groups are chemically altered polyunsaturated fats. The chemical process of hydrogenation has altered them. The hydrogenation process causes a twisting deformation that is an unnatural occurrence in real fats. Numerous baked goods, breads, snacks, and chips have altered fats added to them. The hydrogenation process is one example where altered fats add firmness to the product. These polyunsaturated fats are chemically altered and are more twisted when they stack together. Fats in the body need to be stacked together in the cellular membranes (the lipid bi-layer). The twisted configurations of chemically altered fat means they form awkward fat conglomerates (irregularities) that line the cell membrane.

All other cells in the interior blood vessel lining have a cell membrane made up of fat and interspersed with proteins. The polyunsaturated fats are also chemically reactive with many oxidizing agents that may be in the blood stream (aluminum, fluoride, oxygen radicals, carbon monoxide, ozone and other smog components, etc.). When these fats oxidize, they promote 'Velcro' formations on the inside wall of the blood vessel (chapter 1). This formation summons the macrophages to lay down a temporary patch job that sometimes is never repaired. When LDL cholesterol is high, these macrophages collect fat and grow into foam cells eventually.

Blood vessel health depends on the inner lining layer (the tiles) of blood vessel wall to compose themselves with chemically altered polyunsaturated fats (hydrogenated fats) or healthy fats. This is determined by diet content. Diets consisting of fast food fats, margarine, fried foods, baked goods, and commercial breads will add twisted fats to the lining layers of blood vessels. Diets containing real fats have surfaces in the blood vessel that are composed of less chemically reactive fats (real fat).

Picture two beautiful flowerbeds. In one, there are short stocky stems and in the other fragile, slender stems. The contrast between the two types of stems allows an analogy that elucidates the body fat composition type problem.

Short stocky stems are analogous to blood vessel friendly fats (olive oils, fish oils and canola oils). They are more durable. These fats are only possible when the owner makes good diet choices when consuming fats. Fragile long stems are analogous to chemically altered polyunsaturated fats (found in junk food, processed food, and fast food). They are more vulnerable to numerous oxidizing agents that are present in the blood stream.

Visualize a dog (oxidizing agent) that sequentially runs around in each type of flowerbed. The short stocky stems would endure less damage because of differences in structural characteristics between the two flowerbeds. The oxidative vulnerability in the blood vessels is analogous to what happens in the blood vessel lining cells when unhealthy fat is eaten. The vulnerability of blood vessel lining cells to trampling by the "dogs" being unleashed in the blood stream are determined by the composition of the "stems". In a dirty environment where air pollution, water pollution, and food contaminants prevail, the blood vessel lining cells are overexposed to oxidizing agents (rust producers). The rust producers are analogous to the dog running around in the flowerbed. Real fats versus altered fats are analogous to the durability of the stems in the flowerbed. The more chemically reactive (altered) the fats are, the more they create rust (Velcro formations). The more the lining cells in the blood vessels are composed of real fats, the more durable they are when confronting oxidizing agents.

This consideration gradates the relative risk of different types of dietary fat and their potential to produce disease. The amount of abdominal fat is a clinical marker for diet or lifestyle determined high insulin levels. Men who have a greater abdominal measurement than hip measurement evidence high insulin levels. Women who are greater than 80% in their waist compared to hip measurement evidence high insulin. Until insulin levels are optimal, by diet and lifestyle changes, health is in jeopardy. The higher the oxidant exposure load that operates on a daily basis, the more important it is to minimize consumption of the chemically reactive fats. Owners who are chronically exposed to air pollution, water impurities (fluoridation), and impurities in food will have an increased rate at which the chemically reactive fats oxidize. Chemically reactive fats oxidize when exposed to harmful pollutants. Improving dietary fat choices and avoiding environmental 'rust' producers benefit healing.

Liver Manufactured Fat Clogs Blood Vessels

It has been known for years that LDL cholesterol synthesis rates are controlled by the balance between the levels of insulin and glucagon. The insulin message tells the liver enzyme, HMG CoA reductase, to make sugar into cholesterol. Glucagon message instructs the liver to stop making cholesterol by inhibition of this same enzyme. Glucagon also stimulates the release of fuels into the blood stream. For this reason, healthy, active people with a higher glucagon level will have lower cholesterol levels.

Glucagons will not help people who are sedentary and obese. Glucagon stimulates the dumping of fuel into the blood stream from the liver. In chronically sedentary types, the extra fuel eventually stimulates the release of insulin. This effect is an example of the weight and counterweight system that keeps opposing hormones in balance. People who sit around all day, but eat the right diet initially promote the release of glucagon. They lose the benefits of glucagon when insulin needs to be secreted to manage the extra fuel glucagon directed to be made and secreted into the blood stream.

Extra insulin arises because sedentary owners have no need for increased fuel in the blood stream that glucagon directs. If owners on glucagon promoting diets were to exercise, they would use the extra fuel and need less insulin. Lower insulin relative to glucagon signifies the liver enzyme HMG CoA reductase will stay less active and less cholesterol is manufactured. When this happens, the serum cholesterol level decreases.

Owners have a choice about taking toxic medication to lower cholesterol. It is often unnecessary if they begin a program that tells the liver to work properly. Practices that raise glucagon and lower insulin keep cholesterol within the healthy range for the vast majority of owners. A high protein/good fat, low carbohydrate diet promotes the optimal ratio between insulin and glucagon. The proper balance of these two hormones is difficult for sedentary owners because of the need for increased insulin.

Additional Hormones that are Beyond the Diet, but Influence Digested Foods to Deposit Fat

Most owners who take active steps in daily exercise and dietary decisions (low carbohydrate diets) will notice a dramatic fall in blood cholesterol. The glucagon and insulin ratio have been favorably altered. Adequate message content from other body hormones such as androgen (from adrenals and gonads), estrogens, thyroid hormone, IGF, and cortisol are also important. When these are correctly proportioned blood fat-cholesterol-protein complexes will benefit.

These considerations can be assessed through a complete twenty-four hour urine test that includes a quantitative and qualitative analysis of what hormone levels are manufactured. Healthy owners have optimal amounts of critical steroid and thyroid hormones that are passed into their urine over a twenty-four hour period. Unhealthy owners pass sub-optimal amounts of critical androgen steroid hormones and possibly excessive amounts of stress steroids. If thyroid function is inadequate, the urine is often the most reliable way to detect the deficiency. These hormone considerations are sometimes important when lifestyle and dietary modification fail to improve the cholesterol profile.

The need to use a twenty-four hour urine collection illustrates what science has revealed versus what is practiced. Hormone levels can fluctuate widely in the blood stream. Some hormones have life spans measured in seconds. Most have life spans measured in minutes. When a blood sample is taken, the amount of hormone measured in that sample reflects the instant the venous sample was drawn. This is an accurate measurement only if the hormones are relatively stable in the blood stream. Most hormones vary widely throughout the day in the blood stream. The informational substances convey a programmed message to different targeted cells. Different activities of daily living obligate the release of different hormones that communicate to cells on how to spend energy.

An accurate method to assess hormone tone would incorporate the basic scientific understanding that over a typical twenty-four hours an average amount of hormone output will occur. Urine measurements are useful only when the hormone of interest exits the body via the kidney. This is true for thyroid and steroid hormones and includes the different breakdown derivatives of the different hormones. Urine that is collected in a typical day can measure the types and amounts of hormones present. This sophisticated approach toward an assessment of the hormone status is more appropriate.

Most of the larger hormones composed of amino acid sequences (peptides or proteins) do not pass in the urine. This class of hormones must be measured in the blood stream. Insulin, glucagon, IGF, and some of the larger pituitary and hypothalamic hormones are examples of this class. If a more accurate method for the assessment of hormone status exists, patients have the right to know about this option.

Many physicians are unaware that they are victims of an education that has removed some basic scientific understanding that conflict with profit. There have been numerous instances where a patient brings in a well-run twenty-four hour urine analysis only to be scoffed at by their conventionally trained, but limited second opinion physician. Owners are advised to have a little fun with these types of practitioners. Asking them to explain all the big words that describe the different breakdown products of certain hormones. A good physician at this point will admit that he doesn't understand the results and will look into it. Unfortunately, many physicians that are confronted with what they do not understand habitually resort to attempts to discredit approaches that inquire above their education level. When one confronts the later type of practitioner, it may be time to begin thinking about a new doctor.

Fluids and Electrolytes

Fluids and electrolytes are the water and minerals that make up the various body juices. Digestive juices contain enzymatic machines that are specific to the digestive chamber where food is present. The mineral component of juices and body processes that have an effect on the adequacy of digestive juices will be covered in this subsection.

Good health is possible when adequate juices are secreted and absorbed at the proper time during the digestive process. The digestive system requires the appropriate quality and quantity of digestive juices or degenerative processes to occur. These degenerative processes rob the body of vitality when the quality of mineral content contained in the digestive juices becomes deranged.

Each adult consumes about two quarts of fluid every day. In addition to this fluid intake, the digestive tube itself secretes an additional seven quarts into the meal contents. The digestive tube needs to secrete various digestive juices in order to assimilate the various molecular parts contained in one day's food intake. The total seven additional quarts of digestive juices secreted each day needs to be in properly proportioned amounts. These different digestive juices are secreted into the tube as various chemical combinations designed to dismantle different food types. In the end, the bowel movement contains less than 1 cup of water. A typical digestive tube encounters two and a half gallons of fluid every day. When the digestive tube is healthy it reabsorbs not only most of this fluid, but also usable molecular parts.

The Amount of Digestive Juices Secreted in the Tube

Daily ingested fluid: >2 quarts

Daily secreted juices into the digestive tube from various digestive lining cells:

(7 quarts) salivary glands	> 1.5 quarts
Stomach secretions	> 2.5 quarts
Gallbladder secretions	> 0.5 quarts
Pancreas secretions	> 1.5 quarts
Intestinal secretions	> 1.5 quarts

Total fluid load daily passed into the digestive tube is >9 quarts

Total reabsorbed fluids daily farther down the tube on average is 8.8 quarts or diarrhea manifest itself.

Jejunum	0.5 quarts reabsorbed
Ileum	2.0 quarts reabsorbed
Colon	1.3 quarts reabsorbed

The mineral content of the digestive juices and meal are important determinants of the ability of the body to reabsorb the fluid in the digestive tube before it arrives at the rectum. Diarrhea is the result of too much fluid. Constipation is the result of too little fluid reaching the rectum. Fiber and certain minerals keep water in the tube and promote a loose stool.

Certain minerals or substances pull water with them as they move down their concentration gradient. This process is called osmosis. Osmosis describes a way of predicting which direction water will move. Substances that pull water with them as they move into different body chambers are called osmotically active. These include the digestive tube, intestinal cells, kidney filtration system, etc. When these substances move from one body chamber to the next they pull water with them.

When healthy, the act of absorbing the molecular building parts contained in a meal pulls water back out of the digestive tube. Bowel movements of healthy owners do not contain excessive osmotically active material and therefore, little water is contained in the stool when it exit's the body. Deficiency or excess in osmotically active bowel contents leads to constipation and diarrhea respectively.

Indigestible fiber has a weak osmotic affect that allows sufficient water to stay in the bowel movement and facilitate regularity. Sources of indigestible fiber are vegetables, fruits, and psyllium husks. Some minerals are incompletely or poorly absorbed so they osmotically retain water. Salts of poorly absorbed osmotically active minerals or substances are the salts of magnesium, vitamin C, and some antacids. Part of the task of efficient digestion is to insure adequate mineral absorption. Minerals usually present to the digestive tract in the form of a salt. A salt signifies that positive and negatively charged minerals occur together. The positively charged mineral of the salt is more important and always named first. Examples of commonly ingested salts are ferrous sulfate, calcium citrate, magnesium oxide, potassium chloride, and sodium chloride. When a salt absorbs into the body from the digestive tract it will pull water with it. When a salt is not absorbed in the digestive tract it will retain water.

Calcium and iron are important minerals. The salt they are hooked to (the negative half) will determine how readily they absorb into the body.

Most owners are aware of the importance of obtaining adequate calcium and iron. Often times this opinion results from an effective media campaign. The more important a mineral is, the more potential it has to harm body tissues if the mineral isn't carefully regulated. Calcium and iron illustrate the importance of mineral control within the body tissues.

Calcium can Help or Kill Cells

Calcium intake requirements are on the mind of most owners. Calcium plays an important role in the maintenance of adequate bone mass. Many owners ingest some form of calcium salt on a daily basis. There has been very little attention given to taking too much calcium when certain factors exist. Calcium intake can accelerate the aging process.

Calcium is controlled and channeled in the tissues of the body by an elaborate regulatory system of hormones. Calcium content must be narrowly channeled. Therefore, an elaborate system of calcium regulatory hormones becomes necessary. Calcium can be better understood when one realizes that all cells operate as miniature batteries. Maintaining a concentration difference between calcium and magnesium charges the cells. Calcium is pumped outside the cell while magnesium is pumped inside the cell. Calcium is in high concentrations in the fluid around the cell because of this pumping around the membrane (a ratio of 12,000:1). Magnesium is maintained at a relatively high concentration inside the cell.

Adequate cellular energetics (adequate ATP formation) maintains this electrical gradient between these two opposing minerals. A similar gradient occurs between sodium outside the cell and potassium in the cell. Cells are constantly draining this gradient between these opposing minerals. The energy released is used for cell work. Energy released by the draining process is like any activated battery. In the case of cells, the energetic gradient is constantly drawn upon and used to live.   Simultaneously, the healthy cell constantly recharges the gradient difference by utilizing ATP from the cell power plants. ATP availability is used to recharge the membrane gradient between these opposing minerals.   Specific mineral pumps maintain the concentration differences of these minerals around the membrane. Mineral pumps are in the membrane and require ATP to power them. The higher the concentration differences between the opposing minerals, the higher the amount of energy available for the cells.

The differences in concentration between calcium and magnesium about a cell's membrane allow the performance of useful cellular work. The concentration gradient also prevents harmful ions from penetrating the cell and causing damage within. Healthy cells are able to generate large concentration gradients between calcium and magnesium and sodium and potassium. They achieve this concentration gradient by having highly functional mineral ion pumps in the membrane. These pumps exchange opposing minerals against their concentration gradient.

The large concentration difference between opposing minerals around the membrane creates electrical potential. The energy contained in the membrane is drawn off to perform cellular work. The same principle applies to any battery when it becomes the mechanism for donating energy to power a toy. Also, both types of batteries (the cell and the battery) have to have a way to recharge and prevent depletion.

All batteries, whether living or manufactured, need to keep their mineral content within carefully gated channels. When the channels are circumvented, battery corrosion results. Calcium needs to be channeled into and out of cells by carefully regulated channels. The cell performs work when calcium enters through specific channels. The pumping of calcium outside the cell and magnesium inside the cell requires ATP energy. Sufficient ATP allows the cell membrane to recharge as it depletes.

If calcium gets inside the cells inappropriately (outside the gated channels), it harms intracellular structures (molecular corrosion). Once inappropriate calcium gets inside a cell it is difficult to remove it. As owners age, inappropriate calcium sneaks in and chemically reacts with delicate intracellular structures. If enough calcium gets inside a cell, the mitochondria begin to sequester it. Eventually extra calcium causes the mitochondria to swell and weaken. Weakened mitochondria become less capable in their role as a power plant facility (ATP generation). Inappropriate entry of calcium into a cell irreversibly deactivates enzymes.

When calcium enters a cell through the appropriate channels (gate), it does not have a destructive effect on the cell. The movements of calcium, through these channels, down its concentration gradient releases electrical energy that the cells use to perform the work of living. Processes that accelerate inappropriate calcium accumulation in the cell accelerates aging. Calcium is elaborately contained by a complex interrelated group of hormones. These different hormones occur at diverse entrance and exit sites for calcium throughout the body. Situations that overwhelm or disrupt these regulators of channeling calcium safely through and in the tissues, can cause cellular harm.

Some of the calcium regulatory hormones and proteins are worth mentioning. Calcitonin hormone opposes parathyroid hormone. Androgen hormones oppose cortisol hormone. Active vitamin D hormone opposes inactive vitamin D. Blood albumin content opposes the freely dissolved blood calcium.

Sometimes it is useful to recall the weight scales with a weight and a counter weight. This is analogous to a hormone being secreted and there will always be a counter-regulatory hormone (counter weight). The counter weight hormone always attempts to balance the response. Hormonal imbalance leads to disease due to the breakdown in the balance between the opposing hormones. Loss of balance between the opposing hormones "tips the scale" out of the optimal equilibrium. The loss of hormonal balance within, tips energy usage into unbalanced pathways that lead to wear and tear. Wear and tear manifest in the tissue that is the recipient of this out of balance hormonal state.

Body tissue wear and tear all too often results from poor quality message content that, in turn, results from sub-optimal hormone mixtures. This leads to a disorganized cellular direction on how to spend energy wisely. The balance between the different opposing calcium controlling hormones determines where calcium is channeled. There needs to be a balance between regulatory and counter-regulatory calcium hormones or tissue injury is possible. Inappropriate calcium can enter a cell and injure the delicate intracellular contents.

Minerals Opposition Charges the Cell Battery

The body's system of chemical reactions sustains life. These reactions are powered by the concentration gradient between opposing minerals around the cell membrane. Certain opposing minerals create electrical membrane potential between these minerals. The cell membranes accomplish this difference in mineral concentration by specialized pumps located within the membrane. Each type of membrane pump is powered by the energy contained within the ATP molecule. ATP availability directly limits the ability of a cell to recharge its membrane. The better a cell recharges its membrane, the more energy available for cellular work.

One of the main caloric expenditures of the body involves energy used by these various mineral pumps. They are present throughout all cells in the body. This explains the large amounts of ATP necessary to charge the differential between these opposing minerals against their concentration gradient. The concentration buildup of these opposing minerals can be used in the performance of cellular work.

Magnesium, in high concentrations in the cell, is opposed by the high concentration of calcium outside the cell. This allows an electrical gradient that the cell can harness to function within that cell type. When a car battery discharges in the wiring of the electrical system of the car it powers many gadgets. The cell "battery" (the cell membrane) powers the activities of life. Constant energy is required to power the cell battery maintained by the gradient between calcium and magnesium (also between sodium and potassium). This is similar to a car battery that needs to be recharged while the auto burns fuel. The combustion of protein, fat, and sugar occurs only after processing into a common, combustible derivative called acetate. When acetate is exposed to oxygen within the power plant (the mitochondria) of the cell, the energy released is trapped as ATP. ATP can then be used to recharge the cell membrane by powering the mineral pumps. This describes the process that continually occurs throughout life in the trillions of cellular batteries contained within the body. Energy is contained in the membranes and is created by the concentration differences between the four minerals.

Healthy cells avoid unnecessary oxidation from inappropriate escape of un-channeled calcium inside the cell. Potential trouble always lurks inside the body if calcium is allowed to bind to in-dissolvable anions (the negatively charged half of any calcium salt). Calcium is always the positive part of any salt that it forms. Some salts of calcium prefer to stay in solid form and do not dissolve well in body fluids. Calcium salts outside of bone tissue are of the dissolvable variety in a healthy body. Even under the best of circumstances, cells are confronted with numerous potential precipitate formers (in-dissolvable salts). If not constantly flushed from body tissues they will form solid salts of calcium. Common examples are found in kidney stones, osteoarthritis, bone spurs, and calcium deposits in soft tissues and blood vessels.

Excessive dietary intake of phosphates and oxalates can lead to acceleration of these solid deposits in the tissues. An increase in free water consumption helps the body clear these substances. Soda pop (diet and regular) contains high amounts of phosphate. There is a price to pay for clearing it through the urine. Each phosphate molecule cleared from the blood stream requires an obligatory loss of one calcium molecule. Soda pop not only contains phosphate, but also lacks calcium. In order to remove excess phosphate, there needs to be calcium removed from somewhere else in the body. If it becomes chronic (as in the case of the habitual soda pop user) there is slow leaching of bone calcium to allow phosphate removal. This shows up clinically on x-ray as premature loss of bone mineral content. Mineral deficient bones are known as the disease osteoporosis.

Energetic situations that allow inappropriate calcium into the cell are also a concern. This becomes destructive to the more active cells metabolically (nerve, heart, kidney, etc.). Dr. Salpolsky from Stanford University has documented low blood sugar in the hippocampus.[15] Low blood sugar in the brain leads to low energy in these nerve cells. The 'force field' has diminished and a consequent massive influx of calcium can occur. This vulnerability stems from the brain cells and can only burn sugar for energy needs under most circumstance. Most other cells readily utilize protein and fat for fuel. This makes brain tissue much more vulnerable to low blood sugar. Low energy in a nerve cell, caused by low sugar availability in this situation, allows the massive influx of calcium. It is the massive influx of calcium that irreversibly harms intracellular contents. In these cases, calcium harms cells because the low energy content within the cell membrane allows it to penetrate the cell through inappropriate methods.

The vulnerability of cells in low energy states can be visualized by imagining the star ship Enterprise in an attempt to ward off the attack of missiles. The Enterprise does this by powering up its force field. This is similar to what any cell in the body constantly performs in order to keep out inappropriate ions like calcium. Every cell must power up energetically against the influx of calcium through inappropriate channels. Calcium is an intracellular missile. When it penetrates the cell outside of the appropriate channels (the membrane pumps), it forms solid complexes with cell components.

Other states of cellular energetic depletion occur in situations where the blood or oxygen supply is compromised (drowning or cardiac arrest) or if vulnerable tissue is excited beyond its energetic capacity to maintain adequate cellular membrane energy (seizure). All of these mechanisms injure cells because they allow the depletion of the cell membrane's electrical charge (the force field). When the force field is depleted, a massive influx of inappropriate calcium enters the cell. Excess levels of calcium react destructively with intracellular components.

Calcium's energetic opponent, magnesium, doesn't need the same strict regulatory control within the body. Magnesium doesn't seem to form solids in the tissues, but forms soluble complexes (those that dissolve in body fluids). This difference in behavior, between calcium's chemical reactive properties contrasted to magnesium's, helps explain why the presence of calcium becomes necessarily layered with hormonal protection systems and backup protection systems. Dietary factors can affect the availability of calcium within the body. Different body minerals, which include calcium, are necessary to power up the trillions of cell batteries. The cell batteries are used for the reactions of life and to defend the cell from outside the cell hostile ions. Calcium can be hostile when the body fails to properly regulate its presence.

Iron - Life Giver or Testicle Taker

Iron is a lot like calcium. The access of iron to various tissues must be precisely regulated by the digestive tract. Iron is carefully utilized within the hemoglobin molecules of red blood cells to carry molecular oxygen to the tissues. If the multifaceted protective mechanisms of the body fail to prevent excess iron in certain body cells, tissue is destroyed. Testicles are particularly vulnerable when iron control systems breakdown. Iron is heavily regulated toward balance in the healthy state.

Men lose about .6mg per day of iron and women lose about twice this amount during their menstrual cycle years. A body will carefully attempt to match iron absorption rates to loss rates in order to maintain iron balance.

Phytic acid, phosphates, and oxalates in the diet bind iron in the digestive tube into solid complexes. The excess presence of these types of substances can prevent adequate absorption of iron into the body tissues that need it.

Small amounts of trace minerals are needed. These include iron, zinc, manganese, cadmium, calcium, copper, and nickel. All of these trace minerals need adequate stomach acid to be absorbed. The intestinal power pump requires adequate acid to function. The creator designed a power pump in the stomach that exchanges the trace minerals for one acid proton ($H+$). It is the job of the power pump to maintain adequate trace mineral absorption. Acid deficiency can potentially compromise trace mineral absorption.

Adequate stomach acid also facilitates the less absorbable form of iron ($Fe+3$) to convert to a more absorbable form in the precence of vitamin C. Only when Fe 3+ is chemically reacted upon will it form the more absorbable form ($Fe+2$). It is only the Fe 2+ form of iron that carries oxygen when associated with hemoglobin in the red blood cells. Inadequate stomach acid causes vitamin C to be in its inactive form.

Adequate stomach acid allows iron absorption in the stomach-lining cell. Once iron is inside this cell, a protein, ferritin, designed with iron safety considerations carefully sequesters it. The gut lining cells have a lifespan of only 2-5 days. The body must decide whether it needs this iron or not. If the answer is negative, the iron sloughs off (when the cell dies) into the digestive tube where it is passed in the next bowel movement. This is the first body defense against iron overload that leads to tissue injury.

The next layer of body protection from iron is found in the transport protein, transferritin that orchestrates delivery into the various iron storage depots. If iron is allowed to accumulate to high levels, it is these storage depots that become injured first. The body protects itself from additional iron storage damage by increasing the transferred level in the blood stream. Transferritin levels are sometimes used to measure the risk of this storage problem. Common storage sites of tissue injury resulting from iron excess are pancreas damage, cirrhosis, hepatic cancer, and gonad injury. Iron overload also presents with a tanning effect that result from its deposits in the skin.

Common nutrient and minerals need to be present in the diet for the availability of adequate molecular parts. The common hormone influences on what happens to these raw foods and minerals, once they are absorbed into the body, was discussed. The following discussion centers around how the different digestive juices dismantle the molecular building parts themselves. The body constantly needs reusable molecular components for regeneration and fuel. When raw food is dismantled with precision, there will be reusable components available for absorption.

A Trip Down the Digestive Tube

With the completion of what is ideally contained in the diet, it is time for an imaginary trip down the digestive tube. Imagine shrinking down to the size of a single cholesterol molecule and hopping aboard an indigestible glass ship. The final destination will be the toilet bowel. The trip begins within a bite of food that contains proteins, carbohydrate, fats, vitamins, and minerals. A spinach and squash quiche would contain most of these.

The first thing most travelers notice would be the roughness of the ride beginning in the mouth. Swishing up and down with the salivary juices that are being secreted into this one bite of food. The juices are squirted out from various chambers of the digestive tube and contain precision food dismantling machines (enzymes). All of the digestive juices from each chamber are very

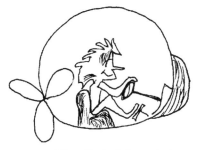

adept at disassembling the architectural framework of the different foods into building block components.

The mouth is the first digestive chemical reaction chamber. In the mouth are the salivary juices that contain enzymes. The salivary secreted digestive enzymes begin the dismantling of fat and carbohydrates contained in this bite of food.

The first juices being secreted in the mouth contain machines (enzymes) capable of breaking carbohydrates down into the simple sugars. There are additional enzyme machines that can dismantle fats into free fatty acids. The disassembly of carbohydrate is rapid. The rate of disassembling fats, by these first machines, is rather slow.

All human digestible carbohydrates break down into glucose, fructose, or galactose. Common examples of indigestible carbohydrates occurring in nature are wood and various plant fibers (lettuce). Simple sugars start to become available for absorption starting in the mouth.

In contrast, fat disassembly is a much slower digestive break down process. One fat molecule is called a triglyceride molecule. One triglyceride molecule is made from three fatty acid molecules joined together by a single glycerol molecule. The act of digestion frees three fatty acids and one glycerol per triglyceride molecule. These are dismantled in the process of digestion. Fat cannot be absorbed until it breaks down into these component parts.

Understanding What Fat is When It is Swallowed

The type of fat swallowed in the bite full of food is important. There are many different types of fatty acids found in nature. Different types of food break down into their own unique fatty acids. Before disassembling fat, the bite of food's fatty acid content has combined with glycerol. Each glycerol can connect to three fatty acids. It is the combination of three fatty acid types that always connect to one glycerol which makes each type of fat (triglyceride). The combination of the different types of fatty acids makes up the fat content type in a particular food. Some fatty acids are called essential because the body cannot manufacture them. These essential fatty acids have powerful effects on the way blood vessels respond to injury, tissue inflammation, and the immune system response to various stimuli. An imbalance of essential fatty acids could tip the scales towards disease (section five).

Fatty acids can be two carbons to twenty-four carbons long. Each carbon binds four times to the same or to different elements at a time. Each carbon atom is bound to something four times. If two of these bonds are used in binding twice to another carbon in the fatty acid chain, scientists call this an unsaturated fatty acid. If the double bond occurs only one time within a given fatty acid it is mono-unsaturated. If the double bond occurs more than one time in a fatty acid it is called polyunsaturated. The more unsaturated (the more times carbon binds twice to another carbon) the fatty acid, two things occur. First the fatty acid twists up in a bulky way. Visualize this as the difference in gathering wood for a campfire when it is all bent and twisted versus the straight sticks. The twisted sticks are cumbersome and awkward. They don't stack well like straight sticks do. Polyunsaturated fatty acids don't stack well.

Second, whenever a double bond occurs more than twice within a fatty acid, it confers a reactivity to rust promoters that may be in the blood stream. If the fatty acid is mono-saturated it reacts less readily to rust promoters than the poly-unsaturated varieties. Stability or reactivity of a bite of food is determined by the fatty acid content present.

Returning to the Voyage Down the Digestive Tube

Back in the glass ship, note that up to 30% of the fat and a slight majority of carbohydrates in this bite of food digests by the saliva containing digestive machines (enzymes). Farther down the tube, different digestive machines are unleashed from the pancreatic secretions that aggressively continue dismantling the remaining complex carbohydrates and fat molecules contained in this food.

Suddenly there is a violent lurch forward and the tiny glass ship moves into the esophagus, traveling at about four centimeters a second toward the stomach. Swallowing is coordinated so that when the food and salivary juices reach the upper stomach valve it is open and permits smooth passage to the acid bath chamber.

Acid Bath Chamber

The stomach is the second digestive chemical reaction chamber. In a healthy stomach miracles occur. There are special cells deep within tunnel like pits that open into the inside of the stomach. These special cells that line the numerous tunnels that exit on the stomach surface are called parietal cells. It is the parietal cells job to make and secrete stomach acid. There is a very good reason these cells lay hidden beneath the inner surface of the stomach underneath the further protection of stomach mucus. The acid these cells secrete is so powerful that it would digest the acid producing cells. Looking out of the glass ship in the stomach chamber, one would see that beneath the mucus layer there are numerous small pits that are poke-a-doted all along the middle area stomach lining. From these pits, acid juices would be flowing out from their source deep below.

There is a second type of cell, chief cells, which occur deep down inside these tunnels. These tunnels also open on the inner stomach surface. The chief cells specialize in the production of one model of protein disassembly machine. The originally secreted version of this enzyme machine for protein disassembly, pepsinogen, is inactive until its 'wrapper' gets pulled off, whereupon they call it pepsin. The wrapper is composed of an amino acid chain that conceals the active part of the protein disassembly machine. To pull the wrapper off of pepsinogen requires adequate acid be present or inactive factory product ends up lying around in the stomach doing nothing.

Adequate acid also is necessary to provide working conditions that this model of protein dismantler requires. Further down the tube the enzymatic machines require the opposite working conditions. These enzyme machines need basic pH (alkaline) to activate. As soon as the food leaves the stomach there must be adequate alkaline juices flowing out of the pancreas or next group of digestive machines will not activate. Different digestive chambers require different pH balance to activate the enzyme machines pertinent to that chamber. Some owners get into trouble because they have not been counseled on ensuring the proper pH balance for the chamber activities in question. In the stomach the pH needs to be sufficiently acid or the digestive enzyme machines will not activate.

Adequate stomach acid also protects owners from the passage of intact bacteria, viruses, fungi, and various digestible protein toxins. It also protects because acid is destructive to these potential invaders. Some toxins are not adequately digested within the digestive tract. Inadequate digestion (disassembly of foreign toxins) can lead to food poisoning. Acid is an important first line defense against opportunistic pathogens. These are pathogens that wait for the chance to enter a body. Very few microorganisms can survive the acid bath in the stomach. This sterilizes the contents entering the small intestine under normal circumstances. If a microorganism makes it into the small intestine, there are many noxious surprises to contend with. It is the job of the stomach to make enough acid.

Acid is needed for three things. First, acid destroys pathogens. Second, acid signals the stomach-esophagus valve to close tightly preventing heartburn. Third, acid is necessary in sufficient amounts to stimulate the pancreas when the food exits the stomach. Only when the pancreas receives adequate acid stimulus will it vigorously release alkali and other powerful digestive machines that the pancreas manufactures.

Various informational substances (hormones) are secreted into the blood stream and into the digestive tube at specific sites as food travels toward the rectum. The stomach chamber is the first digestive chamber where hormones play a role in the strength of secretions. The message content of the hormone, gastrin, stimulates histamine. Histamine stimulates acid release. In a healthy stomach, the informational content released coordinates efficient dismantling and absorption of nutrients in a meal by the acid and enzyme secretion.

A cornerstone principle for healthy digestion is the ability to secrete adequate stomach acid. Paradoxically, many owners suffer from heartburn symptoms because they have a deficiency in their stomach to manufacture acid.

The minority of heartburn patients makes too much acid. In these cases, their stomach problems become amenable to the expensive acid suppressors available. Many patients are incorrectly diagnosed with acid over production when the real problem causing the heartburn results from acid under production. Weak acid accessing the esophagus can still burn a hole and cause painful irritations. Acid does not belong in this anatomical area. Suppressing weak acid output damages other digestive processes.[16]

The stimulus for the stomach-esophagus valve to shut tightly is the presence of adequate acid in the stomach contents. Without adequate acid to stimulate the tight closure of this valve, heartburn symptoms occurs when a patient lays down with a full stomach. Physicians denote this condition as gastro-esophageal-reflux disease (GERD). The mechanism involving under production of acid with consequent reflux backward through an incompetent stomach valve occurs in many heartburn sufferers. There are a few patients who have incompetent stomach valves for other reasons (hiatal hernia).

Another consequence of inadequate stomach acid secretion concerns the diminished pancreas stimulus to secrete juices. The pancreas needs adequate acid to stimulate release of digestive and acid neutralizing juices. Without an adequate pancreatic stimulus, further protein and fat dismantling and absorption is compromised. This becomes clinically noted as patients who habitually avoid high protein meals because of the digestive difficulties that follow.

Acid deficient output diminishes digestion and absorption of critical minerals. Calcium, magnesium, iron, copper, zinc, and nickel all require acid in order for the operation of the 'one for one' exchange pump. The mineral exchange pump in the stomach is responsible for the absorption of trace minerals. These types of mineral absorption pumps need acid (H+) to exchange for each trace mineral absorbed.

Finally, adequate acid production is a powerful protection from the dirty outside world of microorganisms seeking access to the internal anatomy.

There are powerful alternatives available to the standard prescriptions used to suppress acid production in the treatment of heartburn. Healing involves soothing the inflamed tissue (esophagus, stomach, or duodenum). In the cases of stomach inflammation, there is likely diminished mucus production. Mucus production depends on the presence of high quality hormonal fats (essential fatty acid derived). The non-steroidal anti-inflammatory medication like aspirin poisons the hormonal fats. This causes a decrease in mucus production and an increase in stomach irritation.

Certain plants possess the ability to calm and soothe irritated digestive tissues by creating mucus. They are not commonly acknowledged because they are affordable and effective. Licorice root is very effective in soothing inflamed gastrointestinal tissues. Unprocessed licorice root can raise blood pressure by prolonging the influence of fluid retaining hormones made by the adrenals. This fraction of licorice root needs removal. This process is known as deglycerrhization. Enzymatic Therapy Co. makes an excellent product of this root in a powdered form. If an owner takes this processed powdered form when the next attack occurs, relief will be minutes away. The heartburn relief will occur without altering the gastrointestinal physiology. Licorice root powder creates a thick mucus when mixed and swallowed with small amounts of water. Licorice-mucus is similar to the protective mucus made naturally by the stomach and protects against digestive acids. Unlike acid suppression pharmaceuticals, deglycerrhized licorice root has no side effects and allows irritated tissues to heal.

After adequate healing of the inflamed tissues occurs, the next step can be undertaken. The next step involves the supplementation of stomach acid with meals and needs to be supervised by a competent physician. The goal is to restore adequate acid to the digestive process in order to make nutrient digestion more effective. Deficient acid producers are often deficient in secretion of the first protein-dismantling machines called pepsin. It is beneficial to take a supplement that contains acid and pepsin. The product label will say pepsinogen denoting the inactive form. When combined with water and acid it will be activated to pepsin. With successful acid and pepsinogen supplementation patients notice an increased tolerance for high protein meals and the ability to digest larger portions of steak, fish, and chicken, etc.

Typically, acid supplementation should be done during consumption of a protein meal. Adequate fluid should be swallowed with the hydrochloric acid pills as well. The best dose per pill contains approximately 600mg of hydrochloric acid. The dose per mid-meal should be increased by one pill until a warm feeling is noticed. This sensation denotes that the correct dose of acid supplement has been exceeded by one pill. With the next meal decrease the dosage by one pill. If acid deficiency is part of the digestive problem, supplementation will lead to feelings of increased well being following protein meals.

Alternatively, consuming alcohol with meals enhances the digestive process through the stimulation of acid output. Caffeine has been documented to stimulate acid secretion as well. Some of these fluids destroy the mucus lining that protects the stomach from digesting itself. Substances that disrupt the integrity of this mucus barrier are excess alcohol, vinegar, bile salts, and aspirin-like drugs (ibuprofen, aspirin, indomethacin, etc.).

The hormones and nervous control of acid secretion can be complicated. Both of these acid producing mechanisms pathways converge on histamine, which is increased by the activation of the vagus nerve and the hormone, gastrin. Histamine directly causes the acid producing cells to release acid into the stomach. Blockers of histamine release (Tagamet, Zantac, and Pepsin) are commonly used to decrease acid release. The more powerful proton pump inhibitors (Prilosec and Prevacid) act by their ability to poison the acid producing cells in the stomach.

In summary, there are three main determinants of stomach function: The adequacy of acid production, the quality of the mucus layer which protects the stomach lining from digestion, and the quality of the enzyme machines which are released when sufficient acid is present. Looking out from the glass ship into this stomach, all three of these processes are occurring in an orderly fashion.

The next stop in the glass ship occurs upon exiting the stomach through the pyloric valve. Immediately outside the stomach two drains that enter the small intestines are noticed. One drain comes from the gallbladder. The other drain is from the pancreas. There is food trickling out of the stomach valve causing each drain to gush with its own characteristic juice and mixing with the partially digested food

Pancreatic Juices and What They Need to Perform

The pancreas requires adequate stomach acid to be stimulated into releasing its stored juices. Pancreatic juices contain two basic components. The first component contains the acid neutralizing juice. It is needed because the enzymatic machinery works only in an alkaline environment (the opposite of an acid environment). These digestive machines operate in the third digestive chamber, the duodenum. While the partially digested meals' contents seep from the stomach, the pancreatic juices are released. Pancreatic juices contain bicarbonate that reacts with the acid forming carbon dioxide gas and water. When the pancreas is healthy, more bicarbonate than acid is secreted upon food entering this chamber. An alkaline environment is required for the second component of the pancreatic juice to work.

The second component of the pancreatic juice contains unique pancreatic enzymatic machines. These are designed to further dismantle fats, proteins, and, to a lesser degree, the few remaining complex carbohydrates. These juices are only part of the whole complement of digestive juices in the third chemical reaction chamber. The first chemical reaction chamber is in the mouth and the second in the stomach. Each of the chemical reaction chambers requires different work environments (acid or basic). The different work environments are necessary for the enzymatic machines secreted in that compartment to become fully functional.

Just like in the stomach, the enzymatic machines released within this digestive chamber, the duodenum, release with their packages wrapped around them. The enzyme machinery floats around idly and is useless until the wrapper is removed. The wrappers in this chamber are composed of amino acid chains that cover the active site of the protein disassembly machines. The inactivity precaution before secretion prevents the pancreas from digesting itself. The intestinal digestive chamber activation of the enzyme machinery depends on the cells lining the intestinal tube.

The cells that line the intestinal tube contain an unwrapping enzymatic machine. This particular machine activates only one of the pancreatic-produced enzymes. Scientists call this particular enzymatic machine trypsinogen while its still in the wrapper and trypsin when it is unwrapped. It is the enzyme machines produced in the intestinal lining cells that unwrap trypsinogen to trypsin. The intestinal lining cells are protected from digestion by their own layer of mucus. Trypsin in turn unwraps all the other pancreatic digestive machines that are in wrappers. Once trypsin has been freed, it begins to digest any protein that is not concealed behind the protective mucous barrier.

The Intestinal Chamber

The intestinal chamber is the third chemical reaction chamber. It receives chemical concoctions from the gallbladder and pancreas that dump into its proximal portion. The three different successive areas of this chamber reabsorb the majority of the secretions that occur higher up in the digestive tube. These chambers are the duodenum, the jejunum, and the ileum. The cells lining the intestinal tube look like shag carpet. One strand of carpet is composed of millions of intestinal lining cells called a villus. Millions of strands make up the shag carpet and provide maximal absorptive contact with the digested food.

The intestinal lining is called the brush border where the digestive building blocks (amino acids, simple sugars, various fatty acids vitamins, and minerals) are absorbed. Each type of molecular building component is absorbed at specific sites along this digestive chamber. Like the stomach, the cells lining the small intestine tube are protected from digestion by a mucus layer. Each specific molecular part (amino acids, sugars, various fatty acids, minerals, and vitamins) has a specific transport method through this mucus layer. If a molecular part cannot successfully cross through this mucus barrier, it cannot be absorbed.

The short life span of the digestive lining cells (the brush border) illustrates how body molecular parts are recycled and reused interchangeably. The recycling arises because these cell types are continuously being sloughed into the digestive tube every two to five days. This is much like how a snake sheds its skin, but from the inside of the tube. When these cells are sloughed, they are dismantled (digested) into molecular building parts. These mix with the food content contained in the digestive juices. These molecular parts are then reabsorbed by the digestive tract to be used somewhere else. Interchangeability of a molecular part ends only when it becomes damaged. Secretion of dead cells and the eventual re-absorption of the remaining useful molecular building blocks illustrate the interchangeability of the molecular parts that enters and leaves the tube. The interchangeability of molecular parts is an important concept.

Millions of recycled molecular parts move around the body. These same molecular parts build themselves into a structure that later is dismantled into the molecular building parts only to again be recycled into another structure. This occurs constantly at different locations throughout the body. The end to the interchangeability of molecular body parts arises only when they become damaged. Replacement of the damaged molecular parts explains why a continuous supply of new quality molecular parts must be available.

In summary, the stomach allows seepage of its contents out of the pyloric valve and into the small intestine. Vigorous pancreatic contractions release sufficient acid neutralizing bicarbonate. Bicarbonate release occurs in excess of the acid present to produce the opposite (alkaline fluid) work environment. An alkaline pH optimizes the simultaneous release and activation of the unique pancreatic digestive machines. The pancreatic digestive machines are designed to work best in an alkaline environment. In the small intestine chamber the final dismantling process of fats, protein, carbohydrates and the genetic material building blocks occurs. The third digestive chamber is also where these molecular building blocks are absorbed into the body.

Gallbladder Secretion

The gallbladder secretes juice out of the second hole in the proximal duodenum. Fat in the meal forces the gallbladder to simultaneously secrete out of the second drain hole located in the duodenum. Fats need additional molecular concoctions in the intestinal chemical reaction chamber, in order to be dismantled. The gallbladder secretion solves the problem of fat floating on water. The meal content floats in copious digestive juices. Therefore, they do not mix well with fat. The gallbladder secretes salts and acids that will break oil into tiny droplets. This process explains how the dairy industry makes the fat in commercially available milk stay dissolved in the milk. These substances are called emulsifying agents. The gallbladder secretes emulsifying agents made from acids of cholesterol and the break down of hemoglobin salts. In specific ratios, these substances raise the fat absorption from 50% without a gallbladder to 95% with a gallbladder.

The entire contents of the gallbladder are secreted into the upper small intestine (duodenum) and reabsorbed at the end of the small intestine (the ileum). After being reabsorbed, they are quickly re-secreted into the gallbladder at such a rate that they are recycled 6-8 times per day.

Nutritionally - The Owner is only as Good as What He Absorbs

When the owner is healthy the orderly uptake of different building blocks becomes possible and begins to happen as individual parts become available to the brush border cells. There are billions of brush border cells that line the small intestine tube. In this digestive chamber, the quality of juices that come out of the pancreas and the gallbladder significantly affect how the body absorbs nutrients. This concerns the health of the brush border cells and their associated protective mucus.

The small intestine is presented with more than 9 quarts of fluid per day. By the time meal remnants reach the large intestine only 1-2 quarts of fluid remain. By the time they leave the colon in the bowel movement, less than one cup of the original 9 quarts passes in the feces.

Digestion involves the secretion and re-absorption of large amounts of water. The content of the fluid changes considerably as the food moves down the digestive tube. These changes facilitate the dismantling tasks that need to occur. The fluid, salt, and even the enzymatic machinery parts are largely reabsorbed and recycled again and again.

The voyage down the small intestine in the glass ship has seen the absorption of almost all the nutrients that were contained in the meal. The remaining components are indigestible fibers and friendly bacteria that comprise 50% of stool weight. Only small amounts of fat and protein are contained in the stool. The glass ship arrives at the passageway to the next digestive chamber, the iliocecal valve. The next digestive chamber is the large intestine.

Health Cannot Occur Without a Happy Colon

The colon (large intestine) comprises the fourth chemical reaction chamber for the nutritional remnants still in the meal. In addition to finishing the digestive process, the colon is one of six organs that take out the trash (section four). Constipated people do not take out the colon trash very well. On the opposite extreme are those owners who have chronic diarrhea. Chronic diarrhea means that the body discards important minerals, water, nutrients, and vitamins with the trash. On top of this backdrop of colon tasks are the unique requirements of the healthy colon being colonized by helpful bacteria.

The large intestine requires certain bacterial colonies to assist it in performing its many biological functions. If the right bacteria are living in this chamber, good things happen. The right bacteria (mostly acidophilus and bifidus bacteria) re-acidify the meal remnants again. The meal remnants are all that is left of the meal that has finally made its way to the colon.

It is very important for overall body health that the colon contains ample friendly bacteria. These bacteria produce many B-vitamins and vitamin K. The colon-inhabiting bacteria feed the colon lining cells by changing indigestible fiber into carbohydrates. Second and more importantly, these bacteria change some of the carbohydrates into the short-chained fatty acids that are particularly nutritious for the needs of the colon lining cells.

If one of the colon functions isn't working correctly, health consequences occur. It is worthwhile to consider some of these imbalances and the simple ways an owner can return to balance. The first imbalance concerns the colon's role as one of the organs responsible for preventing the fifth path to an old body.

It is important to identify the role of the colon in this path to longevity. The fifth path is about taking out the cellular trash that accumulates daily as the cells function doing their thing.

When certain conditions exist, the colon becomes compromised in its ability to perform the necessary trash removal. The first compromise involves the wrong bacteria or amounts inhabiting the chamber. The second is for trash removal problems to occur when the colon contents are fiber deficient. This prevents helpful bacteria from being able to create butyrate for the colon lining cells nutritional needs. Butyrate is a short chain fatty acid that colon cells prefer for energy. The water retention role that fiber plays in keeping bowel movements soft is of significant importance. Third, involves the chronic retention of feces or constipation that encourages the formation of toxins (putrefaction). Putrefaction results in the re-absorption back into the body of some of these poisons.

The last compromise concerns yeast organisms over growing in the colon chamber. Decreased acidity encourages yeast overgrowth. Sufficient colon acidity depends on adequate amounts of acid-producing bacteria.

Whenever an owner takes antibiotics, there is a risk that these friendly bacteria will die. Friendly bacteria also die from chronic consumption of chlorinated water. When friendly bacteria die, the acidity of the colon decreases encouraging yeast overgrowth. This allows the release of toxins into the system. A careful, laboratory performed stool analysis can identify most of these common problems.

All of the trash removal problems are made worse when certain hormones become deficient in the colon. The primary hormones for colon health are thyroid, cortisol, IGF, and vitamin A. When any of these are deficient, colon health suffers.

Low thyroid function is manifested as chronic constipation because thyroid message encourages energy production in the colon cells. Only through sufficient energy creation can the colon motility and activity be normal.

Cortisol deficiency leads to colon inflammation and mucus abnormalities. Therefore, colitis is very responsive to cortisol medication. Often the patients have a thyroid problem as well.

Decreased IGF levels lead to a decrease in the protective layer of glycosaminoglycans occurring throughout the body. The glycosaminoglycan layer protects the cells that line the body cavities (respiratory tract, gastrointestinal tract), vessels and body surfaces (skin and organs). The IGF level determines the adequacy of the protective layer in the colon. The consequence of the glycosaminoglycan layer becoming deficient enables an increased propensity for toxic molecules to leak into the body. The increased toxic load further burdens the liver.

Vitamin A makes cells grow up. Cancer is a problem of cells not growing up. Some cancer cells do not grow up solely because they are deficient in vitamin A. Sufficient vitamin A is necessary to instruct DNA programs. Vitamin A is particularly important in the same cell types for which the glycosaminoglycan layer forms a barrier. Signs of vitamin A deficiency show up best on the skin. Examples of this include roughened skin, pigmentation spots, and fine wrinkles. When these are present the same tendency exists in the colon. Colon cancer risk can be lowered by adequate vitamin A intake. Vitamin A is found in high levels in carrots, squash and avocados.

Chapter 14

Pancreas

The Hormones That Keep the Pancreas from Killing

The exocrine part of the pancreas secretes digestive juices. This subsection discussion is concerned with the hormonal pancreas (the endocrine portion). The type of hormones that the pancreas secretes is determined by diet and lifestyle. The type of hormones that the pancreas chooses to secrete has a powerful effect on what the liver will do with the fuel supply.

Insulin message dominance leads to one extreme of liver activities involving fuel supply. Insulin that the pancreas secretes, directs the liver to store carbohydrate in the form of glycogen (the minority form of stored body fuel). When the capacity of the liver to store carbohydrate as glycogen becomes filled, insulin directs the liver to manufacture the rest of the carbohydrate into LDL fat molecules. LDL fat is designed as a transport package for the major storage sites of fuel. Next, the insulin hormone direction leads to the release of LDL cholesterol into the blood stream. Clinically, the high production rate of these types of fats can show up as an increased LDL cholesterol or triglyceride level. From the blood stream, the LDL cholesterol moves into the fat storage areas of the body (blood vessel macrophage cells and belly fat).

The other extreme of hormonal direction from the pancreas to the liver occurs when diet and life style direct glucagon message content release. The glucagon message directs the liver to dump its stored sugar and fatty acids into the blood stream. These molecules are readily accessible sources of fuel to power the power plants. Therefore, the glucagon message contains an opposite liver direction information relative to that of the insulin message. When glucagon predominates, fuels are released into the blood stream from the liver for use as fuel in the cellular power plants. In addition, the glucagon message stimulates the liver conversion of amino acids into more sugar.

The insulin message to the liver directs the body fuels to be stored. The process of storing body fuel involves the liver stored varieties and the LDL cholesterol that is released into the blood stream for transit purposes only. LDL cholesterol utilizes the blood stream for transit on its way to fat storage sites (in the blood vessels and fat cells). It is important to consider the balance of message content that the liver receives and how it is directed to deal with fuel. Whether fuel is stored or released is determined by this basic pipeline of information flowing from the pancreas into the liver.

The pancreas is a major source of message content for determining whether the liver stores or releases fuel. When balanced informational content occurs, the pancreas secretes optimal amounts of the opposing hormones insulin and glucagon. Failure to understand this dynamic tug of war between these opposing informational substances leads to unnecessary prescriptions, surgical procedures, and disease complications.

Healthy owners use almost all their pancreas secreted insulin and glucagon instructing the liver how to handle fuel. Ninety percent of the glucagon hormone secreted by the pancreas is used in the liver. The glucagon message directs the liver to release stored sugar and fat into the blood stream. The message of glucagon stimulates the liver to manufacture more sugar from available amino acids within the liver storage houses. Also contained in the message content of glucagon is the cessation of the liver synthesis of cholesterol. The glucagon message content accomplishes this by the inactivation of the enzyme HMG CoA reductase in the liver. Lastly, the glucagon message content inhibits further synthesis of fat in the liver. Overall, the glucagon message tells the liver to maximize fuel delivery into the blood stream that allows more fuel uptake in the cellular power plants when other hormones are present.

Insulin delivers the opposite message to the liver. Healthy owners use up to eighty percent of their insulin message content on telling the liver to store fuel. Fuel is stored as fat and a small amount of glycogen. The insulin message in the liver can be summarized as: stop the manufacture of amino acids into sugar, suck the sugar out of the blood stream and sequester it in the form of glycogen, and when the capacity to store sugar is filled (about 400 grams) it then directs the liver to manufacture extra sugar into LDL cholesterol. The insulin directed increase in the manufacture rate of LDL cholesterol involves the activation of the enzyme, HMG CoA reductase that manufactures cholesterol in the liver. Simultaneously, insulin directs conversion of the extra sugar into fat in the liver. The newly manufactured fat and cholesterol manufactured in the liver combine to form LDL particles. These particles are secreted from the liver into the blood stream and destined for the storage depots. The storage depots are fat cells and macrophage cells that line arteries.

Substances such as caffeine stimulate pancreatic secretion of both insulin and glucagon at the same time. Here the more powerful effect is glucagon as evidenced by a slight increase in the blood sugar level. Owners that have a damaged pancreas, such as the insulin-deficient type diabetic, should take particular note of this induced effect. The extreme blood sugar increase occurs because as the caffeine arrives at the pancreas there is no ability to increase insulin. The consequence in the insulin deficient diabetic, when glucagon becomes unopposed by insulin, results in blood sugar increases.

There is a total of four hormones, including glucagon, that counter the effects of insulin. When one or more of these counter regulatory hormones fail, it leads to unnecessary suffering and disease complications. Many cases of hypoglycemia, poorly controlled diabetes, muscle wasting, and other chronic degenerative diseases result from a failure to comprehend the weight and the counter weights of hormones that affect liver fuel direction parameters. When the liver physiology becomes unbalanced, an altered response to insulin occurs.

The insulin message content desires to direct the liver to suck every sugar molecule out of the blood stream. When the counter response to a high insulin levels at the level of the liver becomes deficient, a dangerously low blood sugar can result. Some owners suffer from a roller coaster like blood sugar brought about by imbalances in their ability to mount an effective counter response to insulin.

There are four main counter response hormones that the body needs in order to keep insulin effects balanced. Insulin serves as the weight in the antique weight scale analogy. For health to occur, it takes all four other counterweights in effective amounts to rebalance the weight scale. The weight scale balances when two processes occur. First, there needs to be an appropriate amount of sugar and fat in the blood stream created by adequate amounts of the four counter regulatory hormones. Second, the need for the presence of adequate insulin-like growth factor type one is necessary. Insulin-like growth factor facilitates entry of these fuels into the cellular power plants outside the liver and fat storage cells.

The counterbalancing hormones that oppose the action of insulin are glucagon, cortisol, adrenaline, and growth hormone. Many poorly controlled diabetic conditions arise from failure to consider the status of the counter regulatory hormones (liver chapter). Other countless owners are misdiagnosed with mood disorders, seizures, depression, and even hypochondria when aberrations in the counter response hormones are the culprit. If these owners better understand this ignored interplay between these opposing hormonal forces then healing becomes possible.

Cortisol as a Counter Regulatory Hormone to Insulin

Above and beyond the opposing message content between glucagon and insulin are the other counter regulatory hormones. Cortisol is a level one hormone. It will have powerful message content directed at liver cell DNA programs. The DNA programs activated by cortisol in the liver, involves the ability of the liver to recognize the glucagon message. This important fact is often skirted around in the medical textbooks. In these textbooks, in a disorganized and fragmented way, there is an acknowledgment that cortisol is necessary for the liver to respond to the glucagon message. The liver cannot recognize the glucagon message content without enough cortisol to direct the manufacture of the receptors of glucagon through DNA program activation.

Cortisol is the heavy weight to insulin in regard to blood sugar level. The adrenal glands make cortisol. Owners that have weakened adrenal function have brain 'fog' symptoms thirty minutes to three hours following a carbohydrate meal. Carbohydrate intake increases the need for more insulin secretion from the pancreas. There then needs to be an adequate ability to manufacture and release increased cortisol from the adrenal to counter the increased insulin desire to lower the blood sugar in the blood stream below optimal. Adrenal deficient owners experience low blood sugar because a high carbohydrate diet necessitates an increased insulin release. Unless adequate counter regulatory hormones effectively counter the increased insulin release, the blood sugar will fall. Cortisol is the main counter regulatory hormone to insulin's blood lowering effects.

Cortisol is the primary hormone necessary to develop in the liver machinery necessary to counter the insulin message. Cortisol counters the insulin message by instructing liver cells DNA programs. Cortisol instructs liver cell DNA programs by involving the manufacture of the glucagon receptors necessary for the liver to respond to glucagon. The pancreas releases glucagon during times of low blood sugar. There are many owners who suffer from low blood sugar because no one evaluates their adrenal ability to increase cortisol production in the presence of high insulin levels.

Adrenaline as a Counter Regulatory Hormone to Insulin

Adrenaline saves lives when the adrenal glands ability to release sufficient cortisol diminishes. Adrenaline message content is also dependent on cortisol to direct the liver DNA programs to manufacture adrenaline receptors. It needs to serve as a counter hormone to insulin only when something goes wrong and the blood sugar gets too low. In non-diabetics this occurs when they consume a high carbohydrate diet and there is insufficient presence of the counter hormone cortisol.

When the adrenal releases adrenaline to counter a drop in blood sugar, there are the side effects of pounding heart rate, anxiety, and sweating palms. Many unsuspecting owners that love to binge out on carbohydrates develop these wide swings in blood sugar and fail to understand the anxiety like symptoms that follow. These symptoms result from the blood sugar falling and then being rescued from death by a massive outpouring of adrenaline.

Nutritional adequacy is the concern of the fourth principle. Some unfortunate owners have weak adrenals and therefore poor cortisol production. The problem magnifies when there is the additional disaster of poor nutrition. These owners have an increased risk for seizure disorders because their blood sugar falls father than most (section VI).

Both cortisol and thyroid are needed to manufacture a mature adrenaline receptor. Thyroid is a level one hormone. Thyroid message content is also needed to direct liver cell DNA programs in the synthesis of part of the adrenaline receptor (thyroid chapter). Deficiency or excess in these interrelated hormones cause a sub-optimal human experience. The sub-optimal experience occurs because the mature adrenaline receptor manufacturing process requires direction by both of these level one hormones.

Growth Hormone is the Most Misunderstood of the Counter Response Hormones to Insulin

The most misunderstood and neglected role of the counter response hormones to insulin is growth hormone (GH). This neglect occurs because its name leads owners down an erroneous mental image path.

Growth hormone's protein conservation message content explains where its name originates. Protein conservation is a pre-requisite for growth to occur. Growth hormone, other than its stimulatory effect on cartilage cell growth, has few direct effects on the tissues. One direct affect, concerns its ability to act like modified glucagon at the level of the liver with two exceptions. First, involves the fact that unlike glucagon, growth hormone has powerful protein sparing effects. Growth hormone in the liver inhibits the conversion of amino acids into sugar. The second difference from glucagon involves the fact that GH directs the liver to release a special hormone called insulin-like growth factor type 1. Like glucagon, it stimulates the release of sugar stored as liver glycogen into the blood stream. Also like glucagon it stimulates the liver to release stored fats into the blood stream for fuel.

Insulin-like growth factor type 1 (IGF-1) can only be released with the direction of growth hormones presence. Confusion arises from the fact that the affects of IGF-1 message content, directly opposes the initial fuel release effects of growth hormone. IGF-1 release occurs simultaneously to the growth hormone directed liver release of sugar and fat into the blood stream. If one sees the overall effect in the sequential release of growth hormone followed by IGF-1, this begins to make more sense. The more IGF-1 released, the less insulin needed.

Growth hormone stimulates the release of fat and carbohydrates from liver stores into the blood stream. The second part of the effect involves the simultaneous release, from the liver, of adequate insulin-like growth factor (IGF-1) into the blood stream. The IGF-1 hormone in the peripheral tissues (blood stream) behaves very much like insulin does in the liver and body fat cells. The body needs less insulin when the liver secretes adequate IGF-1. When adequate growth hormone has stimulated sufficient IGF-1 release into the blood stream, the peripheral tissues, like muscle, are facilitated to procure fuel (carbohydrate and fat). This is the insulin-like effect of IGF-1.

Sufficient release of insulin like growth factor negates the initial increase in blood sugar and blood fat caused by the presence of growth hormones message to the liver. Mechanistically insulin like growth hormone behaves like insulin in the peripheral tissues. IGF-1's presence instructs the peripheral tissues to take up the fuel released by growth hormones presence.

Many clinicians fail to appreciate this sequential arrangement that operates in the healthy population. Both IGF-1 and insulin bind to the same cell receptors. This makes sense when one realizes their similar message content in regards to their instruction of different cells within the body to take up fuel out of the blood stream.

Different cell types have different affinities for IGF-1 and insulin, and different cell receptor concentrations for either insulin or IGF-1. For example, the liver and fat cells have the highest amount of insulin receptors of any other cell. There are about 200,000 insulin receptors per fat or liver cell. Insulin directs these tissues to store fuel. In contrast, the IGF-1 receptors are found throughout most of the rest of the cells. IGF-1 blood levels, in healthy owners, occur at levels one hundred times that of insulin levels. Many disease processes have their origins in a falling IGF-1 level. When the IGF-1 level falls, insulin needs to be secreted in abnormal amounts. Increased insulin has health consequences that increased IGF-1 does not share.

A major advantage of adequate IGF-1 to that of higher insulin is that insulin levels determine the amount of body fat. Fat is the major stored fuel type because there is a limited ability to store sugar as glycogen. Total storage capacity for glycogen is about 500 grams (about 2200 calories). About four hundred grams are stored in the liver and the other one hundred grams are stored in the muscles. Sedentary and well-fed owners have little opportunity to draw down these stored forms of sugar. The more sedentary and well fed the owner, the more carbohydrates will be channeled into the production of liver fat and pathway of cholesterol making machinery. Insulin directed pathways are designed with fuel storage in mind. The major fuel storage sites occur in arterial macrophages and the fat cells.

Certain genetically predisposed owners have a higher insulin secretion (on a daily basis) with a similar diet, compared to normal owners. The increased insulin responding owner means these owners create more message content directing their livers to make carbohydrates into LDL cholesterol. In these same owners, practices that increase growth hormone will result in increased IGF-1 release. Increased levels of IGF-1 share essentially none of the liver stimulation effects that lead to increased LDL manufacture. This will help lessen the need for insulin secretion by facilitating the cells to uptake sugar from the blood stream, beyond the liver.

When an owner is healthy most of his insulin production is used at the level of the liver following a meal. This situation allows low insulin needs because these owners produce sufficient growth hormone in counter response to rising insulin levels. Insulin levels rise whenever an owner consumes carbohydrates. Less insulin is needed when there is the increased presence of IGF-1 because it facilitates the removal of sugar from the blood stream. Unlike insulin, which has a major effect on the liver and fat cells ability to remove sugar out of the blood stream, IGF-1 has effect in the periphery cells (muscles and organs). IGF-1 competes with insulin as to where the extra nutrition is sucked. Higher IGF-1 favors increased nutrition procurement for muscle and organs cells. Higher insulin levels favor the uptake of nutrition out of the blood stream by liver and fat cells.

There are two major stimuli for growth hormone release. IGF-1 release in a normal liver occurs whenever growth hormone levels rise. The GH releasing stimulus results from fasting and intense exercise. Both of these conditions produce a decrease in blood fuel level. This decrease causes an initial rise in growth hormone that initially directs the liver to release IGF-1, sugar, and fat into the blood stream. The released IGF-1 acts like peripheral insulin in facilitating the peripheral uptake of the released fuel from the liver. In this way, the body has a mechanism for ensuring that appropriate amounts of fuel are in the blood stream between meals and when physical exertion draws down the blood fuel.

Exercise has a powerful contributory effect on the amount of growth hormone released and hence, IGF-1 levels. This release does much the same thing in the periphery that insulin does in the liver and fat storage cells. However, low blood sugar effects are prevented because growth hormone also directs the liver to dump sugar into the blood stream while the liver is releasing IGF-1. The design of IGF-1 facilitates the peripheral cells uptake of fuel out of the blood stream that, in these cases, growth hormone started. Where growth hormone production falls off as well as IGF-1, there is the need for increased insulin production. In these unhealthy situations, insulin is forced to pick up the slack in the periphery (muscles and organs). This is one of the mechanisms for insulin resistance (liver chapter).

Increased IGF-1 levels occur for the opposite reasons of increased insulin levels. The increase in IGF-1 in the exercising or fasting state facilitate cellular uptake of the growth hormone stimulated liver release of sugar and fat into the blood stream. However, the fuel storage in the liver depends on enough insulin directing the liver to suck up nutrition for storage purposes following a meal. Without sufficient insulin, there would be no stored fuel to release when GH directed the release of fuel and IGF-1 from the liver. In this way, the healthy body balances the blood fuel supply following meals and between meals. Insulin and IGF-1 remove nutrients from the blood stream following meals. Insulin directs nutrients into the storage pathways that occur in the liver and fat cells. Conversely, IGF-1 directs nutrients into the vast majority of other cell types. The healthy body having at least one hundred times more IGF-1 than insulin in the blood stream evidences this fact.

Increased insulin becomes necessary to shore up lagging growth hormone with the consequent diminished IGF-1 output. There are three subtle, but dangerous consequences to a body that relies on increased insulin production. First, the stimulation of the appetite center leads to an increased tendency to gain weight. Second, increased insulin stimulates the liver in the manufacture of LDL cholesterol. Third, there is increased reliance on cortisol and adrenaline to keep the blood sugar elevated, between meals, when growth hormone levels fall. The consequence of normalizing blood sugar levels between meals with elevated cortisol and epinephrine is a loss in protein conservation. Only growth hormone helps retain body protein when fasting. Less body protein leads to less muscle mass and organ size. These are some of the major characteristics of the onset of aging.

Growth hormone release occurs from regular exercise, low normal blood sugars, glucagon, the low secretion rate of serotonin in the hypothalamus, and when the hypothalamus neurons secrete dopamine. There are other details, but if one keeps these five determinants in mind it encourages making better choices.

The above discussion gives a mechanistic explanation for why couch potatoes tend to develop insulin resistance. Increased insulin resistance will eventually exhaust the genetically determined ability of the pancreas to increase insulin production. When this happens, it exhausts the pancreas beyond its genetically determined capability manifesting in adult onset diabetes.

Making things worse is the fact that when GH secretion rates fall the protein content in the body decreases proportionally. GH is a fundamental requirement for the conservation of body protein between meals. Without adequate GH between meals the body increases the secretion rate of cortisol, glucagons, and epinephrine in order to maintain blood sugar levels. All three of these will activate the liver machinery that converts protein stores into sugar.

The other extreme of health contains highly trained athletes who secrete high levels of IGF-1 secondary to increased growth hormone secretion. Increased growth hormone secretion occurs because exercise increases fuel delivery requirements. GH is one of the main hormones that raise the liver secretion rate of fuel into the blood stream and body protein content is spared from breakdown. In contrast, the other three fuel increasing hormones, cortisol, epinephrine, and glucagon make protein fair game. Another benefit of high IGF-1 levels is that less insulin is required. The highly trained athlete needs very little insulin for efficient fuel delivery into exercising muscle cells because of the high IGF-1 levels. For this reason, exercise lowers LDL cholesterol levels. The decreased need for insulin results in a lessened stimulus to manufacture LDL cholesterol in the liver.

It has long ago been known that growth hormone levels decline with age. A sedentary life style accelerates this decline. Conversely, regular exercise increases IGF-1 levels secondary to increased growth hormone release.

These facts unite several health consequences of insulin resistance into a common thread of causality. There is sequential decline of growth hormone and IGF-1 levels with certain diets and lifestyles, with aging. The decline of these two hormones explains some of the insulin resistance occurring with advancing age and sedentary lifestyle. It also explains how regular exercise remedies insulin resistance by raising growth hormone and IGF-1 levels. Applying this association could save owners the unnecessary complications of diabetes and the acceleration of aging. Lastly, the fall in growth hormone levels brought about by a sedentary lifestyle explains why muscle and organ mass are lost. Growth hormone conserves protein content. Unless owners have processes operating in their lives that encourage GH secretion, they will lose protein. Insulin increases when the GH decline leads to decreased IGF-1 levels. This can create more body fat.

IGF-1 differs functionally from insulin in the blood stream by binding to a carrier protein. In contrast, insulin circulates unbound in the blood stream. There are six different carrier proteins for IGF-1. One carries 95% of all insulin-like growth factor. Clinical application occurs because one of these carrier proteins provides a crude index of how much insulin-like growth factor operates in a body. This one carrier protein binds about 95% of all insulin-like growth factor (binding protein 111) in the blood stream. The levels of IGFBP type 111 are a crude index for the ability to deliver fuel to many cells (other than the liver and fat cells). Many labs are now able to check this value in the blood streams for the cumulative hormone report card.

What Patients Teach Physicians

The uniqueness of each owner allows an accumulation of insights with the passage of clinical practice. Most physicians are driven to learn and curious about the inner-workings of life. Sometimes the societal situation beats down the doctor- patient partnership and the sacred bond of trust becomes stretched. In the current western system of doctor patient interaction, many doctors feel a feeble ability to provide the healthcare they envision in the best interest of their patient. They feel caught in the teeth of a system largely devoted to the wasted energy of bureaucratic busy work that has nothing to do with healing.

It wasn't always this way in the western world of medicine. There have been times when a more loving friendship participated in the decision making process. Healing is more effective when the physician is allowed to concentrate on how to heal. Focus has a direction that facilitates insight into a given patients uniqueness. In contrast, organizational and bureaucratic medicine has doctors caught in self-perpetuating lose of the medical complex economy.

Some physicians are now committed to breaking free of the complex's 'shackles'. One movement, 'Keep It Simple', has origins in Seattle, Washington. The basic tenant is that a large proportion of health care expenditure goes to paperwork and time devoted to feeding the government and insurance bureaucracy. Physicians that participate in this movement have decided that good health care is facilitated when these interests are eviscerated from their workday. They no longer recognize insurance or government programs and can reduce the cost of an office visit. In addition, they are freed intellectually to study and learn about the latest scientific paradigms.

Greater momentum would be realized if more owners understood the consequences to their doctor's ability to continue learning as long as they continue to jumps through bureaucratic hoops. Valuable energy expenditures in these wasteful pursuits leads inevitably to less time for one to follow their curiosity hunches to their logical conclusion.

A clear insight into the consequences of a medical system run by the profit interests of the complex is analogous to junk food. Although junk food taste like food, it will harm the body if it is continually ingested. Owners are continually bombarded by clever methods of advertisement that encourage consumption of these injurious ingredients. Most owners know that these junk foods are harmful, but everyone else does it and they feel better. Slowly but surely more owners have become aware that environmentally contaminated foods, which are full of chemicals, toxins, and hormone mimics, will injure body functions. The food industry complex still touts the latest clever come on, but there are less gullible owners with each passing year.

The strategies of the profit driven health care system are becoming suspect. Many astute owners have cultivated an awareness of the need of the medical industrial complex to sensationalize what is for sale. Profit driven healthcare will remain partial to the expensive and symptom control medicine because there is no incentive and in some cases a disincentive to discuss the holism of what science has revealed. Inexpensive solutions to health problems hurt profit margins that, when lowered, the tax that the government collects is lowered. Healing is bad for the economy and the government's ability to collect money.

Movements like 'Keep It Simple,' are a start to allow some physicians time to rediscover the passion for healing. They have begun to discuss among themselves radical new ideas that are more consistent with the scientific evidence that has been revealed.(Cont.)

(Cont'd) In many cases, the bond among physicians is stronger than the pigeonholes of the complex hierarchy. Good things are happening and many brave patients can be thanked for the help they have provided in stimulating doctors to learn. Patients often bring fresh ideas because they have had less brain washing history. Physicians often become vulnerable to narrow thinking because of their extended educations funded by the complex. Many still possess the spark of curiosity that led them to their life's work. These are the physicians who are able to listen with an open mind to successful encounters of patients with alternative healing modalities. Alternative methods for healing begin to make mechanistic sense when some of the old scientific truths are re-included in the analysis. This can occur when the holism (commonly eviscerated from mainstream medical educations) of scientific revelation reunites with the pieces of disjointed medical thought so prevalent in the complex today.

Chapter 15

The Torture Chamber Diet

There is a complete lack of attention to the consequences from abnormal hormone levels that the ADA diet creates in the adherent's feeding behavior. Abnormal hormones exaggerate feeding obsessions. The torture chamber effect describes the feeding obsessions that result from this official diet. This diet is the place where abnormal hormones create a perpetual preoccupation for the next feeding event. As long as the American public is led to believe in the diet, endorsed by the American Dietetic Association, there will be continued economic need from the complications of obesity. Examples of these complications are high blood pressure, diabetes, and heart disease. The ADA diet is easy to expose when some basic missing facts are included in the analysis.

There is a narrow band of truth in the ADA diet that occurs for one type of physique. The only physique for which this occurs is in an athlete who is at ideal weight and/or peak performance. Peak performing athletes are at optimal weight and have achieved optimal physical fitness. Through training, genetics, and/or age, they have the right balance of hormones.

Owners that are at ideal weight and physically fit have properly proportioned hormone message content. This allows the proper appetite stimulation and exercise motivation to continue. They can handle increased carbohydrate intake that necessitates only a slight increase in insulin production. The increased insulin is tolerated because their lifestyles and/or genetics allow an operational message harmony of counter hormones. The counter hormones successfully counter weights the fat building message of insulin. Most owners are not endowed with superior amounts of androgen (section two) and growth hormone.

There has been little acknowledgement of basic scientific facts about the relationship of dietary choices and hormone consequences to feeding behavior. Some notable exceptions are found in the Drs. Atkin's, Schwarzbein and Sears diets. There have also been fewer acknowledgments about the circular trap that feeding behavior dictates the consequence of which hormones are secreted. This explains the vicious and circular trap overweight owners find themselves in, despite the earnest attempts to diet.

When obese owners adhere to the ADA diet's tenants, powerful hormones are released. These stimulate a preoccupation with the next feeding and a decreased ability to shed fat. It is a travesty to withhold acknowledgement that the ADA diet creates a virtual torture chamber of emotional desires in the owner who attempts to make positive health changes when the attempts to change are doomed. They are destined for defeat by unfavorable hormones.

Dr. Atkins was one of the first physicians to recognize the powerful role that hormones play in feeding behavior. He did this by reviewing what was known about the hormone, insulin, in basic medical physiology textbooks. He studied cultures that do not have high rates of obesity and obesity related diseases. Dr. Atkins first began to apply what was known over twenty years ago about hormone levels and consequent feeding behavior. He correctly reasoned that insulin levels that are allowed to reach higher than optimum levels act as a powerful appetite stimulant. This creates an obsessive preoccupation for the next feeding event. He understood that insulin has a dramatic effect on the ability of the body to manufacture fat. He understood how insulin prevents the body from accessing fat reserves.

Health benefits from lowering insulin levels are receiving renewed interest. Lowered insulin levels will decrease the stimulation in the appetite center of the brain and also increase the ability to use fat for energy. Obesity is on the increase in America and it can rarely be curtailed without an improvement in feeding behavior hormones.

It is important to extend the work of Dr's like Atkins, Sears, and Schwarzbein. Their important contributions allow consideration of other obesity hormones (section two). Other hormones, in addition to insulin, that need to be normalized before weight loss occurs are cortisol, androgens, estrogen, IGF-1, epinephrine, and thyroid. The normalizing of these hormones provides an extension of these authorities work.

The importance of real food versus processed food also needs to be added into the plan. Real foods provide the mineral nutrition necessary for maximum avoidance of the complications from obesity related disease. The real food component of successful dieting explains why the opposite approach to dieting has some success. These diets for which Dean Ornish and Nathaniel Pritikin are most famous do a better job about expressing the importance of real food in place of processed food. However, these diets failed their adherents because of the high insulin that results. In the end both diet camps on the extremes have some success, but each fails in success by ignoring either the hormones or the importance of real food.

Consuming real food helps avoid ingredients that are easily missed in the high protein diet. High protein dieters need to take care not to consume high protein sources from processed food.

The diet that has the least success in the long haul is the ADA diet. The ADA diet takes the worst features from both diet extremes. It advises consumption of 50-60% of total daily calories from carbohydrates. Carbohydrate consumption in this proportion of total daily calories is destined to condemn the obese owners into the vicious torture chamber cycle. Weight gain consequences occur because of the obligatory rise in insulin levels. There is also a degree of other hormone imbalances.

A discussion of the additional hormones involved in obesity brings up a concept that Dr. Atkins calls metabolic resistance. Metabolic resistance denotes those women for whom the low carbohydrate diet is slow to effect weight loss. The high protein diet approach fails to acknowledge that many of these women need the added benefit of androgen. Androgen deficiency explains some of the cause for this phenomenon quite well, as it is androgens that oppose fat gain. Fat gain is accentuated in some female owners because they have less androgen compared to men. The removal of the ovaries and the onset of the menopause can exacerbate androgen deficiency. Consideration of the twenty-four hour urine test for steroid production will identify this type of metabolic resistance caused problem.

An additional cause of metabolic resistance is the increased production rate of the stress hormone, cortisol. High cortisol levels in the urine identify other owners who have trouble with weight loss despite strict adherence to a low carbohydrate diet. High stress will increase cortisol release. Increased cortisol in a setting of mental stress will elevate blood sugar inappropriately and will only come down with exercise or increased insulin secretion. It is the increased insulin secretion brought on by stress occurring in a sedentary lifestyle that leads to obesity. Intensity of the problem is because their adrenal glands are particularly adept at cortisol production when they feel stress. These obese owners make more cortisol with the same amount of life stress as a non-obese owner. Increased cortisol causes an inappropriate increase in blood fuel that has nowhere to go in a sedentary owner until insulin is released. Only exercise and stress management will provide a way to stop this hormone cycle in the torture chamber.

Thyroid hormone levels need to be carefully evaluated. The thyroid gland determines the rate at which calories can be burned in the cell power plants.

Estrogen levels when high, as occurs in pregnancy and birth control pill usage, exacerbates the obesity problem in some female owners. Environmental estrogen problems can occur in men and women (section two). High estrogen levels stimulate growth hormone release, but inhibit IGF-1 release. This aberration leads to insulin resistance. Increased insulin is needed to bring the blood level back to normal. The higher the insulin levels, the more the liver fat making machinery is geared up to make fat and more fat is then available for storage sites in the liver, arteries, and fat cells.

Epinephrine release is an extension of the stress response. Like cortisol it contains message content that instructs the liver to elevate fuel in the blood stream. When stress is mental in nature there becomes little need for the extra fuel in the blood stream. Insulin needs to be released to normalize blood sugar. Increased insulin leads to an increased fat making message in liver and fat cells.

There is the 'tug of war' between the hormones that help shed fat and the hormones that make fat. It is worthwhile to assess whether these interrelating hormones are in excess, deficiency, or are present in the optimal amounts needed for a healthy body.

Thin people who eat as much as they want are not always fine specimens of raging androgen production. Deficiency in muscle mass usually is a clue that increased androgen may not be the reason for perpetual thinness. Emaciated skinniness in the presence of increased caloric intake can be due to poor digestive absorption of critical nutrients. Some owners are unable to manufacture extra insulin in a setting of increased carbohydrate intake. They never develop diagnosable diabetes because their pancreas limps along with just enough insulin and IGF-1 output to keep it from spilling over into the urine.

All of the Popular Diets Today Are Missing Vital Consideration for Weight Loss (each has part of the puzzle, but not the whole picture)

Two different extremes in diet philosophy have been introduced. Each has a part of the puzzle that will help shed fat. Each also contains an impediment to weight loss. The best science in each diet approach is needed, while avoiding the downside.

High protein and fat with low carbohydrate diet plans are incomplete in their effectiveness because they do not contain the right mineral ratios. Their incompleteness sheds light on how some of the other diets have a weight loss effect. Some other diets have a weight loss effect because they inadvertently partially address mineral balance. The omission of the mineral balance creates the hormone imbalances (higher insulin) that the high protein diet philosophy attempts to avoid. Mineral imbalance will occur any time a processed food is preeminent in the diet.

On the up side, the high protein diet leads to lower insulin levels. In contrast, the upside of the fresh and raw food dieters is that they contain properly proportioned minerals that will better help with hormone balance. On the downside these diets are higher in carbohydrate so the insulin need is higher. Higher insulin levels are counter-productive to any diet effort. Mineral intake balance is important to the obesity hormones that result.

The Mineral Design Conservation Features are Obsolete in Face of the Processed Food Diet

The human body was designed for a natural mineral ratios intake. This would be a minimum of three times as much potassium as sodium and there should be sufficient magnesium to counter calcium. The sodium and potassium ratio is more than reversed when one adheres to a processed food diet. Magnesium intake is commonly deficient as well.

In prehistoric times there was a survival advantage for anyone who could retain sodium. Natural food is relatively deficient in sodium content compared to potassium. When natural food is eaten the potassium to sodium mineral ratio is greater than three to one.

Processed food has a drastically altered mineral content (mineral chart chapter 3). Processed food diets have greatly diminished potassium and magnesium content. At the same time a processed food diet has a greatly increased amount of sodium added to preserve the shelf life of the product. This combination causes a chronic imbalance between potassium and sodium.

The same owner types that once had a survival advantage now have a disadvantage if a processed diet is chronically consumed. These owners retain sodium inappropriately and have reversed mineral content included in the processed food diet. Around middle age owners on a processed food diet will develop a whole range of health consequences. This leads to six obesity related health consequences. These owners who are predisposed to health consequences from the high sodium and low potassium diet were the genetically superior human design machines of prehistoric times. In modern times as long as they adhere to a processed food diet, they are on a rapid self-destruct program.

Six Ways Obesity is Propagated – Mineral Imbalance and Middle Age
1. Insulin resistance
2. Increased fat and cholesterol synthesis in the liver
3. Loss of protein content
4. Decreased steroid biosynthesis to keep blood pressure normal
5. Slower metabolic rate
6. Stress exacerbates the mineral imbalance and weight gain

All six of these factors need to be circumvented if an effective weight loss rate is desired. If one optimizes all six hormones (section two) that lead to obesity and corrects their mineral imbalance, their diet plan is more complete because they are now applying the best from the different diets available. They are also concurrently omitting the obsolete components of these diets in light of new scientific understanding. These are important if one really wants to know what makes them fat. When owners know what makes them fat they can progress. After all, getting better is what healing is all about.

Chronic Mineral Imbalanced Diets are a Major Cause of Insulin Resistance

The chronic consumption of a mineral imbalanced diet will lead to the need for increased insulin secretion. Increased insulin becomes necessary because insulin needs sufficient potassium to get sugar into the cells. One potassium is needed to take one sugar molecule out of the blood stream and into a cell.

The chronic ingestion of reversed ratios between potassium and sodium leads to a decreased availability of potassium for insulin directed sugar removal out of the blood stream. The delay of the blood lowering effect of insulin leads the pancreas to secrete more insulin.

The delay of potassium availability occurs after many years of consuming reversed mineral ratios. The blood stream amount of potassium contains only 2% of body potassium. The other 98% of potassium resides in the cells. It is the potassium in the cells that donates itself to keep the smaller potassium pool constant in the blood stream. Owners that eat processed foods will inevitably deplete their total potassium. The potassium in the blood stream can be thought of as the 2% 'tank' of potassium content. It is the very last tank to become depleted. The standard test at the doctor's office measures the blood stream level only. The blood stream value will only change when the larger tank has been severely depleted. The larger tank, containing 98% of potassium, resides in the numerous cells. Cells will sacrifice their potassium content in order to keep the blood levels in the normal range.

Here lays the deception occurring in America today. Physicians wrongly reassure their patients about the potassium levels in their blood stream while they have not inquired about the status of the larger tank. Failure to consider the consequences that ensue when the body becomes chronically deprived of the correct ratios between potassium and sodium intake leads to chronic degenerative diseases. Insulin resistance related disease is only one of several consequences of diminished potassium to sodium content.

Examples of chronic degenerative diseases that result from imbalanced potassium to sodium intake are adult onset diabetes, high blood pressure, high cholesterol, obesity, fatigue, and anxiety syndromes.

Insulin resistance can eventually progress into adult onset diabetes (liver chapter). The accompanying signs of obesity and an abnormal cholesterol profile often are associated with adult onset diabetes. The mineral balance between potassium and sodium dramatically affects all three of these processes. Misery is propagated when this important relationship is ignored.

Insulin resistance is caused by a chronic imbalance between potassium and sodium intake. As the mineral imbalance increases more insulin is secreted to normalize sugar intake because adequate potassium is needed to bring sugar into most cells. For each sugar transported into most cell types, one potassium is needed. The trouble arises from the fact that the body conserves the blood stream potassium level when potassium is in scarce supply. The needed potassium is then acquired at the expense and sacrifice of the potassium content of other cells.

The pancreas senses that blood sugar is still elevated and more insulin is secreted when there is a delay in lowering blood sugar. The increased amount of insulin needed to do the same job for a specific sugar amount is termed insulin resistance. When an owner's pancreas is exhausted in its ability to produce insulin, then adult onset diabetes results and blood sugar begins to rise. There are many people who are able to keep making more and more insulin and therefore they do not get diabetes. However, it is the high insulin levels that make both of these types of owners obese and have abnormal cholesterol levels. The only difference between the two types of owners is in one the pancreas reaches exhaustion and blood sugar rises.

It is the high insulin that promotes the blood vessels getting clogged with fat. The ability of insulin to lower the blood sugar is potassium dependent. Less potassium availability will delay the ability to lower the blood sugar level. The pancreas senses this delay and more insulin is secreted as the body cells sacrifice the potassium necessary for insulin to work. The end result is the peripheral cells receive less nutrition. They need adequate potassium to bring sugar aboard. In contrast, the liver uptakes a higher amount of sugar and processes it into more fat and cholesterol than is healthy.

Blood vessels get fat and people get fat when the fat maker message is present. The fat maker message is always delivered by insulin. If there is no insulin, there is no fat. With high insulin there will be more body fat. Insulin resistance is often caused by potassium depletion in middle age.

Increased Cholesterol and Fat Synthesis in the Liver

An increased message content in the liver to make more cholesterol and fat occurs when there is insulin resistance. Cholesterol and fat are made from the sugar that is not entering other cells because of diminished potassium content. Diminished potassium content impedes the ability of the peripheral cells, muscle cells, to uptake carbohydrate nutrition. The increased blood sugar becomes more liver accessible. The liver does not need potassium to suck sugar out of the blood stream and make fat and cholesterol. All the liver needs is adequate message content from insulin and it begins sucking out the blood sugar. The liver needs adequate potassium, like other cells to store sugar as glycogen. Glycogen storage requires fixed amounts of potassium to sugar. Without adequate potassium the liver is only able to make cholesterol and fat. Next, the increase in availability of sugar in the liver and the increased insulin message in the liver accelerate the liver manufactured cholesterol and fat particles, LDL cholesterol. LDL (triglycerides) cholesterol is a hallmark of high insulin. This mechanism explains the potassium deficient diet's contribution to this problem.

In the insulin resistant state, at the level of the liver, the low carbohydrate diet can fail to protect the owner because no one has counseled them about their potassium deficiency. Potassium deficiency will lead to increased insulin production (insulin resistance) even on a low carbohydrate diet. If these owners restore total potassium content, their insulin needs will drop dramatically over time.

Many owners on low carbohydrate diets are not correcting their potassium deficiency that causes an increase in insulin levels. The increased insulin levels direct the liver to produce huge amounts of LDL cholesterol. When LDL cholesterol levels increase there is an increased risk for blood vessel disease and obesity. It is the increased insulin level that is directing both of these disease processes.

When one increases potassium content then they will be able to tolerate more carbohydrates without the abnormal increase in insulin levels. Obese owners are warned to initially curtail carbohydrates dramatically to decrease the appetite center activation that insulin directs. The more normal the weight becomes then the more carbohydrates from real food that can be consumed.

The reason adequate potassium content in the body is so important for controlling cholesterol is because of its ability to help normalize blood sugar with less insulin. Less insulin means less fat and cholesterol synthesis in the liver. The liver is a faithful servant that does as the message directs.

The tug of war between glucagon and insulin in the liver was discussed. The low carbohydrate diet, in the presence of adequate body potassium, will have more glucagon message content. More glucagon message content will, in physically active owners, curtail fat and cholesterol synthesis. This explains why owners on high protein and fat diets with low carbohydrate intake have decreased cholesterol levels.

The fact that adequate potassium is needed for the body to hold onto protein has been known by science for over fifty years. Decreased protein content results in shrinking muscles, organs, skin, and bones.

Mineral Imbalanced Diets Lead to Loss of Body Protein

Owners that arrive at middle age with a history of consuming processed food diets will experience chronic protein depletion in their tissues. These bodies sacrifice cellular proteins in order to obtain sufficient potassium for the blood stream. This process takes many years to manifest. Even though the depletion rate is slow, eventually these middle-aged victims begin to look typical as in an increased middle area from fat accumulation and smaller muscles in the limbs and chest areas. The protein depletion also shrinks the size of their organs.

The protein depletion process occurs because potassium in the cells stabilizes the proteins. When a cell loses potassium the protein content will decrease. Little muscles, little organs, and shriveled skin are the result of mineral imbalanced diets because of processed food that contains an altered mineral content.

Less body protein translates to decreased cell function in the affected cells and less need for cell energy. Less energy equates to fewer calories needed to gain weight. Less energy also means less ability to participate in what life has to offer. The cycle of obesity is broken when a middle-aged owner begins to understand how to regain mineral balance. The first step of this process involves a commitment to real food diets that restore mineral intake in proper proportions.

Mineral Deficient Diets Reduce Steroid Production to Have Normal Blood Pressure

The body, which is chronically fed altered mineral ratios faces a difficult choice in middle age. It can try to maintain steroid production, but the side effect is an increase in blood pressure. Alternately, some bodies decrease steroid manufacture, but blood pressure normalizes.

Owners that eat a real food diet can secrete optimal amounts of aldosterone without raising blood pressure because they are consuming the right ratios of minerals. Owners that eat processed foods are consuming mineral ratios that are destructive to body functions. These altered minerals eventually strain the ability to keep an appropriate mineral balance.

The altered mineral balance causes the middle age problem in both cases. Some bodies increase blood pressure to continue manufacturing adequate steroids that depends on adequate aldosterone production in the adrenal (adrenal chapter). Other bodies diminish aldosterone production, but have a normal blood pressure. Aldosterone gives the message to the adrenals and gonads to increase steroid production. Owners do not tolerate increased aldosterone levels with mineral imbalances between potassium and sodium. Potassium and sodium imbalanced owners will conserve excess fluid when aldosterone becomes elevated. Excess fluid leads to blood pressure elevation.

Mineral Imbalances Lead to a Slower Metabolism

The diminished protein content slows the metabolic rate. Protein content comprises the active fraction of body tissue metabolically. Proteins, like enzymes, consume energy and therefore metabolize calories. Metabolism also slows with mineral imbalance because there is less electrical potential across mineral depleted cell membranes. Mineral imbalance slows metabolism because it diminishes cellular charge (section five). When the body is resting the majority of energy is spent in recharging the trillions of cell membranes (the cellular force fields). These can only recharge adequately when the right mineral ratios are opposing one another.

Each cell uses the cell membrane charge energy to sustain life. There is less membrane energy content when the minerals are altered in their proportion. This is similar to what would happen to a car battery that had its mineral content altered. Car batteries function better when manufactures directions are followed adding the proper fluids.

The food industry is not cognizant of this basic body design feature. Magnesium and potassium are depleted from food when it is processed. Next large amounts of sodium are added to processed food in order to retard spoilage. This altered formula of mineral ratios is dumped into cells year after year. Around middle age feeble cell batteries lead to diminished calories burned and weight gain.

Stress Exacerbates Mineral Imbalance

Stress will increase the need for insulin. Increased insulin leads to an increased fat making message content. There is an additional way that chronic stress makes fat by involving the extra potassium loss that was increased by cortisol. Increased cortisol causes increased sodium retention and increased potassium loss. This aldosterone effect of cortisol occurs because cortisol at high levels will create message content that is similar to aldosterone in its sodium retentive effects. Sodium retention and potassium wasting are not a problem with normal levels of cortisol. Cortisol at normal levels is weak in message content to retain sodium and excrete potassium.

Surgeons are well aware of this fact in post surgery states. The body cannot survive the stress of surgery unless there is a massive output of cortisol from the adrenal. The increased cortisol excretion rate depletes potassium. Surgeons routinely give intravenous potassium postoperatively because the owner's body will secrete increased cortisol in order to survive the stress of surgery. The increased potassium in the IV prevents a precipitous fall in potassium. With mineral balance in mind the real food diet that allows this is contrasted with the processed food diet.

Two Diets on Opposite Extremes in Mineral Content

Real food is high in potassium and magnesium, but low in sodium and unprocessed.

Fresh vegetables	Fresh fruits
Eggs	Fresh meat, chicken and fish
Low salt cheese	Brown sugar and honey
Unprocessed rice	Unprocessed grains
Unprocessed nuts	Unprocessed beans (dry or fresh)
Potatoes	

Processed food is high in sodium content, but low for both magnesium and potassium

> Anything that comes in a box
> Anything that comes in a can
> Anything from a fast food restaurant
> Anything that has more sodium content than potassium content
> Watch the amount of sodium added to frozen foods
> Store bought bread with a few exceptions

A word of caution becomes necessary for those owners that are already overweight. Overweight owners need further dietary restriction within the real foods that are high in carbohydrate content. Even though some foods are real foods, when an owner is already overweight, the high carbohydrate foods need to be further restricted. Carbohydrate curtailment allows insulin needs to drop. A lowered insulin need is the primary move for exiting the torture chamber. Once one moves outside the torture chamber, they can begin to lose weight. Weight loss accelerates when both the carbohydrate intake and the mineral imbalanced components are correct. As a normal weight approaches, there will be increased tolerance for more carbohydrate. Every owner physiology differs and needs the counsel of a competent physician for sustained weight loss to occur.

A good place to start involves the almost complete elimination of carbohydrate contained real food and all processed foods. The high carbohydrate containing real foods are potatoes, rice, beans, grains, brown sugar, honey, and pasta. Following this initial approach will counter the IGF-1 deficit occurring in obesity by requiring less insulin-produced side effects. Once the target weight, mineral balance, and hormone balance are achieved some carbohydrates, from real food sources can be allowed. Physiology is unique to individuals and the counsel of a competent physician is necessary.

Summary of the weight loss considerations:

1. Hormone levels for insulin, cortisol, androgens, estrogen, thyroid, epinephrine, and IGF-1
2. Exercise program to counteract cortisol and increase growth hormone
3. Stress management
4. Real food diet that provides a balanced mineral intake

Case History (application of principles)

Jack was a forty four year old professional that began to notice weight gain over the last several years. This weight gain occurred despite a vigorous work out schedule that was often 1-2 hours long for each session. Workouts included a run in the mountains; strenuous uphill climbs, and prolonged mountain bike rides. Despite the commitment to fitness training, he continued to notice a slow, but progressive 'fat tire' around his midsection. He attempted to follow the ADA diet and was always hungry. Food was constantly on his mind. He was in the torture chamber. Hormones drove an excessive feeding behavior.

Eventually Jack came across Dr. Atkins book and figured it would not hurt to give this contrary advice a try. In the book it was explained how to get insulin levels down and how this will greatly diminish the preoccupation with the next feeding event.

Jack eventually went on to learn, through his doctor's counsel, about several other hormones that affect feeding behavior and the tendency to gain weight. He also began to understand the hefty contribution of insulin to his high cholesterol. To Jack's credit he exercised regularly, which increases testosterone production and secretion in the gonads. Testosterone counteracts the desire of insulin to make fat. He understood that middle age leads to a tendency for decreased testosterone production even with regular exercise.

Jack began to understand how increased carbohydrate consumption increases insulin secretion that eventually tips the scale, in the setting of falling testosterone, for increased fat manufacture.

There is a genetic variability in how much insulin is needed to stimulate abnormal LDL cholesterol formation to abnormal levels. A general rule is that if LDL and/or triglyceride levels are too high then suspect high insulin as the culprit. Remember that both diminished thyroid function and very rare genetic defects can cause the same abnormalities of increased blood fat of this type. Strict adherence to the outlined diet will dramatically lower LDL cholesterol in most people. It is important to assess the status of other hormones (thyroid, androgen, cortisol, IGF-1, estrogens, and adrenaline). Finally, mineral balance and its influence on insulin levels need to be optimized if weight normalization is to be realized.

Individuals with high testosterone (athletes, young adult males, and body builders) can tolerate a higher carbohydrate intake. Likewise, an owner with mineral balance between sodium and potassium can handle more carbohydrate intake. In both cases less insulin is needed to move sugar into cells. Less insulin correlates with less fat manufacture.

It is the high testosterone and growth hormone, with consequent IGF-1 increases, combination occurring in youth that allows a decreased insulin requirement. The growth hormone levels increase IGF-1, which facilitates sugar uptake out of the blood stream without the fat manufacture message content contained in the insulin hormone.

Once fat begins to accumulate the body hormones must change in order to return to a trim physique. This summarizes what happened to Jack before he realized this fundamental fact in the attainment of a more youthful physique again.

When the optimal weight is achieved some increased (tailored to activity level) carbohydrate intake is allowed. Owners like Jack need to understand that decreasing the insulin and cutting back on carbohydrates, will decrease the stimulation of the appetite center in the brain.

Owners, as they head into middle age are destined to failure if they adhere to the ADA diet. Failure usually manifests as a slow, but steady increase in abdominal obesity measured from one year to the next. The torture chamber always wins until a hormonal harmony facilitates weight loss.

Knowledge provides power to take action in the destiny of the physique. This is what happened in Jack's case as he applied basic hormone knowledge his 'middle aged physique' began to rejuvenate to a closer version of his youth. He also noted a dramatic decrease of total cholesterol and LDL cholesterol (triglycerides). This means that Jack will have to watch carbohydrates more closely than others because a return to unfavorable cholesterol will always result if insulin levels increase.

This dramatic improvement in Jack's LDL cholesterol and triglycerides occurred despite his eating four eggs with extra cheese every morning for breakfast. This effect explains the ability of the high protein and fat diet to raise glucagon while lowering insulin. The change in the hormone ratio will turn down the rate of liver synthesized cholesterol.

Jack had an added weight loss advantage by regularly engaging in aerobic exercise that burns calories, but also stimulates gonads to manufacture and release increased androgens. The ratio between glucagon and insulin will improve with regular exercise. Glucagon turns off cholesterol synthesis in the liver and increases this fuel in the blood stream. The increased fuel that the glucagon message directs, without adequate exercise will eventually require more insulin. Viewed in this way, it is easy to see why regular exercise is one of the biochemical advantages of health.

Later in the workup process, Jack's doctor noted high stress operating his life. Prolonged stress depletes adrenal glands and affects the adrenal itself. It also increases cortisol release that directs energy away from cellular rejuvenation and into survival. When stress is prolonged it shifts the optimal ratio between DHEA (an adrenal androgen with testosterone-like activity) production and into cortisol production. Increased cortisol is one of the hormones that direct the gonads to manufacture and release less androgen. The increased amount of cortisol also directs the liver to dump sugar into the blood stream. Modern stress is usually of a mental nature. This extra sugar is not used by physical activity. When this sedentary stress occurs, insulin is released to bring the blood sugar back down to normal.

When stress is the operational emotion there needs to be consideration about the message content to raise blood sugar even when no carbohydrates are eaten. Now this discussion is flipping things on their head. As cortisol increases, the reoccurring body theme about hormones needing to be balanced comes into play. The only difference is that stress creates a situation where cortisol is the weight that needs the counter weight of insulin to put the breaks on the increase in blood sugar. This is another mechanism for creating a torture chamber within if prolonged stress occurs. The fact that cortisol raises blood sugar makes sense teleologically when remembering that in survival situations prehistorically (as in running from the jaws of some large animal) a rapid rise in blood sugar confers a survival advantage by increasing alertness and facilitating muscle fuel. The problem today occurs because many stresses are psychological. The predominance of psychological stress means that no flight ever comes. The stress molecules circulate directing valuable energy inappropriately. One of the inappropriate consequences of mental stress is an increased blood sugar.

The final point about Jack was the hardest part for his physician to realize. Mineral imbalance in middle age is a substantial cause of fat production. There is little understanding about mineral balance and fat. This information is not in many diets offered today.

Jack eventually began to appreciate the many similarities between car batteries and his cells. He began to realize that he would not alter the mineral composition of a car battery any more than he would his trillions of cells. This relationship helped him to understand that unless he took in mineral ratios similar to body design, his many cell batteries would become depleted. When minerals are consumed in the proper design ratios the cell batteries can charge. Only a body that has fully charged cell batteries can sufficiently liberate enough potassium into the blood stream to help sugar enter cells. Adequate potassium lowers insulin requirements dramatically. The mineral determinant is the fifth determinant of how much insulin a body needs to normalize blood sugar. All five determinants were eventually improved in Jacks life.

The five basic determinants of insulin requirements are:

1. Carbohydrate load
2. Mental stress load
3. Exercise level
4. IGF-1 levels
5. Mineral ratios of intake within the diet.

When these five basic determinants are optimal an owner will have a normal insulin level. There are other factors, but these are the central players of fat making potential in a body. They need to be reconciled first and the other factors can be worked on later.

This section concerned itself with how to supply and absorb molecular replacement parts. In the colon section, the concept behind the fifth principle was introduced. The fifth principle of longevity concerns the adequacy of taking out the cell trash.

SECTION IV

TAKING OUT THE TRASH WATER

Principle 5

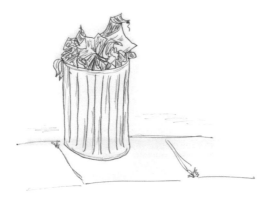

Some people collect trash in their yards, houses, and cars. Grime is everywhere. So it is with certain owner's cells that collect trash water within their body tissues and chambers. These cells are crying out for someone to take out the garbage. Dirty cells lose functional ability. The most powerful trash remover, water, needs the help of certain body organ systems. These organ systems filter out the trash water or recycle it after being purified.

The trash collectors of the body, filters and purifying plants fall under the domain of six organ systems, the lungs, kidneys, liver, skin, colon, and immune system.

A common factor occurs, besides water, that determines the functional ability of the six trash removal organs. All six of these organs need adequate thyroid message content. The thyroid message is among the most powerful hormone class (level 1 hormones). Only the most powerful hormones can directly instruct these organ's cellular DNA programs (genes). Thyroid message content facilitates infrastructure development activities in the cells of these six organ systems. Failure to recognize this central determinant for trash removal systems has significant health consequences. All six of these organ systems need adequate thyroid message content to function. Inadequate thyroid message content results in prematurely old bodies. This fact underscores the relationship between the fifth and third (optimal informational message content) principles of healthful longevity.

Diminished thyroid function in these six-trash removal organs manifest:

1. In the lungs as decreased ability to increase oxygen delivery under physical stress. Thyroid hormone, in lung tissue, is a determinate of the ability of the lung to respond to increased adrenaline message content.
2. In the kidneys the thyroid level determines infrastructure investment activities of kidney cells. This keeps the kidney tissue from succumbing to filtration pressures, which desire to inflict

harm on the delicate epithelium which lines the functional unit of kidney; the nephron.

3. The liver cells are dependent on thyroid message content to direct the investment in the rejuvenation of the liver cell.

4. When thyroid content falls at the level of the skin cell, there are many deleterious changes that ensue includeing:
   a. Dryness, scales, the puffiness of myxedema, and yellow discoloration.
   b. Hair is thin with additional premature grayness and brittleness.
   c. When these clinical signs occur in the skin, the less obvious role of the skin in trash removal is also diminished.

5. Low thyroid at the level of the colon manifests clinically as chronic constipation that causes backward absorption of many putrefaction molecules. These leaking back into the body can eventually overwhelm the ability of the liver to detoxify them and they can spill into the general circulation.

6. In the immune system, diminished thyroid message content decreases the ability of immune type cells to consume (phagocytize) unwanted cells (cancer, bacteria, virus's, and debris).

Failure to take out the trash, which continuously generates within the cells, can lead to some chronic degenerative diseases such as certain types of arthritis, tumor growths, degenerative skin changes, diminished organ function, and some of the mental deterioration syndromes.

The body has an ongoing problem caused by the toxic waste that spews out of the trillions of cellular factories. Owners who practice habits that improve waste removal strategies have an advantage in the maintenance of physical youth. Owners who stuff their cells with waste begin to look like they feel. Waste products build up in the cells, around the cells, and in the blood stream. External sources of trash add to the internally generated accumulations and increase the overall waste removal burden. Examples of these external trash generators are the increased air pollutants, water pollutants, food adulterants, and toxicities from prescription breakdown products.

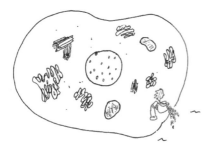

A useful metaphor that addresses trash accumulation is found in the rivers, deltas, and lakes of the earth. Only when the river that feeds the deltas and lakes is clean, can downstream entities remain pristine. When factories dump waste into streams and rivers, not only the river is polluted. The downstream deltas and lakes are contaminated as well.

The ongoing problem of cellular trash removal has many of the same challenges. Pristine mountain lakes are similar to young cells in the non-polluted state. The wilderness river deltas with their delicate ecosystems that depend on clean water are like the spaces between the cells (the interstitial space). The rivers are the recipients of the clean and the polluted tributary waters. River purity and blood stream purity become compromised when 'factories' are allowed to dump toxins into them. The actions of life create waste that constantly dumps into the blood stream. Unlike the physical world of rivers, deltas, and lakes, the body has elaborate cleansing systems built into the waterway system. These elaborate cleansing systems remove toxins and purify wastewater. The ability to remove the ever-generating waste depends on the health of the six organ systems.

Healthy cells are much like pristine mountain lakes. As cells accumulate trash water, secondary to a failure of these trash removal systems, they become similar to polluted lakes. This process also describes what happens to water that surrounds cells and fluids in the waterways (plasma, lymph, and cerebral spinal fluid). Failure of the trash removal systems in the cells, around the cells, and in the blood stream causes trash water accumulation. Many health problems arise simply because no one helps these owners heal their six trash removal organ systems.

Body composition is normally (approximately) 67% water. Generous supplies of clean water bathe tissues. Adequate clean water allows the toxins to flush away. Ongoing trash removal enlivens continued health. Some owners accumulate trash water because the capacity of their trash removal systems is diminished. Each of the six trash removal organ systems has unique contributions and abilities. An interrelationship occurs between these sanitation and recycling facilities.

This new principle describes where the cellular trash comes from and how the body is designed to dispose of it. The different types of cellular trash and how they are generated will be considered. Kidneys are the first trash removal organs that will be discussed. Some other functions of kidney maintenance and health are included.

Chapter 16

Kidneys

The kidneys are the filters of fluids that pass through the blood stream. Their job is to decide what to keep and what to discard when the blood passes through the filter. The kidney comprises one of the main trash collectors for the small and electrically charged 'dust' particles. Electrically charged 'atomic dust' particles are produced as a result of combustion of foods. When food metabolizes certain charged particles are created and become the waste product of the cellular factories. This is one type of cellular waste that discharges into the waterways.

These charged particles include acids generated in the process of the combustion of carbohydrates, fat, and some proteins. The lungs remove the majority of acid produced during combustion. The kidney is the only place where certain types of acids can exit. When the ability of the kidneys diminishes these acids begin to build up in tissue.

The amount of acid in tissue plays a role in determining:

1. How well the enzymatic machinery can function.
2. How vulnerable the cellular architecture is.
3. The energetic charge of the cellular battery (force field).
4. The ability to generate energy.

The kidney filters two types of 'atomic dust' particles that need to be carefully regulated. The first is the acid content (H+ protons). The second is that the kidney carefully attempts to regulate the mineral concentrations. The main minerals that are regulated are sodium, potassium, magnesium, and calcium.

Diseases like high blood pressure often result from a failure in the mineral balance of the kidney's trash water removal strategies. If the reason the kidney has inappropriately wasted or conserved a specific mineral is identified, healing can begin.

Cellular Discharge of Organic Acids and the Solution is the Responsibility of the Kidneys

The first part of the kidney's trash removal role concerns the importance of acid removal. Acid content is about the amount of positively charged hydrogen protons separated, in space, from their negatively charged halves. All acids have hydrogen as their positively charged half, but can have numerous negatively charged halves. The ease with which the positive (hydrogen proton) separates from the negative half in a fluid determines the strength of the acid. The more these dissociations occur, the stronger the acid. Separation is determined by the molecular qualities of the negative half. Weaker acids separate less readily from their positive and negative halves. The amount of acid content in living tissue determines its energetic capabilities, the functional abilities of the enzymatic machinery, and whether components dissolve or solidify in that tissue. Health is impossible without the right acid content in the different tissues.

Different body chambers have specific acid content requirements for optimum functioning. The stomach requires adequate acid production as a prerequisite for the ability to turn on its enzymatic machinery to full capacity. After the food exits the stomach and trickles into the duodenum, the opposite conditions occur. These conditions depend on the release of the acid neutralizing juices delivered from the pancreas. This is only possible when the pancreas manufactures this type of juice and secretes it into the duodenum chamber. The enzymatic machinery, designed to finish what the stomach started, requires a much higher alkalinity (less acid) for optimal function. A little further down the digestive tract in the colon, the food remnants must be sufficiently acidified or yeast over growth occurs. None of these chambers specific acid level requirements can be maintained without the kidney faithfully regulating certain types of total acid content.

The kidney allows other tissues to maintain the right amount of organic acid content similar to the catalyst that allows the right electrical charge to occur. The right electrical charge keeps life energy unfolding. It is the job of the kidney to either excrete or conserve certain acids that it constantly filters.

Understanding the chemistry of opposing ions is important in the role of the kidneys in taking out the trash. The physical world revolves by opposing molecular forces. All molecules are composed of atoms that are drawn together by these forces seeking relative stability once united. Some atoms have more strength than others that is measured by the electronegativity of an element relative to all other elements. The stronger the electronegativity of an element, the more force of these elements to gather negative charges. Negative charges are gathered by the stronger elements from the electrons they steal from the weaker electronegative elements. There are an equal number of positive (protons) as compared to negative (electrons) charges in the universe.

Chemistry involves the study of combinations of the atomic elements that occur. Also the science of chemistry involves an interest in the energy contained within these associations and in the energy released when they break apart. The natural world (the physical world of nonliving things) moves in the direction of more stable molecular arrangements. In the process of achieving more stable molecular arrangements these changing molecules give off energy much like a battery that runs down. This process is the fundamental law of entropy.

Living things somehow violate the basic law of entropy because living things are able to trap energy in usable packets after combusting food with oxygen. These energy packets are used to build complex molecular machines, power up the energy of cell factories and membranes, and manufacture architectural structures at the cellular level. Life energy somehow moves simple molecular arrangements in the opposite direction and creates more complexity (section six). The life process of complex molecular creation is not possible without a strict control of the acid and mineral content in the fluids which baths cells. It is the kidney's job to maintain optimal acid and mineral content so that the body stays balanced.

In the process of cellular combustion of foodstuffs, large amounts of acid are generated. Having just the right amount of acid ensures that the biological molecules are in the right configuration. The right amount of acid allows the molecules to possess the right electrical charge consistent with optimal function. Different body chambers have their own optimum level of acid content that creates the most efficient work environment for the enzymatic machines designed for that chamber.

The body requires that the right amount of hydrogen protons be in body fluid. These protons are sufficiently distanced from the negatively charged half, and this creates the electrical milieu that will optimize other molecular charges. Acid excess or deficiency in tissue leads to energetic, electrical, molecular, and structural aberrations. It is the job of the kidney to remove the trash that is constantly generated called organic acid. The organic acids are constantly discharged from the cells into the blood stream. One of the kidney's roles regards the ability to excrete organic acids.

There is a requirement beyond the need for right amount of acid to be present. There is a requirement for proper amounts of essential minerals (calcium, magnesium, sodium, potassium, chloride, bicarbonate, and others). The proper amount of these minerals is not possible without the kidney excreting excess minerals and conserving deficient minerals. When acid and mineral requirements are actualized an optimal electrical environment is created throughout the remainder of the body for each cell type. It harmonizes the multiple electrical charges of the bulky molecules (proteins, phospholipids, mucopolysaccharides, and nucleic acids). The kidney is responsible for taking out organic acid and mineral trash.

The right electrical charge occurs with balanced acid and mineral content. The kidney needs to remove the organic acids that cellular factories constantly generate and ensure the proper balance of essential minerals. The minerals are continually lost or accumulating. The kidney sorts out what needs excretion and what needs to be conserved. Performance of this task is a determinant of the overall health.

There are two main types of acid in the body, gaseous acid (carbon dioxide) and organic acids. There is more carbon dioxide generated than organic acid. Much of the acid generated from the cellular factories is removed in the lungs as carbon dioxide except organic acids, which is mostly the responsibility of the kidney. One example of an organic acid not removed by the kidney but processed in the liver is lactic acid. Examples of organic acids created by the reactions of living cells are acids of sulfate, phosphate, nitrate, carbonate, and ammonia. These waste acids are generated from the cellular factories up stream and filtered by the kidney, which also removes or conserves the mineral content

Mineral Balance and Other Organs that Help the Kidney

Each human kidney is composed of 1.3 million complex and vibrating filter machines each called a nephron. The nephron is often thought of as the functional unit of the kidney. At rest 25% of all the blood volume circulates through the kidney. Before the blood can leave the kidney it must pass through the filters contained in the nephrons, the glomerulus. Kidneys know what is needed and what is trash.

The kidney in cooperation with the lungs removes the majority of acid generated in the body and is a primary regulator of the mineral content. Healthy owners maintain stable amounts of the essential minerals and acid content that is unique for each cell type.

Two main things need to happen if the total concentration of these minerals is to remain at optimal levels (sodium, chlorine, potassium, calcium, magnesium, bicarbonate and phosphorous). First, there needs to be an adequate intake in the diet and a digestive tract capable of absorbing what is offered (section 3). Second, there needs to be the right amount of message content delivered to the kidney that instructs excretion or conservation of minerals. In living things message content is determined by how much and which hormones is delivered to the tissue in question. When these two processes occur the owner is in mineral balance.

Some other organ systems interrelate to the kidney in the task of acid and mineral balance. Similarly, the lungs are responsible for removing the gaseous acids generated in cellular factories. Lungs are minimal players in regard to mineral balance. Two other organ systems, the colon and skin, help the kidney with mineral balance. They are involved with the maintenance of mineral balance when adequate supplies are present. There is some backup between the trash water removal organs. In all cases, of acid and mineral balance, these organ systems need the help of the most powerful medicine of all, water.

Mineral Balance – Proportions of Minerals in the Diet

The most common diseases that originate in the kidney result from the chronic ingestion of imbalanced minerals in the diet. The typical situation is one in which an owner eats predominately processed food. These food groups have a drastically altered mineral content from their natural state. It is the natural proportions of minerals that occur in real food that are needed. Food processing diminishes magnesium and potassium contents and increases sodium content.

Natural food has natural mineral content intact and unaltered. Real foods are fresh vegetables, fruits, meats, chicken, fish, and grains, beans, and seeds before they are processed (ground into flour or butter). These foods all contain excellent mineral ratio content and when fresh, are high in potassium and low in sodium.

The foods that are green or seeds are also high in magnesium. Magnesium and potassium deficiency are quite common in America because Americans consume large amounts of processed foods. Owners who subsist on processed foods develop mineral imbalance diseases. More pertinent to the trash water removal functions is how altered mineral intake eventually curtails the ability of the kidney to remove excess minerals. Minerals in excess are a form of kidney trash. There are situations that arise when one mineral is deficient and the excess mineral is allowed to build up. The processed food diet favors this scenario.

Many prescription drugs become chronically necessary because clinicians ignore sub-optimal mineral intake inherent in the American diet. Altered mineral intake patterns result in many types of high blood pressure problems, fluid retention, body wasting syndromes, and many different syndromes of mineral excess and/or deficiencies.

Mineral Balance depends on the Quality of the Message Content

In the kidney's, as in the other organs, there is a recurring theme. The quality of the message content is a central determinant of the functional ability in the target organ. The quality of the message content determines how the kidney is directed to spend energy.

The science that unites these two vital concepts (message content and minerals) is well developed. The trouble begins in the clinical setting from the fractured medical thought among the specialties. As medicine becomes increasingly ultra -specialized there is a trend toward disjointed and incomplete reasoning in light of the holism that science has revealed. Holism often leads to healing. Many times healing from disease is a matter of understanding where the imbalance began. Imbalanced acid and minerals lead to extra trash water and high blood pressure. Healing from high blood pressure is a good example of the importance of scientific holism.

When the Trash Removal Systems in the Kidneys Fail High Blood Pressure can Result

Ideally, when owners first head toward mineral excesses or deficiency, high blood pressure, arthritis, or fluid imbalance, the trash water would be thoroughly evaluated. Trash water evaluations include attention directed at the quality of the hormone message and mineral content arriving in the kidney. Early diagnosis of high blood pressure is easy to heal when the mineral deficiency is quickly identified and corrected. In most cases, which involve chronic potassium deficiency and sodium excess, the kidney becomes damaged with the passage of time and elevates the blood pressure. Low potassium diets damage the kidney function. Before kidney function becomes permanently damaged the correction of the potassium and sodium imbalance will heal the problem. This fact provides an example where symptom control medicine has the consequence of needing a permanent prescription. The kidneys were damaged because symptom control medications were administered rather than a diet that included balanced mineral content.

Symptom control medicine usually affects a disease symptom by poisoning some enzymatic process. One example of poisoning an enzymatic process is the common prescription class called the angiotensin converting enzyme inhibitors (ACE inhibitors). ACE is used to activate angiotensin 1 to angiotensin 2. Unfortunately, when one targets the kidney content of this enzyme machine, it is not possible to avoid poisoning the same machines found in other parts of the body. Two additional locations for this enzyme are the lungs and testis. In the lungs ACE is used to control inflammation. In the testis ACE is needed to promote adequate steroid synthesis.

In some cases this may be the only way to lower blood pressure to a safe level. In the majority of cases, there are safer ways to cure or prevent high blood pressure. Actually one of the main beneficial effects of this type of blood pressure medication, the ACE inhibitors, is their ability to help conserve potassium content. If owners were counseled on this fact before kidney damage was permanent, they could start a real food diet (section three).

Most high blood pressure problems are the result of the kidney failing to remove trash. Blood pressure can be lowered to safe levels if one addresses the cause of trash water accumulation. Rather than poison an enzyme to bring blood pressure down, consider the four common kidney derived causes of blood pressure elevation: insulin excess, magnesium deficiency, inadequate potassium intake relative to sodium intake and cortisol or aldosterone excess. In each case the ability of the kidney to remove trash water is compromised. When trash water accumulates in the pipes the pressure elevates.

These causes can be traced back to hormone message content mismatch. This results in the wrong hormones being delivered to the kidney and this misdirects it on how to spend energy. Additionally, the deficient or excess minerals cause high blood pressure because the kidney cannot remove trash properly. The kidney responds to whichever hormones deliver message content. Message content determines how the kidney is directed to spend energy.

The kidney can send out appropriate or inappropriate message content to distant tissues via the secretion of its own informational substances. The types and amounts of hormones (informational substances) that the kidney excretes determine whether it is helpful or exacerbating for an imbalance.

A holistic approach to blood pressure control includes an assessment of hormone tone (the quality of informational substances). It also includes attention to mineral balance. The science exists for an accurate assessment of the major hormones and minerals for an owner. It is time to implement what is known so that healing opportunities are not missed. Blood pressure elevations can begin in the kidneys with dysfunction of the trash removal of minerals. High blood pressure can be thought of as a consequence of the kidney failing to take out its share of waste. An assessment of insulin excess, magnesium deficiency, potassium imbalance, and excess cortisol and/or aldosterone is appropriate. This is preferred before committing to symptom control medicine.

Insulin Caused High Blood Pressure

Often blood pressure lowers when owners commit to a diet that reduces the need for insulin since the counter response to insulin is largely cortisol. Cortisol has powerful fluid retaining side effects when it rises above low levels. Recall the antique weight scale and picture the more insulin one has to secrete (the more carbohydrates, the more insulin), the greater the need for larger counter weight, cortisol. The body needs more cortisol to oppose the desire of insulin to suck every sugar molecule from the blood stream. Cortisol is one of the main counter weights to insulin, but because cortisol elevation promotes fluid retention it can elevate the pressure.

Insulin authorities like Bernstein and Atkins believe that insulin has a direct effect on the kidney that promotes blood pressure elevation. To really know how insulin interacts with the kidney further research is needed.

A Stanford researcher, Dr. Gerald Reaven, has coined the term Syndrome X that describes excess insulin, which causes high blood pressure. Syndrome X also includes symptoms of owners who are on an accelerated path toward heart disease. These owners seem to have an excessive oxidation (rusting phenomena) rate in their tissues. Insulin excess is one of the main aberrations that allow Syndrome X to work on body destruction (blood pressure chapter). Syndrome X starts with high insulin and ends in fluid and sodium retention.

Excess fluid and sodium retention become trash water that the kidney should remove. Some authorities believe that insulin excess is responsible for half of all high blood pressure states. A lowered carbohydrate intake will decrease the need for insulin. When high insulin causes high blood pressure then attention here is warranted.

Magnesium Deficiency Caused High Blood Pressure

Another group of high blood pressure patients can be helped by high quality magnesium supplementation. Magnesium is a powerful smooth muscle relaxant. Smooth muscles are plentiful in the arteries.[17]

Magnesium supplements occur as salts that contain a positive and negative half that separate when dissolved in water. Like acids, salts in the body fluids in the right amounts create the proper electrical milieu that allows life processes to continue. They charge the system.

The similarity between a salt and an acid is that both are made with a positive and a negative half. However, with acid there is always hydrogen in the positive half. In contrast, salts contain different types of positively charged halves. Usually these are minerals, but never only hydrogen as the positive half. Both acids and salts can have the same types of negative halves. When a salt contains the same negative half as an acid it's called the salt of an acid. Lastly, minerals are always on the positive half. Magnesium is a mineral.

The body charges trillions of different cells electrically by the manipulation of the potential differences between the various minerals across a membrane. On opposite sides of the membranes the concentration differences between the salts and acid content creates potential energy. The cells to power life actions can use the potential energy contained in these membranes. These mineral differences are constantly being recreated so the membrane energy is not depleted. The process is similar in the car battery that always needs to be recharged when the motor consumes fuel. When the cell burns fuel it creates ATP to constantly resupply the energy content contained in the membrane. The membranes re-power from the mineral pumps contained within that exchange magnesium for calcium. Other pumps exchange sodium for potassium. The power contained in cell membranes is created by the difference in concentrations across the membrane of the various minerals. Excessive minerals behave as trash because they alter the proper proportion of balanced opposing minerals. Mineral deficiencies can also alter the proper proportion between opposing minerals. Magnesium deficiency commonly results from eating a processed food diet.

The positive and negative halves of salts are separated in spatial arrangement. This allows positive and negative charges to exist in body fluid. It is the difference in the concentrations across different membranes that exist between different mineral types (magnesium, calcium, sodium, potassium, hydrogen ion, chloride, bicarbonate, etc.) of charged particles that allow electrical work.

Electrical work occurs when opposing minerals flow into their concentration gradient. The release of these minerals toward equilibrium releases energy that the cell can use. When minerals flow toward equilibrium they discharge the energy contained in the membrane. The membrane is recharged by the continuous supply of ATP provided by the cell power plants. ATP is utilized to pump minerals back up their concentration gradient. Magnesium is one of the minerals that charge the membrane. The typical American diet is largely deficient in magnesium content. Magnesium deficiency in the blood vessel elevates the blood pressure.

All magnesium supplemental salts are not created equal. Some save their manufacturer's money, but have nasty side effects that are mild when compared to the best prescription drugs. Choosing intelligently between the many brands on the health food store shelves requires some knowledge. Other brands lack sufficient magnesium content to effectuate a response in lowering blood pressure. They are weak. Magnesium is only part of the salt. Any weight stated on the bottle has only a fraction of this weight as true magnesium content (the salt is made up of positive and negative halves). Magnesium forms the positive half. Both halves have weight. If one looks carefully at the label there is the exact weight per tablet of magnesium content called the elemental weight. The salt weight will be the weight per tablet (100mg, 200mg, etc.).

All magnesium salts are not created equally because the negative half, which is not magnesium, has properties of its own. Magnesium citrate is a powerful laxative. Citrate is named second denoting it to be the negative half by chemical nomenclature convention. Most owners can do without this powerful laxitive effect unless they are evacuating their bowels for surgery or medical procedures. Magnesium oxide is another salt sold over the counter. It is poorly absorbed and possesses potential as an oxidizing agent (chapter 1). The oxide component of the salt is ingesting trash in pill form, which needs water to remove. Most store bought magnesium salts are composed of oxide, which is a tissue oxidant and has no useful purpose. Oxide is body trash.

Examples of the best absorption and the safest second half (the negative half) are magnesium amino acid chelate, magnesium aspartate and magnesium malate. Many companies offer magnesium preparations that are too weak unless swallowing the entire contents of the bottle each day. This is where alternative medicine can undeservedly get a bad name. Weak and ineffective preparations of various herbs and supplements abound. For the best strength and quality of magnesium, the Source Naturals brand is safe.

If one chooses to begin a trial of magnesium supplementation to lower blood pressure, the support and competence of a knowledgeable physician is necessary. The effective dosage is between 300-1000mg of elemental magnesium a day. This total daily dosage should be divided between meals. Magnesium is a mineral and needs adequate stomach acid for absorption. Owners who have healthy gastrointestinal tracts will secrete maximum acid that follows a high protein meal. This becomes an important consideration when attempting to absorb this much magnesium each day (digestions chapter). Lastly, in some types of kidney disease magnesium supplementation is ill advised.

Potassium Deficiency and High Blood Pressure

When potassium is consumed at a sub-healthy rate compared to sodium, high blood pressure can be a consequence. The ability of the kidney to remove excess fluid depends on having adequate potassium compared to sodium. The healthy body maintains an optimal ratio between the two. When dietary choices diminish this ratio, high blood pressure results in susceptible owners.

Before the days of processed food this problem was much less prevalent. Processed food encourages this problem due to the sodium that is routinely added and the removal of potassium and magnesium. This relationship is not discussed straightforwardly in the medical physiology textbooks, but has been observed clinically. It is included here to plant a 'question mark' for the possible solution to blood pressure problems caused by imbalance between potassium and sodium.

An imbalance here, leading to high blood pressure, makes sense in light of the huge amount of sodium that the food processing adds. This alone upsets the delicate balance between these opposing minerals. Natural food diets result in a greater than three to one ratio of potassium compared to sodium. A processed food diet reverses this ratio.

In the case of magnesium and potassium, a deficiency of natural foods in the diet sets the stage for these minerals to unbalance. Unprocessed meats, nuts (unsalted), vegetables, whole grains, dried beans, and fruits are examples of real foods that contain balanced amounts of minerals. In contrast, when food is processed the mineral ratios reverse.

Sodium is critical to extend the shelf life of food. Fast food is usually loaded with added salt. The act of processing food depletes magnesium and potassium content. Some bodies are not equipped to deal with this deviation from the natural way that food is grown. Excess sodium retains water and trash. When this occurs high blood pressure results.

Mineral imbalance can lead to elevated blood pressure. Stress affects the mineral content in the body. This ties together, the four mechanisms for blood pressure elevation at the kidney level. The stressed owner is a trash water retention machine.

Steroid Message Content - A Determinant of Blood Pressure

The fourth example of how the kidney can misdirect trash water removal and lead to high blood pressure is found in the overall message content of the steroid hormones that the kidney receives. A high quality steroid mixture that interacts with the kidney and directs use of energy occurs only in the healthful state. As the quality of the steroid mixture that reaches the kidney decreases, there is an increase of health consequences.

Many women just before their period experience the effects of lower quality steroid hormones reaching their kidneys. Premenstrual bloating and fluid retention (trash water accumulation) evidence this fact. Just before menstruation the content of natural progesterone falls off dramatically. Synthetic progesterone does not count here because it does not behave like natural progesterone in the promotion of fluid loss. The dramatic fall of progesterone causes the sudden loss in informational message content which directs the kidney to dump extra body fluid (diuresis).

Men and woman when subjected to chronic stressors of various types have fluid retention. If the process becomes chronic it can lead to high blood pressure because of the increased fluid in the pipes. Stress that elicits a change in the hormone message content reaching the kidney effectuates a change in the energy expenditure of the kidney. The western medical standard often ignores these basic hormonal mismatches that lead to disease. They employ symptom control medicinal approaches, which do not restore hormone quality. These are attended by the consequent side effects. Sometimes prescription medication is warranted. Many toxic and dangerous side effects are avoidable when the holism of what science has revealed are included in the workup.

These first four fixable causes for elevated blood pressure are only the beginning of what is known when the holism of science is included in the treatment. There are many effective, non-toxic ways to treat high blood pressure early in the disease process. This can only occur if an owner is informed and motivated to heal. Tying together all four factors that contribute to the kidney allowing trash water accumulation and consequently high blood pressure is critical.

Stress and Dead Food Consumption Combine All Four Reasons for High Blood Pressure in an Inter-connected Web

When avoiding real food and adding daily stress, blood pressure elevation is likely because the four processes lead to trash water accumulation. When physicians are not taught this fact they end up dutifully prescribing medications that peripherally alter the trash water imbalance. These approaches always have side effects. Side effects lead to more prescriptions and medical procedures. Some of these scenarios can be avoided. When the goal is avoidance of symptom control approaches, these four interconnected determinants need adequate consideration - insulin level, stress hormone level (cortisol), potassium intake relative to sodium intake, and magnesium content.

Chronic stress elevates aldosterone and cortisol output from the adrenal glands. High cortisol and aldosterone accelerate potassium loss and sodium retention. When the kidneys have high sodium relative to potassium in the diet there are problems. An high sodium relative to potassium mineral intake is found in processed food. Chronic stress leads to an exacerbation of fluid retention and an accelerated loss of potassium while retaining sodium. These two effects result from the kidney being directed by stress hormone to misdirect water and minerals.

Around middle age when the potassium deficiency has become more pronounced the kidneys begin to deteriorate (hypokalemic nephropathy). The longer the potassium deficiency causes injury, the more likely the need for permanent blood pressure medication. When the kidneys suffer damage, medication is required to keep blood pressure normal. It is imperative that physicians begin to counsel their high blood pressure patients early on in the disease process before permanent kidney damage occurs. When patients implement the advice to increase potassium relative to sodium in the diet they will diminish the tendency toward high blood pressure in stressful situations. Blood pressure stabilizes because they now have a more proper amount of sodium compared to potassium in the kidney filter. Water will be less likely to accumulate because with less sodium intake sodium retention exacerbated by stress becomes less significant.

An overlooked consequence of a low potassium diet concerns a long known fact. When potassium is low more insulin is necessary to do the same job (insulin resistance). This creates a vicious hormonal cycle. High insulin necessitates higher cortisol to keep blood sugars normal (the antique weight scale) and powerfully stimulates fat cell growth. Lastly, these people with increased insulin are thought of as the typical Syndrome X types.

The syndrome X owners are on an accelerated tract to an old body. Their fundamental defect involves elevated insulin levels in a setting of increased stress. Low potassium and low magnesium diets with elevated sodium intake makes the owner's disease process worse. A high stress hormone output explains, in part, how Syndrome X patients age so quickly and have high blood pressure. Elevated cortisol output chronically communicates the emergency message helping explain the increased catabolism associated with this syndrome. When the body perceives an emergency energy is directed into survival pathways (catabolism). The survival pathway becomes the norm instead of rejuvenation. Trash water removal is a rejuvenation activity.

When the body directs energy into survival pathways, wear and tear becomes more likely secondary to the lack of cellular repair. Adequate repair is necessary to slow aging. Syndrome X owners' age quickly because they have high insulin and cortisol derived diseases.

A huge contribution to the severity of the Syndrome X clinical outcome involves the mineral imbalanced diet. Syndrome X owners add to their problem by consuming processed foods that exacerbate mineral imbalances. Chronic mineral imbalance intake around middle age eventually overcomes the kidney's ability to correct altered mineral content.

The last of the interconnected four basic causes of elevated blood pressure is magnesium deficiency. This deficiency is common in Americans who consume processed food. Excess sodium intake, in a setting of chronic stress, makes the magnesium deficiency worse. The two mineral deficiencies usually occur together. When potassium is depleted often times the kidney will excrete magnesium instead.

Assessing Hormones Contribution to Trash Water Accumulation

Often times if an accurate twenty-four hour urine test discloses imbalances in steroid hormones it may be unnecessary to manipulate the hormone mismatch directly. Using the holism of science can effectively counter the mismatch. In the case of elevated stress hormone secretion, supplements like magnesium and potassium, with sodium restriction, allow for an effective counter regulatory response promoting fluid removal. In other cases it becomes prudent to facilitate a more harmonious steroid profile.

Each owner is unique in their kidney appropriation of water and minerals in relation to blood pressure. This uniqueness will present itself in the diagnostic workup. Part of the workup needs the inclusion of unraveling the hormonal mess that causes a kidney-derived problem. The twenty-four hour urine test will provide the relative excretion rates of the important minerals.

The Inter-relationship Between Cortisol, Insulin, and Blood Pressure

The message content that the kidney receives determines the resultant blood pressure. This relationship is important because it emphasizes the interrelationship between cortisol and insulin. Insulin is secreted when carbohydrate is absorbed from dietary sources. Death would shortly follow because insulin would direct the liver and fat cells to suck every sugar molecule out the blood stream if an effective counter response was not mounted quickly. Healthy owners can do this by secreting effective amounts of cortisol from the adrenals that raise blood sugar.

The opposite sequence of hormone release occurs when mentally stressed. Stress causes cortisol to be released, which directs the elevation of blood sugar inappropriately. Eventually insulin needs to be secreted to return the blood sugar to normal. The extra insulin is necessary because in mental stress no physical challenge ever comes and the extra fuel is not needed. When healthy, the overall effect is to keep a constant amount of sugar in the blood stream.

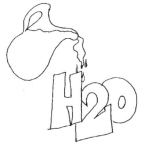

Glucagon, growth hormone, and adrenaline are also part of the counter response to insulin. Around middle age growth hormone becomes less involved in the prevention of low blood sugar compared to cortisol (section three).

There is a subtle, but important clinical point often missed in the relationship of cortisol and insulin. Cortisol is one of the main counter-weights to insulin. The more insulin that weighs down on one side of the scale, the larger the counter weight amount of cortisol that needs to balance the scale (normalize the blood sugar). A vicious cycle of response and counter response is created when the owner is eating high amounts of carbohydrate and under stress. Mental stress raises blood sugar and this requires more insulin to bring it back to normal. This produces a cycle of disease that begins when either one of these opposing hormones isn't optimal.

Most patients are capable of making some life changes and habit cessation if they understand that it will help in healing. Many patients appreciate an opportunity to heal, even if it requires effort and commitment on their part. It involves helping patients understand that when the hormone message content within is chaotic, their behavior as well as health will deteriorate. Health deteriorates when the kidney receives the wrong message about what to do with trash water. Trash water will accumulate when the stress response initiates.

In the case of Syndrome X, cholesterol elevation, and high blood pressure a careful analysis of the 'antique weight scale' situation between insulin and cortisol will help the motivated patient. In all three of these conditions improvement occurs if the physician and patient work together to unravel this vicious cycle.

In summary, the kidney's role in organic acid removal, mineral balance, and blood pressure control have been reviewed. The last section of this chapter was complex, but necessary if one is going to have a better understanding in the full healing abilities of the most powerful medicine of all, water. The body's ability to cleanse itself becomes hopeless when inadequate supplies of pure water occur. The mineral proportions in the diet and the quality of the hormones that are directing the kidney influence taking out the trash water.

The Most Powerful Medicine of All

Water is the most powerful medicine of all. Five of the six taking out the trash organs require ample water to carry out their waste removal functions. The sixth, the immune system doesn't directly engage the services of water, but their work is increased without the adequate supply of clean water. The colon requires sufficient clean water or constipation and backwards absorption of putrefaction molecules occurs. The lungs need adequate water in the respiratory secretions or thick mucus plugs the airways. The kidney's need water to remove xcess minerals and water-soluble toxins. The skin needs adequate water content to prevent wrinkling. The liver needs adequate water in bile secretion to prevent stone formation in the gallbladder.

With a clean water deficiency, salt retention in the form of waste and mineral excesses occur. As these accumulate, the body begins sequestering the waste that eventually injures delicate tissues because there isn't enough water to remove the toxins.

The sequestering site depends on the toxin type. Uric acid is stored in the big toe areas and in gouty tophi (hard bumps) formation. Salts of calcium are stored in the kidney's drain system and form kidney stones. Imbalances between serum phosphate and calcium concentrations cause the chemical solidification reactions that precipitate calcium salts in the blood vessel walls, the joints, and create osteophytes (bone spurs). Other organic acids that are not disposed of can react with the molecular structural components and lead to deformation injuries.

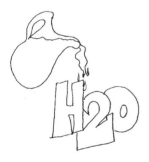

Some water supplies have diminished usefulness because they already contain toxins. Toxins accumulate in the water supply from industrial, agricultural, and automobile gaseous emissions. Some beverages act as drying agents or diuretics. Diuretics cause more water to be eliminated when they are consumed than the water they contain. Commonly consumed diuretics are coffee, tea, and alcohol. Unless adequate supplemental clean water is taken along with these beverages the body will sequester toxins.

The chronic consumption of soda pop beverages has a unique damaging effect on the skeleton. Carbonated beverages contain phosphates without calcium forcing the body to use its own calcium to eliminate phosphate from the system. Chronic soda pop abusers are at risk for developing a calcium deficiency in their bones. Fortunately, the universe was constructed so that beer is free of phosphate and will not damage the bones like soda pop.

Some air supplies require increased clean water consumption such as environments where each breath inhaled contains acids. Smog is the most common source. Some of these acids are absorbed through the act of breathing and the kidneys eliminate them. The kidney will fail without abundant pure water.

Physicians from antiquity thought of old age as a drying out process. In many ways this is true. Now additional understanding of how the decrease in essential hormones leads to the drying out of body tissues comes into play. Dry body tissues become brittle and weak. Altered minerals ingestion accelerates hormonal decline and the drying effect. The proper hormones within, proper mineral intake, proper activity level, stress management, and adequate supplies of clean water all help the kidney prevent the shrinkage into old age.

Proper Garbage Removal Allows the Kidneys to Facilitate the Cellular Force Field

The body is an electrical system that is maintained by properly proportioned and appropriate concentration of opposing minerals. Water content allows proper concentrations in the different tissues. It is the kidney's job to maintain the water content at 67% of the total atom weight content, remove waste products, and maintain the ability of the cells to generate an optimal electrical charge. The quality and proportion of the minerals (electrolytes) used by the cells to power the cell batteries are dependent on the kidney. The kidney responds to this after the digestive tract makes minerals available.

After the digestive tract extracts the minerals from a meal, the kidneys evaluate which minerals are retained and which are eliminated as waste. The kidney responds to the hormone message that it receives. Healthy owners have high quality message content that directs the kidneys in the use of its energy. Healthy owners choose optimal mineral content in their diet so that the correct ratios of minerals become available to the kidney. These are then distributed at the cellular level. Only when these processes occur can an owner make it past middle age with appropriate mineral balance. Much of the feeling of getting old comes down to the loss of the cell's charge abilities and diminished function.

The kidneys oversee that mineral balance is maintained. That depends on the quality of the message content (type and amounts of hormones delivered), the adequacy of nutritionally balanced mineral intake, the functional abilities of the digestive tract, and the adequate supply of clean water. Attention to these four variables can have powerful effects on regaining health from diseases like arthritis, high blood pressure, fluid retention, and osteoporosis.

Excesses and deficiencies of the minerals constantly confront the kidney when a processed food diet becomes the norm. With healthy kidneys, elimination and conservation is accomplished through elaborate workstations along the nephron (the functional unit of the kidney). At rest, the kidney receives 25% of the blood flow in the body. Every 24 hours it filters over 180 liters out of the blood. It then processes it and, on average returns 179liters of this fluid back into the blood stream. The 180 liters of filtrate squeezed out of the blood each day contains vital minerals, sugar, amino acids, fatty acids, and hormones along with the trash needing to be removed. It is the kidney's job to constantly decide what is waste and what needs to be conserved.

The Interrelationship Between the Kidneys and the Liver

The kidneys are in partnership with the liver in taking out certain types of trash. The liver begins detoxification of a water insoluble trash by making it soluble. Many vitamins and cofactors are needed for this process such as vitamin C, glutathione, the methyl donor system of vitamins, glucuronic acid, etc. The liver then transfers many of the inactivated molecules to the kidney for elimination. The liver inactivates other toxins and then excretes them into the bile for removal by a bowel movement (liver chapter).

Significant amounts of ammonia are created everyday from the digestion of the 20 different amino acids being used for energy creation (gluconeogenesis) and from other nitrogen containing molecules. The liver removes ammonia from the circulation and converts it into urea. The urea manufactured in the liver is delivered into the blood stream where it travels to the kidneys for excretion in the urine. To a point, adequate urea levels allow the kidney to conserve water. Urea facilitates the ability of the kidneys to concentrate the urine. Higher specific gravity becomes possible when dehydration forces are prevalent. There is some evidence that urea has important immune stabilization effects that are not yet clearly understood. This shows that sometimes a toxin, if allowed to build up, has biochemical usefulness within normal parameters. The liver and kidney trash removal partnership is used for the removal of urea.

Another class of substances dependent on the kidney-liver partnership causes the urine of healthy owners to foam. The amount of urine foam depends on the quantity of steroids and the liver tags them with glucuronic acid. Glucuronic acid is necessary to make steroids water-soluble so the kidney is able to excrete them in the urine. When steroids combine with glucuronic acid they make foam in water. A crude index of the steroidal adequacy can be obtained if one notes the amount of suds created in urine when it is shaken up. Who knows? Maybe steroids combined with glucuronic acid is just one of the clever ways to make soap that washes off the kidney's tubule dirt that collects over time. If this turns out to be true, it will show another example of the perils of scientist thinking inside the box.

Chapter 17

The Lungs

The cellular factories deposit acid in body fluids. The lungs remove the majority of this acid load in the form of carbon dioxide gas. The kidneys remove the organic acids that these factories produce. The lungs are incapable of this task. The kidney is unable to remove carbon dioxide as gas. These two organs work together for the removal of toxic acids. Lactic acid is the one exception because the liver removes it (liver section).

Diminished acid removal is the last function of the lungs to be compromised when they are diseased. Long before acid buildup occurs, the ability of the lung to deliver oxygen decreases. Initially, diminished oxygen delivery occurs only when demands increase.

The fact that an automobile air filter (oxygen delivery) is more vulnerable to malfunction (lung disease) than the exhaust system (carbon dioxide removal) offers an illustrative analogy. Initially diminished oxygen delivery through the air filter only occurs when the gas pedal is floored. Later, oxygen intake diminishes as the air filter becomes further compromised. Finally, late in the deterioration of engine performance, inadequately combusted fuel begins to belch out of the exhaust pipe and buildup in the engine.

The reason oxygen delivery falls more quickly than carbon dioxide removal when the lungs are diseased is that oxygen has less affinity to enter the blood stream compared to the ability of carbon dioxide to leave it. Filling the oxygen sites as a unit of blood passes through the oxygen chambers in the lungs is a critically timed event even in the healthiest of lungs.

The consequence of this, as various processes injure the lungs, then is that oxygen entry into the body falls off before carbon dioxide builds up. Oxygen entry falls off because there wasn't much wiggle room to begin with. Oxygen entry into the body at high levels only occurs in the best of lungs.

The analogy holds for a car's air filter size and design. Auto manufacturers design each type of air filter with the assumption that the car owner will change the filter regularly before airway delivery diminishes. If the auto owner fails to change the filter, performance will fall dramatically. Damaged air filters diminish performance for the same reasons that lung air exchange chambers performance will fall. There is decreased oxygen delivery to both the car engine and the cell fuel combustion chamber (cell mitochondria). When a dirty air filter in an auto causes decreased ability to burn gasoline, so to are diseased lungs affected in their ability to deliver oxygen to the many cellular combustion chambers. Cells contain combustion chambers (mitochondria) that burn fuel vigorously only in the presence of adequate oxygen. Imagine that owners who have diminished oxygen are those who also have weak burning power plants in their cells.

It takes a sick lung before carbon dioxide buildup can happen because carbon dioxide moves from the lungs more readily than oxygen enters in the body. The important exception occurs when the lung allows carbon dioxide to build up in order to compensate for another disease process that drains away body acid.

Better life decisions are necessary here if the body is going to have maximal oxygen delivery. Effective oxygen delivery into the tissues serves as a hallmark of youth. Conversely, as owners' age, oxygen delivery systems coincidently fall. Diminished oxygen delivery leads to an increase in cellular trash because cell power plants burn in a 'soot-like' manner without it.

Consciously induced hyperventilation is a way to understand the importance of having the right amount of acid in the body. Ten to twenty rapid deep breaths usually will produce the earliest manifestations of acid deficient disharmony. The breathing rate and depth are carefully regulated by the autonomic nervous system. Rapid breathing in excess of metabolic demands rapidly decreases carbon dioxide content (a major source of body acid). Contrast this to running for a train. There is an increased demand for oxygen and increased production of carbon dioxide gas. The body needs just the right amount. Too much acid and too little acid produce internal disharmony.

Cells need to have the right amount of acid to create the proper electrical environment. Too little carbon dioxide creates the symptoms of light-headedness, numbness around the mouth, and tingling in the fingers. Accelerated breathing (anxiety) is responsible for much of the misery caused by the loss of carbon dioxide. Anxiety stimulates the autonomic nervous system inappropriately leading to an accelerated breathing rate that exceeds demand.

Carbon Dioxide Leaves More Readily Than Oxygen Enters

Carbon dioxide leaves the body with less effort than oxygen enters the body. Two factors contribute to this phenomenon. First, gases move from a high concentration toward a lower concentration. There is a dramatic difference in the atmospheric concentrations of oxygen compared to carbon dioxide. There are greater than 500 oxygen molecules for every 1 carbon dioxide molecule at any elevation. This is contrasted to the waste gases of expiration where the concentrations of oxygen and carbon dioxide are about the same. Venous blood entering the lungs for expiration is depleted of oxygen after delivery to the tissues. At the same time it is rich in the waste gas, carbon dioxide, that leaves cells and goes into the capillaries. The concentration of carbon dioxide when it reaches the lungs becomes many times higher than the atmospheric concentration of the gas. The body has more difficulty obtaining adequate oxygen inside the body compared to the ease of expelling carbon dioxide out of the body.

The rate of movement of a gas is proportional to the difference in the concentrations between the chambers. Living cells are constantly generating carbon dioxide gas. There is approximately 100 times more atmospheric concentration of this gas when it reaches the lung chambers. Oxygen however occurs in less than a one to four concentration difference between the amounts in the venous depleted lung chambers compared with the outside air. In the lungs, oxygen and carbon dioxide move in opposite directions. Carbon dioxide gas occurs at a higher concentration in the lungs compared to atmospheric levels and moves out of the body. Similarly, higher oxygen atmospheric levels suck oxygen into the body because oxygen is at a lower concentration in the lungs.

A useful construct to understanding the difference in the rate of carbon dioxide leaving and oxygen entering occurs when visualizing concentration differences as the 'steepness of the road'. The steeper the road, then the faster the gas moves. Carbon dioxide has a greater difference in concentration in the body compared to the atmospheric concentration of carbon dioxide. It moves more quickly down the 'steeper road', whereas the road for oxygen is less steep and moves slower.

The second advantage for the ease of movement for carbon dioxide relates to the fact that different gases have different affinities to dissolve in fluids. Carbon dioxide dissolves in the blood stream much faster than oxygen. The more a gas can dissolve in a liquid (the blood stream) the more quickly it can enter the liquid.

Lastly, the hemoglobin protein contained in the red blood cells increases the oxygen and carbon dioxide carrying abilities of the blood stream many fold. As hemoglobin sucks oxygen out of the liquid component of the blood stream a continuous concentration difference is created while the blood flows in the lungs. Healthy owners are able to fill their hemoglobin carrying sites in the short time it takes for the blood to pass through the gas exchange chamber (the alveoli). Aging occurs when there is a decreased ability to fill the hemoglobin with oxygen in the specified time.

Healthy lungs preserve health, but there are common lung diseases that occur when there is dysfunction. Diseases that originate in the lungs lead to diminished oxygen transport. Diminished oxygen content leads to an increased likelihood of toxin accumulation. Toxins accumulate when there is less energy available because cells cannot burn toxins as fuel without sufficient oxygen in their combustion chambers (the mitochondria). This is discussed in terms of aerobic (with oxygen) contrasted to anaerobic (without oxygen) fuel combustion. Without oxygen, lactic acid begins to accumulate quickly in the cells.

Lactic acid is damaging. It does what other acids do to delicate cellular structures when allowed to accumulate in excess. Too much acid or too little acid alters the electrical properties of the different and delicate intracellular contents. Examples of cellular contents are structural proteins, enzymatic machines, and charged ions. Lactic acid accumulation doesn't move out of the cell with the same ease of carbon dioxide gas. Gases are wonderful. They move with ease from high concentrations to low concentrations. Lactic acid is not a gas. Cells have a limited opportunity to release lactic acid once it begins to accumulate. Excess lactic acid forms with certain nutritional deficiencies (chapter one) and when there is not enough oxygen around to meet metabolic demands.

In exceeding exercise ability, the cells can go down the dead end road of burning sugars anaerobically. The ability to burn sugar anaerobically is limited by the amount of lactic acid the body can handle. Lactic acid forms from anaerobic metabolism. In contrast, aerobic metabolism consumes oxygen and involves a process where carbon dioxide gas forms as the waste product. Carbon dioxide gas can exit through the lungs. Lactic acid clears more slowly by processes in the liver and cannot exit through the lungs. Death or the intervention of common sense limits the amount of lactic acid production that the body will allow. Clinically, lactic acid accumulation evidences itself as sore muscles. It is the job of the liver to remove lactic acid from the blood stream (liver section).

Anatomy of Lung Vulnerability

Understanding the vulnerable areas of the lung is enhanced if some basic anatomy is reviewed. There are 300million balloons (alveoli) in each lung held in a basket of capillary vessels. Capillaries are the smallest of all vessels and so small that only one red cell can fit through them at a time by squeezing forward from the rhythmic pressure created by the heartbeat. These vessel walls are only one cell thick, which allows for the smallest of distances between the gas chamber (the balloon) and the red blood cells. Upon entering this chamber, the red blood cells are loaded with waste gases and deficient in oxygen content. Each red blood cell has on average only .7seconds to change by dumping off of carbon dioxide and loading up of oxygen on the billions of hemoglobin carrier sites. Each red blood cell needs to accomplish this before heading out for another transport trip. The transport trip for each oxygen ends when it arrives at a distant, hungry cell where lower oxygen content allows it to get sucked off its carrier protein, hemoglobin. This distant cell location is also one of increased waste gas, high concentration allows hemoglobin to begin gathering waste gas for the trip back to the lungs. One way or another, lung disease interferes with the blood becoming fully oxygenated during its .7-second time allotment in the gas exchange chamber, the alveoli.

The Lung Disease Industry

Asthma illustrates the limitations and toxicities of mainstream medicine's approaches for one of the most common lung diseases. Healing will make sense when looking at the other side of the story of what science has revealed. A diminished ability to deliver oxygen to the trash removal organ systems is the byproduct of asthma. With out adequate oxygen, all trash removal systems are compromised. Learning how to heal diseases like asthma develops the lungs ability to improve all six of the trash removal organs.

Asthma - An Example of Symptom Control Versus Healing

Asthma is a good place to contrast the symptom control medical approach with the holistic approach. Cause and effect treatment strategies have healing potential. The contrast of these two different philosophies, with asthma care as a prototypical example, can show how doctors in training often only receive partial information.

The omission of key scientific facts that regard the asthma disease process leads to unnecessary medication and side effects. There are a small percentage of asthma patients who will still need many of the more toxic strategies. A minority of asthma patients will need the patentable prescription medications to control their symptoms. The majority can be helped by a more holistic strategy.

The conventional explanation for causalities of asthma is considered as one or more of three interrelated processes. First, concerns the process of over reactive airways (bronchial tubes). These airway tubes internal diameter contract in spasm for various reasons. Spasm of the air tube (the bronchioles) leads to the musical wheezing wounds of asthma. Second involves the process of excessive mucus plugging. Many asthma sufferers are not diagnosed because they lack the characteristic wheeze of reactive airways. The mucus buildup can also diminish the diameter of the airway tubes. Often these lung exams are remarkable by there subtle decrease in breath sounds. Lastly, the process of the airway tubes themselves swelling and decreasing the internal diameter of the tube. Swollen tubes, like spasmodic or plugged tubes, are less able to move air back and forth. Like mucus the swelling of airways can fool physicians because wheezing may be absent.

The wheezing symptoms of asthma are supposed to be from excessive spasm in the airways, swelling of these airways, and concurrent mucus overproduction. These three processes lead to the increased effort of moving air back and forth. These three processes lead to blood traveling into the lowered oxygen content lung chambers and carry a diminished amount of oxygen in the red blood cell. Red blood cells that are not fully loaded with oxygen when they exit the lungs cannot deliver oxygen as efficiently. These three mechanisms of developing asthma are very real. A deeper inquiry into the reason airways would spasm, collect mucus, or swell often leads to healing.

The cause of asthma at a deeper level sometimes involes these owners who have adrenal dysfunction, that causes wheezing, mucus plugs, and swelling in the airways. A significant number of asthma cases are caused by a dysfunction in one of the six links in the adrenal health chain (adrenal chapter). Consequently, without an adequate inquiry as to health of adrenal function, these patients will be condemned to symptom control. Failure to recognize how healing happens from asthma causes these owners to suffer unnecessarily. Those patients who have asthma symptoms from other causes lead these patients into receiving the highest doses of toxic medicines available.

Some asthma patients have bronchospasm, swelling and mucus plugging from nutritional deficiencies and digestive malfunction as the primary cause of breathing difficulties. Non-toxic restorative approaches are available for them instead of the more conventional and toxic medications.

Asthma care in America today exemplifies the consequences of treating symptoms rather than causes of a disease process. Symptom control always has side effects and toxicities. The mainstream treatment of asthma usually includes some or all of the following prescription medication types: patentable derivatives of cortisol (a glucocorticoid), patentable forms of adrenaline derivatives, patentable forms of caffeine (the xanthine class that is usually theophylline or aminophylline as the prescribed form), the membrane stabilizers, and leukotriene inhibitors (inflammatory hormonal fat inhibitors). All of these drugs have some utility and circumstances where they are indicated. However, there are often safer ways to heal from asthma that are largely free of side effects. They treat the imbalance that causes asthma more centrally.

A holistic approach will include nontoxic airway relaxants (salts of magnesium), herbal or hormonal mucus dissolvers (lobelia and/or correcting inadequate thyroid function), substances that keep the balloons open because many asthmatics have an unrecognized tendency towards balloon collapse (surfactant deficiency), attention to adequate stomach acid, and the nutritionally derived airway spasm promoters (sulfites, phenols and others). Additional common causes of asthma are: diminished function of the adrenal system (any of the six links in the adrenal system chain), lowered adrenaline (epinephrine) to nor-adrenaline (nor-epinephrine) ratio (methyl donor deficiency), diminished thyroid and/or vitamin A, and the imbalances between certain vertebrae, the skull, and the sacrum that impair lung function (craniosacral therapy considerations).

Holistic Considerations - What Causes Asthma?

1. Deficiency of magnesium that leads to airway spasm
2. Inadequate stomach acid production with consequent decreased magnesium absorption
3. Increased mucus production from inadequate hormone levels

4. Inadequate surfactant production
5. Diminished adrenal system function
6. Diminished thyroid and/or vitamin A activity that decreases the ability to respond to epinephrine's message content to relax the airway
7. Methyl donor deficient
8. Craniosacral therapy indications when there has been some sort of back trauma
9. Dietary determinants like, phenols, sulfites and sulfates

Magnesium - An Airway Relaxant

Many asthmatics respond to aggressive magnesium supplementation because it relaxes airways for the same reasons it lowers blood pressure. Arteries and the airways are composed of a rich supply of smooth muscle. Magnesium relaxes smooth muscle. The smooth muscle layer in the arteries and airways reduces the internal diameter when they contract. In the case of contracting arteries, blood pressure rises. When the smooth muscles contract in the airways, the flow of air out of the lungs diminishes. When encountering extremely cold air the airways should contract to facilitate adequate warming of the inhaled air. However, inappropriate airway contraction causes wheezing.

Holistic physicians have observed the therapeutic effect of intravenous magnesium administered during acute asthma attacks. This has led many to make this their preferred acute intervention. Johnathan Wright MD and Alan Gaby MD have developed an acute asthma intravenous protocol that contains high doses of magnesium.[18] They named this formulation the "Meyers Cocktail". It contains magnesiumt, vitamin C, and high doses of many of the B vitamins, emphasizing B6 and B12. This preparation, when administered properly, can halt the most severe asthma attacks. Close follow up and monitoring are indicated because intravenous repetitions may be needed. Ideally this would be included in the protocols at the emergency rooms.

In contrast, mainstream medical protocol treats acute asthma attacks with high doses of the patentable cortisol type steroids. Synthetic (patentable) versions of cortisol type steroids are always accompanied by side effects. The side effects occur because by changing the shape of the cortisol hormone to get a patent the message content changes. It is the shape that carries the message contained in a hormone. Altered message content changes the way that the body is directed to spend energy at the DNA level. The altered DNA activity that results leads to altered structural and enzymatic protein production. These alterations produce their own side effects that need other prescription medications to curtail.

Intravenous magnesium on the other hand is relatively free of side effects. The exceptions regarding side effects are the occasional Viagra-like effects in woman and rectal fullness sensations in men. There is the additional need to monitor blood pressure because magnesium is a powerful anti-hypertensive. Magnesium also promotes regular bowel movements and some people experience this sensitivity. Unfortunately, traditionally trained physicians probably have not heard about magnesium usage in the treatment of asthma.

Much lower doses of DHEA and cortisol need to be given in the acute setting when the magnesium approach is used as the primary initial intervention. This approach recognizes the difference between physiologic replacement dosages, with real hormones, and the supra-physiologic dosing consequences of synthetic hormones. Side effects will occur with either real or synthetic hormones when body need is exceeded (adrenal chapter).

Adequate Stomach Acid in the Prevention of Asthma

Adequate stomach acid is a prerequisite for proper mineral absorption to occur (digestion chapter). The inability of the stomach to produce sufficient acid results in the failure to procure adequate magnesium from the diet. Many asthmatics fail to manufacture adequate stomach acid and develop an imbalance between calcium and magnesium. Asthma is a consequence of this problem and results in excess calcium. This tends to promote smooth muscle contraction.

The airways are lined with a smooth muscle layer and are vulnerable to spasm when there is inadequate magnesium. The contraction properties of calcium are not counterbalanced by magnesium when magnesium absorption becomes deficient. Magnesium depends more on adequate stomach acid production than calcium for absorption. Here lies the mechanism for imbalanced magnesium to calcium in the smooth muscles. Clinical practices that attempt to reliably measure stomach acid secretion abilities are procedurally cumbersome. Trying acid supplementation is often undertaken without insisting on the documentation of a deficient output (section three). Acid deficiency can contribute to the development of asthma.

Excess Mucus Plugs the Airways of Asthmatic Lungs

The normal lung tubes continuously secrete a sticky film that traps dust and foreign invaders. The airway tubes are lined with motile hairs (cilia) that transport the trapped dust and invaders toward the trachea. To function properly, adequate water is the necessary mechanism for taking out the trash. The cilia need sufficient water content in the sticky film that coats them. Cilia movement is only possible when the viscosity in this film is exact. Thick mucus begins to develop when the water content diminishes. Certain hormones and plants help to ensure that the water content of this sticky film is increased sufficiently. Only when sufficient water is available in the respiratory mucus can the cilia continuously remove the film and debris out of the lungs.

Substances that increase the water content of mucus are called mucolytics. Examples of common mucolytics are lobelia, ginger root, and licorice root. Excess mucus commonly plagues the asthmatic lung. Lobelia inflata is a plant that has the benefit of helping in the dissolution of the over production/accumulation of mucus. Ginger root is also a consideration for a natural way to decrease mucus thickness. Licorice root often has a beneficial effect on the over production of thick lung mucus.

Often the thickness and production rate of lung mucus is a problem of abnormal hormones. Some asthmatic lung tissue does not recognize thyroid message content even though they secrete adequate thyroid hormone amounts. Thyroid message content is important for lung cells in their ability to keep the mucus production rate in check. Low thyroid function causes increased mucus throughout the body. One of the places mucus collects when thyroid function is low is in the breathing tubes. This situation commonly occurs in the thyroid resistance syndromes (thyroid chapter). When a physician tests for this problem in the thyroid in the conventional manner, the blood tests will come back deceptively normal. Where thyroid resistance is one of the causes for asthma, the physician will need to look clinically for other clues of thyroid deficiency (thyroid discussion-section two). The inter relationship of thyroid hormone with vitamin A needs consideration. As does the possibility that thyroid deficiency at the cell level will lead to increased mucus accumulation.

Surfactant Attention is Warranted when Balloon Collapse Causes Asthma

The alveoli in the lungs function like balloons. Collapsed balloons (alveoli) cannot contain oxygen so the blood in the baskets surrounding these flattened balloons enters and leaves without exchanging gases. The more balloons collapse, the less oxygen that is delivered to the cells. Only in the most extreme cases will waste gas build up in the body.

The mechanism for balloon collapse has been understood for quite some time in caring for premature infants. The same mechanism that causes balloon collapse and breathing difficulties is ignored for anyone beyond infancy. Breathing difficulties result in these little patients because they are not producing adequate surfactant. Surfactant deficiency also causes breathing difficulty in other age groups.

Surfactants have the property of forming suds (foaming agents) when in a liquid and shaken. The lung balloons are kept from collapsing by the presence of surfactant. Surfactant deficiency is one of the causes of asthma.

The surfactant's ability to keep the balloons open is better understood when visualizing an ordinary rubber balloon. Anyone who has attempted to blow up a balloon noticed that the hardest part involves the initial expansion to begin distension. After this initial expansion, it becomes much easier. Now add the problem to 300 million alveoli once the gas content has been expired. These spherical structures want to collapse purely from physical forces. Inflating them, once collapsed, becomes analogous to the difficulty in getting that first bit of air into a rubber balloon times 300 million.

In healthy infants and adults the body addresses this problem by continually producing fresh surfactant in the millions of balloons contained in each lung. When the interior of the balloons contains adequate suds (surfactant), breathing becomes easier. The property of surfactants (the ability to keep balloons open) is surface tension reducers. This is secondary to the law of lapace as it refers to spherical bodies and the forces that want to collapse them.

Surfactants are made up of modified fats attached to sugars that facilitate suds formation. The suds keep the chambers from collapsing. The lung chambers (alveoli) produce just the right amount of surfactant. Surfactant deficiency in clinical practice is mostly recognized in premature infants. The quality of surfactant production in adult and pediatric asthma patient is often ignored. This leads this type of asthma sufferer down the road to receiving the highest doses of prescription medications. These patients have a sub-optimal response secondary to ignoring the central problem of needing foaming agents (surfactants). There is a group of asthma patients whose cause is surfactant deficiency.

The science behind the consequences of surfactant deficiency has been recognized in the care of premature infants. Typically, aggressive use of patentable cortisol derivatives is administered in this surfactant deficient group of pediatric asthmatic patients. These medications are effective because synthetic corticosteroids are one of the hormones that increase the production of surfactant. Adequate surfactant levels lower the work of breathing.

After infancy the mainstream medical protocols ignore the consequences and causality of surfactant deficiency as it relates to the disease process of asthma. This practice occurs despite the long known association of surfactant deficiency and the development of emphysema. Most asthmatics develop emphysema in their later years. This association makes mechanical sense because when a balloon is collapsed it will die off secondary to continued oxygen deprivation. Surfactant deficiency, along with lung cell atrophy, will result when certain hormones are deficient. Then a more thorough inquiry is warranted. Emphysema is the medical name denoting loss in the total number of balloons that each lung contains.

There is a need to look at surfactant deficiency at a deeper level. This deficiency is often a biochemical marker of a more central deficiency. Certain growth factors are needed by the lung tissue to remain healthy (thyroid, vitamin A, DHEA, and cortisol). Many asthma sufferers have abnormal twenty-four hour urine output of one or more of these hormones. Science has revealed the consequences of surfactant deficiency and some physicians have begun to argue for its inclusion in the management strategies of this lung disease.

The majority of surfactant is composed of modified fat that confers an electrical charge on the inner surface of the balloon. The charge increases as the balloons collapse. As these chambers deflate with expiration, the charges become closer to each other. Like charges repulse each other. Each one of these modified fats has a positive charge and when these charges get closer together there is an increasing electrical repulsion. The electrical force created in the alveoli as it contracts generates a propensity for the alveoli to inflate with the next inspiration. Deficiency of this electrical force occurs when there is a deficiency of electrically charged fats. It is important to evaluate whether or not an asthmatic has a surfactant deficiency.

An interesting aside consideration is the properties of adequate surfactant and the different ways that this can be achieved (toxically versus non-toxically). The traditional medical theory states that corticosteroids (cortisol-like medications) are so effective in the long-term maintenance of asthma care because they alter the inflammation process that is supposed to be occurring in refractory asthmatic cases. What they often fail to mention is that science has long ago revealed that cortisol like medications directly stimulate surfactant production.

Patentable versions of cortisol-like medications stimulate surfactant production, but there is a big price to pay. The practice of chronically hammering owners cells with synthetic cortisol-like prescriptions can lead to health consequences (altered immune function, decreased cellular rejuvenation activities, obesity, adrenal gland atrophy, etc.). Leaving out a real possibility of why steroids (cortisol types) improve breathing in these asthma patients covers the scientific tracts that can lead to healing. The trail to healing these patients is further concealed by medical physiology textbooks alluding to the fact that attempts to increase surfactant delivery through oral intake have proved ineffective. The truth is more accurately stated as: endogenous surfactant production cannot be increased until improving the hormones that direct its production. There are hormones that will lead to improved surfactant production. However, it is important to touch on how certain plants can help in certain cases.

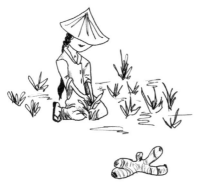

Encouraging results have been achieved with high quality ginseng. Panax ginseng root, that is at least 7 years old, possesses a class of substances called the glycosides. By definition all glycosides possess the ability to form suds (foam). In order to avoid confusion, ginseng is best thought of as a steroid contained in a package. While this steroid is still in its 'package', it possesses properties of the surfactant class. The intelligence of the body decides whether it needs ginseng as the glycoside or as the broken down (package removed) weak steroid building block for the production of other steroids.

An interesting degree of inconsistency in the medical literature occurs, when inquiring into the utility of the plant glycosides as surfactants. Medical dictionaries and textbooks go on about how all plant glycosides are not orally absorbable. They further go on to caution the reader that if given intravenously they lead to rupture of cell membranes. The inconsistency of this statement is revealed when understanding that a very important heart medication being used for over 2000 years comes from this class of plant substances. When looking up the class of drugs coming from the foxglove plant that make the various digitalis derivatives, it is stated that they are from the class of substances called the glycosides. It is further stated that absorption of most glycosides is almost 100% orally. There is nothing about the need to worry about these drugs causing cell membrane rupture.

Assessing the Adrenal System in Asthmatics

The adrenal gland is responsible for adequate secretion of DHEA and cortisol. One or both of these hormones secretion rate is often abnormal in the asthmatic owner. An imbalanced antique weight scale represents the hormonal imbalance operating in asthmatics. The majority of these owners have a DHEA and/or cortisol deficiency. DHEA and cortisol deficiency shows up most efficiently in the twenty-four hour urine test. Western-trained physicians do not routinely check this. The few that do check for DHEA levels, often find it to be diminished. Correlating with this finding is the tendency for other lung problems to be associated with adrenal insufficiency. Therefore by not treating the adrenal deficiency it may allow asthma patients to suffer unnecessarily (adrenal chapter). Conventional physicians are trained to treat only one side of the antique weight scale in an asthmatic patient, the cortisol side.

Compounding the problem, conventional physicians often treat asthma owners with both supra-physiologic doses and synthetic versions of cortisol. These approaches have unnecessary side effects. Only when real hormones (real cortisol and DHEA) are used in amounts sufficient to correct the deficiency can healing occur with no side effects.

Cortisol needs to be appropriately counter balanced with adequate DHEA. When these two hormones are in oppositional balance lung health can occur. Healthy adrenal glands secrete both DHEA and cortisol, appropriately. This happens in an optimal ratio and at the same time. In some cases, asthma becomes a disease of diminished adrenal output of DHEA and cortisol. This relationship provides an explanation for how medicinal plants like ginseng help in the treatment of asthma. These plants provide a source of steroid precursor that could be the reason that the weakened adrenal gland then increases its production of these hormones. The antique weight scale comes into balance again concerning these two opposing hormones.

The advice and monitoring of a competent physician is invaluable in helping an owner's return to balance in the safest way possible. Asthma disease often involves adrenal dysfunction. The evaluation for how the adrenal system can fail is important (adrenal chapter). The challenge is to discern where the basic defect lies that leads a patient to suffer from asthma.

Thyroid, Vitamin A, and Lung Health

Healing asthma requires an understanding of thyroid and vitamin A message content in the lungs. These hormones deliver their instructions at the level of the lung cells DNA program (genes) and deficiency at this DNA level causes disease. These hormonal effects are in addition to the message content of both cortisol and DHEA directed at the lung cell DNA. All four of these level one hormones are necessary in order for the DNA program to activate the proper protein synthesis. Only lung cells containing the appropriate proteins can be healthy. Unhealthy lung cells sometimes manifest as asthma and the resolution of this disease needs to include an assessment of level one hormones production rates.

The importance of adequate thyroid hormone in the lung, colon, kidney, liver, immune system, and skin has been known for over one hundred years. Experiments on dogs that had their thyroids removed established at autopsy what the cell consequences were in these organ systems. In the lungs, kidney and liver the changes were striking. These organs had a marked increase in scar tissue (fibrosis). Thyroid is a central growth factor for these tissues and without it these organ systems cells begin to atrophy (die). When scar tissue forms where there was once viable tissue, the organ has diminished function. Here emerges a recurrent body theme that cells need direction on how to spend energy. The loss of thyroid message content leads to a diminution of rejuvenation. Scar tissue replaces functional cells that die without adequate directions for rejuvenation.

Vitamin A is similar to thyroid in that it is a necessary growth factor at the level of lung cell DNA programs. Its message content provides instruction on developing the growth maturity of the cell (differentiation). Only when cells mature can they produce the cell product, which is inherent in that cell type. The cells that line the lung air passages need to make many secretion products, surfactants, and mucus. Many asthmatics that receive conventional treatment are never counseled on these scientific facts? The lack of nutritional education in conventionally trained physicians is equally problematic in other nutritionally based causes of asthma.

Nutritional Deficiencies Present as Wheezing

Nutritional deficiencies can contribute to the severity of an asthmatic tendency from an imbalance between the forces in the blood stream versus the forces in the autonomic nervous system. This tug of war occurs in blood vessel tension and breathing tube tension. These same nutritional deficiencies cause many cases of curable blood pressure problems (blood pressure chapter) as well.

Basic physiology textbooks teach that when the sympathetic nervous system activates, the airways should open up. This major message for the airways is from the sympathetic nerves stimulating the adrenal medulla to release epinephrine. Part of the asthma problem centers on inadequate epinephrine release because of nutritional deficiencies. Nor-epinephrine released by the adrenal into the blood stream is weak at relaxing the airways. The majority of release from the adrenal medulla should be epinephrine. Epinephrine can only be manufactured in the adrenal medulla when there is a nutritionally intact methyl donor system. The major airway relaxation occurs from stimulation of the sympathetic nerves to the adrenal glands to release 90% epinephrine and only 10% nor-epinephrine. The optimal ratio of adrenal medulla release is important in the prevention of wheezing when stimulated by the sympathetic nerves.

Above and beyond the simple opposition of magnesium and calcium, only epinephrine message content in the blood stream is powerful enough in its ability to relax the air ways. Owners who suffer from nutritional deficiencies in vitamin B6, vitamin B12, methionine, folate, serine, tetrahydrobiopterin, SAMe, and/or vitamin C will not be able to manufacture epinephrine in their adrenal glands. The much weaker nor-epinephrine will tend to be released, but with progressive deficiencies this will diminish and these owners will wheeze. These nutrients make up the methyl donor system except for tetrahydrobiopterin (partially made from folate) and vitamin C.

Owners who eat a processed food diet are likely to become deficient in one or more of these nutrients. Bodies respond to a methyl donor deficiency in different ways. Some experience wheezing as the primary manifestation of methyl donor deficiency.

Epinephrine synthesis is only possible when all the nutritional cofactors are present. A deficiency could be another cause for asthma. Supplementing with some of these nutritional factors in the Meyers cocktail (intravenous route of administration) leads to an improvement in breathing. Including all these specific nutrients would probably make the Meyers cocktail even more effective.

Maintaining adequate epinephrine levels leads to an improved breathing ability. This is why the patentable inhalers like Alupent and Proventil have an epinephrine-like molecular structure. It is also probably why Chinese herbs like Ma Hung get bad press almost daily from the official view of the universe. Epinephrine at normal dosages tends to not raise blood pressure significantly. It increases blood flow to the heart, muscles, and liver. Whenever blood flow increases in these three areas, the total body blood pressure decreases despite epinephrine decreasing blood flow to other areas of the body. This excludes the brain where the blood flow is constant. Ma Hung has a similar effect on both blood flow and airway caliber as epinephrine does.

In contrast, nor-epinephrine decreases blood flow everywhere (except the brain). Nor-epinephrine dramatically raises blood pressure. There is a fixed amount of blood in the blood vessels. The pressure will go up when these vessels contract and will go down when they relax. Nor-epinephrine is very weak in its message content toward relaxing the airways. These two differences between epinephrine and nor-epinephrine are important when attempting to balance airway tube caliber.

The difference of the blood pressure effects between nor-epinephrine and epinephrine explains a lot about patentable bronchial- dilators. The patentable bronchial dilators tend to be closely related to an epinephrine-like molecular structure. If a pharmaceutical company marketed a nor-epinephrine-like bronchial dilator two things would happen. First, the bronchial dilator with nor-epinephrine-like molecular shape would be very weak. Second, blood pressure would tend to rise and this is an unacceptable side effect. Pharmaceutical companies are smart enough to know the importance of avoiding this side effect. Strokes are not good for their bottom line.

The active ingredient contained within Ma Hung is ephedrine. Ephedrine is structurally very similar to epinephrine. Taken orally, under the guidance of a knowledgeable physician, this will be more effective.

The eventual goal is have the adrenal glands make epinephrine in adequate amounts. This is best accomplished by taking live food sources of the B vitamins. B vitamins taken this way are more readily absorbed. Tetrahydrobiopterin is best obtained from royal bee jelly or its precursor, folate. Vitamin C is best in powder form. The amino acids serine and methionine can be obtained in health food store or by eating eggs daily.

Another effective method for correcting methyl donor deficiencies involves the use of intravenous vitamin replacement therapies. Naturopathic physicians are a good source for these treatments. The Meyers cocktail intravenous preparations are one example of how naturopathic physicians can help. These physicians are very good at intravenous vitamin replacement protocols. The intravenous route will often jump start a nutritionally deficient body. This approach allows time to sort out possible absorption problems that are common in asthmatic owners.

Asthma-Influenced by Energy that Heals Versus Energy that Maims

There is another consideration for healing asthma that is probably the hardest one for the western owner to grasp. When energy problems are the cause of asthma, craniosacral therapy has dramatic benefits. It has to do with the emerging understanding of the energetic and rhythmical pulsation occurring from the bones in the skull down through the spine and on down into the sacrum. When this energy isn't flowing properly or has blocked areas, there becomes either a deficiency or excesses of these energies within the organs. The wrong energy pulsation will throw the recipient organs out of balance. This is where the chiropractic technique called craniosacral therapy has achieved some dramatic benefits.

Some cases are never forgotten. A 17 year-old asthma sufferer tried all the above approaches only to fail. Fortunately, her father took her to a competent chiropractor where this craniosacral technique was used and just in two office visits the patient's asthma was cured. This young patient had fallen while skiing several years before. This led to a jamming of the energy pulsation within her spine. This fixation for reasons that are not explainable in the officially sanctified view of the universe led to the symptoms of asthma.

Phenols, Sulfates, and Sulfites Sensitivities and Asthma

Sulfite sensitivity is known to be associated with asthma. A possible explanation for this common observation involves the known association of asthma and DHEA deficiencies. The connection of these two facts allows a thread of understanding between sulfite sensitivity and asthma. DHEA, when attached to sulfate or sulfite, is relatively off limits to tissues like the lung. There are numerous enzymes in the blood stream that constantly trap DHEA with available sulfite or sulfate. The higher the levels of sulfate or sulfite, the more likely it is to trap DHEA. Since some asthmatics have a diminished DHEA level already, adding sulfites in the diet will further decrease the DHEA availability. This is an explanation for why some asthmatics are sulfite and sulfate sensitive. The twenty-four hour urine test is applicable here to help discern why some owners have asthma.

The lungs are one of the organs that help take out the trash water. Lungs remove trash water in two ways. They exhale waste gas, carbon dioxide, from the blood stream. They deliver oxygen to the tissues that is necessary to incinerate the constantly generated trash in cells. The disease of asthma results in the diminishing ability of the lungs to exchange gases. Asthma treatment strategies were contrasted between symptom control and cause and effect modalities. Cause and effect is always preferable to symptom control. Paradoxically, in the treatment of asthma, there is little attention devoted to the cause of this disease.

Chapter 18

Skin

The skin is the largest organ system of the body. The skin not only removes certain types of trash, but also protects the body from outside trash entering. The skin is a protective barrier and a trash water excretion organ. The organ is composed of two distinct layers of cell types. The deepest layer, the dermis, lies over the subcutaneous fat. The dermis is the last layer that contains blood vessels. The hair shafts and sweat glands are imbedded in this layer. On top of the dermis is the epidermis that has no direct blood supply. It depends on the lower level dermis for the diffusion of nutrients and oxygen. On top of the last living layer of epidermal cells are approximately twenty-eight layers of dead epidermis. The integrity of these dead layers is a crucial determinant for the protection of the lower skin layers. Processes that alter this protective coating will increase damage to the lower layers. What the skin does and how it is harmed are instrumental in this chapter. Once harmful skin conditions are identified, common solutions are presented.

Looking at the needs and dilemmas of the typical plant leaf on a hot summer day facilitates an understanding for the needs of healthy skin. Shriveled, crinkled plant leafs result from similar causes that leads to sagging and wrinkled skin. Processes that facilitate continued plant leaf vitality also tend to promote youthful skin.

Plant leaves, like skin, need a vapor barrier to trap moisture content in the cells. A vapor barrier prevents rapid water loss in the dry environmental conditions. Maintaining optimal water content in the skin and leaf cells heavily depends on the integrity of this vapor barrier.

A plant's vapor barrier is derived from secreting a wax layer onto the surface that covers the cell. Wax is a slightly modified fat. Without adequate fat to form a layer over skin cells, they become deficient in their ability to make an effective vapor barrier. Fat provides an important deterrent to water loss. Adequate fat allows the top skin layer of dead cells to remain water filled.

The importance of having adequate fat intake in the diet becomes cornerstone for minimizing the dehydrating forces. Dehydrating forces occur in two common environmental extremes. First adequate fat on the skin surface prevents water loss on a hot summer day. Second, adequate fat prevents water loss in the middle of winter when the heater has taken optimal humidity out of the air. Excessive wind and the low humidity of some locales lead to the fast track approach for the development of the withered skin look.

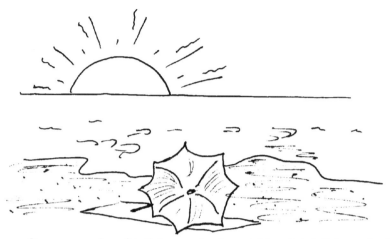

Owners on a low fat diet prematurely wrinkle. Fat deficiency leads to acceleration in the crinkling forces of the skin. Crinkling forces accelerate when the body lacks sufficient dietary fat (oils). Dietary fats are necessary for the development of a vapor barrier formation. The most pronounced wrinkles usually begin as deep creases beginning at the inferior lateral margin of the nose and extend downward toward the lateral border of the mouth.

Instead of counseling owners on ways to maintain an effective skin vapor barrier, western medicine has been preoccupied with avoiding the ultraviolet rays of the sun. It is true that total exposure levels accumulated during a lifetime are one determinant for how fast skin ages. However, leaving out other major factors in the formation of an effective strategy to promote skin youthfulness promotes an incomplete view of what science has revealed. Preservation of healthy skin comes with knowledge.

When the skin stays healthy, it facilitates the kidney's job of toxin removal through the act of perspiration. Perspiration allows the kidney to obtain backup help for the removal of the many toxins and mineral imbalances. Daily perspiration is good for these reasons. There is the added hydration that perspiration adds to the outer skin layers. Added moisture in these outer layers adds to the youthful appearance of skin.

Ultraviolet Radiation

Knowledge is often ignored regarding the needs of the skin and its relationship to the role of ultraviolet radiation and skin damage. Depletion of the ozone layer over some locales on the planet has led to a dramatic increase in skin cancers. There has been little inclination by the industrialized countries to curb the destruction of this important life-protecting layer. Refrigerators and air conditioning units slowly leak ozone-depleting molecules. Increased radiation reaches the planet as this protective layer diminishes and leads to skin that becomes exposed to radiation damage. This damage occurs by its ability to knock electrons off of biological molecules in the upper layers of the body. As was discussed in chapter one this is how biological oxidation (rust formation) begins. The avoidance of the increased radiation contained in the thinner atmosphere is one determinant of skin vitality.

Mainstream Medicine's Mystery Determinant of Skin Vitality

The message content which reaches skin is a powerful determinant of who will age gracefully versus who will age quickly. Yet, for reasons that are not clear, this consideration is omitted from clinical consideration. Skin cells depend on direction from the different hormones. The messages provided from the different hormones tell skin cells how to spend their available energy. Quality message content that arrives at the skin cell gives maximal rejuvenating stimulation to cell infrastructure investment activities. Quality message content that induces skin rejuvenation results in the production of a highly functional vapor barrier, adequate water sucking molecules, the glucosaminoglycans, and the formation of sufficient skin protein (keratin).

Graphic evidence of the skin's dependency on the proper hormones is witnessed in adolescents that are plagued by excessive acne. Acne formation provides a clinical sign of a high androgen steroid message content in the skin that leads to excessive production of skin oil (vapor barrier). Their clinicians encourage these adolescent owners by mentioning that later in life they will have more beautiful skin than their peers. Beautiful skin comes from optimal steroid message content reaching the skin layer. The amount of skin oil produced is directly proportional to the androgen message content. The quality (hormones in types and amounts) of the message determines how a cell spends available energy.

Acne formation may occur due to excess androgen levels or an improper proportion between DHEA and cortisol. William McKenzie Jefferies MD describes in his book, *'Safe Uses of Cortisol'* how adolescents with acne have this problem. Dr. Jefferies points out that healing these patients' centers on two things. An accurate steroid hormone profile assessment and the treating physician also needs to be aware of the difference between supra-physiological and synthetic steroid replacement as contrasted with natural steroid replacement. The natural steroid replacement needs only to correct the deficiency and avoid side effects. Individual attention to the uniqueness of each acne sufferer will allow healing for the majority.

Skin cells possess unique abilities and have unique needs when compared to other cells. The top twenty-eight layers are dead cells that have been filled with three important molecular components. The dead cells are full of the protein keratin. Second, these dead skin cells contain adequate fat to protect the skin from water loss. Third, the inflationary architectural framework allows skin cells to remain filled to the brim with water content. The framework is composed of mucopolysaccharides. Mucopolysaccharides have the property of attracting water inside cells. When this framework begins to crumble, another mechanism for shrinking cellular forces comes into play. The adequacy of this support framework is another determinant for the ability of a skin cell to remain inflated with water (section five). In contrast, fat allows skin to remain inflated by decreasing water loss from above.

The Role of Level One Hormones and Skin Health

There is only one small group of hormones that are powerful enough to directly interact with the DNA program of cells that instructs it on what to turn off or on. There are a few other hormones that can influence the cellular DNA program by indirect means. Most hormones cannot affect the DNA at all. The membership of these powerful hormones with direct DNA interacting ability includes all of the steroids, vitamin A, and thyroid hormone.

Vitamin A plays a powerful role in overall skin health. Adequate vitamin A at the skin cell level allows for the proper message content in the DNA program to activate the production of proteins necessary for a healthy skin cell. Vitamin A is found in yellow vegetables.

The Epidermis is Vulnerable – It has no Blood Supply

The top twenty-eight layers of skin are dead cells that are filled with keratin. There is also an water sucking support framework in the skin cells. Lastly, all of this is covered with oil (fat).

Approximately, below the twenty-ninth layer of the epidermis is alive. The skin and cartilage cells have no direct blood supply and. nutrient delivery and waste removal is particularly vulnerable. These two tissues types need optimal conditions to prevail. Without a direct blood supply, the skin becomes vulnerable to environmental oxidative damage, as well. This occurs from toxins in the air, bathing water, and from chemical hazards that contact the skin. The realization that these processes occur helps owners devise ways to minimize ongoing oxidative damage.

This is why cigarette smokers often develop prematurely aged skin. Cigarette smoke contains carbon monoxide that lowers the oxygen carrying ability of the blood (chapter 1). The outer living layers of skin cells have no blood supply and are more vulnerable to a fall in the oxygen content in the blood. Less oxygen lowers the energy available for use in cellular rejuvenation. Nicotine contained in cigarette smoke compounds this effect because it constricts the blood vessel supply in the lower skin layer (dermis). Lastly, cigarette smoke contains many rust producing substances (oxidizing agents) that further compromise skin cell health.

Bald Men Have Nice Skin

Hereditary male pattern baldness is generally thought to occur from increased concentrations in the scalp of the powerful androgen, dihydrotestosterone (DHT). High levels in the genetically sensitive male direct energy out of the hair follicles causing a dormancy hair type formation. It's as if so much energy is directed toward the skin that the build up choke off the surrounding hair follicles nutrient supply. Once a hair follicle is deprived of its nutrient supply this leads to a very small dormant hair. The dormant hair takes the place of a normal hair.

Men with male pattern baldness usually have youthful skin. This provides another clue to the inner workings of androgens in the body. Androgens direct energy into the skin and a youthful quality results. There will always be examples of secondary processes robbing men of their hair. In these cases the nice skin rule may not apply. In general, the majority of men who develop male pattern baldness have extremely nice skin.

The youthful skin observation ties into the old adage regarding adolescents with excessive oily skin. The youths with excessive oily skin tend to have increased acne. The oily skin is known to lead later in life to the nice skin that is the envy of peers.

These observations have a biochemical basis. Increased androgen content in the skin directs the cells to perform cellular rejuvenation. The excess androgen of adolescence leads to increased acne, but as this level falls with age it becomes less of a problem. Deficient androgen message content, at the skin level, leads to thinning, shriveling and sagging skin.

Gray Hair

What happens when a hair turns gray? One by one the gray hairs form eventually condensing into the many.

Understanding the building blocks of hair coloring leads to insights into the possibilities. Pigment producing cells in the skin and hair are melanocytes. Melanin is the pigment they make. The darker the hair color or skin color, the greater the amount of pigment each cell makes. Blonds and red heads have the least total pigment so they have the least amount of melanin stores. Conversely, darkly pigmented peoples have the most reserve of this pigment.

Intense and prolonged stress has long ago been noticed to accelerate the loss of this pigment leading to gray hair and mottled skin. By understanding the building blocks that make up this pigment the first clue into the process is provided. Melanin is made up of two amino acids occurring in equal amounts and strung together in an alternating sequence that forms long chains. The two amino acids are tryptophan and tyrosine. Each of these amino acids is modified before being linked together in a way that produces the light trapping properties of melanin.

One possibility is that the demands of stress activate the central nervous system in a way that there is a tremendous increases in the need for neural transmitters. Some of the brains main neural transmitters are epinephrine, norepinephrine, dopamine, and serotonin. The first three neural transmitters are made from the amino acid tyrosine. Serotonin is made from the amino acid tryptophan. This could explain the mechanism for diverting pigment producing building blocks. They could then be used to make more neural transmitters during prolonged stress.

The second clue comes from the knowledge that cortisol production rates increase in stressful situations. Cortisol is known for its ability to direct cellular energy out of infrastructure investment and into survival. Skin cell pigmentation production is infrastructure investment and is turned off during prolonged stressful situations. The chronic elevation of cortisol tends to deplete DHEA production. Any owners suffering from a diminished pigmentation pattern should inquire into their DHEA levels with a twenty-four hour urine test. DHEA levels reflect pigmentation levels in the skin.

Prolonged stress under the direction of increased cortisol production directs energy out of the melanocytes for making tyrosine and tryptophan molecular building blocks into melanin. These cell types are consequently deprived of the needed synthesis of melanin for hair and skin pigment. Instead these building blocks are diverted into increased production of neural transmitters that are needed to survive stress. Deprived of their growth factors (DHEA), some of the melanocytes begin to die and will never again make pigment in that area.

The master hormone (ACTH) that directs the adrenal to release cortisol comes out of the brain with a companion molecule with the misleading name of melanocyte stimulating hormone. This name leads one to predict that with increased melanocyte stimulating hormone that coincides with increased cortisol more pigment will be produced. This is only true in specific areas of skin. All other observed effects of prolonged stress lead to an increasing tendency for gray hair formation and blotchy skin. Owners have skin changes under the influence of increased melanocyte stimulating hormone (MSH). The increased MSH occurs only when the master hormone, ACTH is increased. The skin changes which result after the chronic elevated release of cortisol, ACTH, and MSH are increased pigmentation over the neck and creases in the hands and feet. There may also be an increase in liver spots in the facial area.

An explanation for this conundrum is found at the level of the adrenal gland itself. Normally when ACTH activates the adrenal gland, it releases adequate DHEA and cortisol at the same time. Chronic stress changes this ratio with time to more cortisol and less DHEA. DHEA seems to be a necessary growth factor for healthy skin and hair pigmentation. Conversely, excess cortisol hastens the re-direction of energy out of rejuvenation and into survival.

> The purpose of this discussion on gray hair formation is how some scientific thinking is inconsistent. Inconsistent science limits the bigger picture. The bigger picture involves what may be occurring in how the different body hormones are directing energy usage patterns. Changes in energy usage patterns alter the nutritional status of cells. Once the nutritional status of cells, like the pigment producing cells in the skin and hair follicle is altered functional changes occur.

Steroid Pressure

The skin, joints, and the bones serve as excellent examples regarding the consequences of falling steroid content and a decrease from optimal types of steroids (falling steroid tone). These tissues are all on the periphery of receiving a share of the nutrition and energy. Steroid pressure is another useful construct that facilitates a deeper understanding of the unique properties possessed by the steroid class of hormones.

The steroid class of hormones (plus vitamin A and thyroid hormone) concerns the ability of the steroids to access any body tissue. These types of informational substances can penetrate the fat lining of the membranes. They are limited only by their initial concentration, which is determined by their secretion rate. The secreation rate of these informational substances has two determinants. First involves the rate of generation at their sites of manufacture (the gonads, adrenals, and thyroid). Second concerns the amount of stored informational substance available for secretion in these storage sites with the addition of the liver stores of vitamin A.

Much like smoke in a room the informational substance concentration moves from a high concentration to a low concentration. The rate of this movement relates to the initial release rate from the manufacture and storage sites. When the pressure of generation drops in these tissues, the periphery cells suffer first from this deficiency. Cells on the periphery are the skin, the joints, and the bones. The periphery cells deteriorate first when arrival of these substances drops.

A concept arises that underscores the importance of the steroids total body access and the initial rate of release. Steroid 'pressure' denotes both of these determinants of the steroid-like message content adequacy to a cell. The periphery cells are most vulnerable when the steroid pressure falls. Steroids, vitamin A, and thyroid hormone are the only hormones that are powerful enough to switch on or off the DNA programs directly. A complete DNA program is contained in every cell type except the red blood cells and germ cells. The type and amount of steroids that are accessing an owners DNA program is a big first determinant for the functional integrity of a cell. All other hormones act indirectly, if at all, on the DNA program.

The steroid pressure can be visualized as the smoke in a room. It travels from a high concentration to a low concentration and eventually dissipates. It helps to envision this type of situation occurring in the body as the gonads and adrenals are responsible for creating more smoke (steroids). Where smoke is initially released it goes from a high concentration to the low concentration periphery obeying physical laws of the universe. The quality of the type of steroid manufactured and the amount are two determinants of overall health in the cells. The first fact occurs because different steroids, by virtue of their precise shape, instruct the DNA differently on how to spend energy. The second fact concerns the total amount of a certain steroid reaching a cellular DNA program (steroid pressure).

The peripheral tissues are most vulnerable to falling quality of steroid types (decreased steroid tone) and overall amounts (a fall in steroid pressure). The fall in steroid tone and pressure has predictable consequences that occur first in the periphery of the body. The periphery for nutritional supply and waste removal is found in skin, joints, and bone tissues. Looking at the skin in the mirror evidences falling steroid tone around middle age.

Skin appearance and texture is dependent on the maintenance of adequate steroid tone and pressure. Skin is on the periphery and a fall in either of these two cell youth determinants will show up here first. Healing the skin begins with an assessment of hormone levels in the body. Steroids are powerful determinants of how the cell DNA is working and a assessment should be included in the routine office exam.

The skin of physically fit owners will possess high quality and optimal amounts of the different steroids. Conversely, unhealthy owners will have a diminished quality of steroids as well as diminished amounts in their skin. Understanding the need to have high steroid tone and high steroid pressure operating can summarize one of the cornerstones of the healthy skin. There are other hormones that affect skin health by their timing and amount, but it is the steroid-type hormones (including vitamin A and thyroid) that are the most important. Understanding how to attain optimal steroids in the body will expedite healing.

There is an important skin hormone that facilitates the message of the level one hormones. Although the steroids instruct the DNA programs to make cellular proteins, it is the responsibility of IGF-1 to allow nutrient uptake by the cells. An owner can have great steroid tone and pressure, but an insufficient regeneration response because of a nutritional deficiency in the cell (liver chapter).

Even those owners with extremes steroid mismatch states can begin healing once the deficiencies and/or excesses have been identified from a laboratory evaluation (100,000 mile exam).

To grasp the concept of steroid tone, think of its quality ranging from a cellular melody (highest tone states) in healthy extremes, all the way down the continuum of varying levels of cellular noise. Noise creates a chaotic message and is therefore unhealthy in regards to the steroid message directing the cell how to spend energy.

Building on this concept is the construct of steroid pressure that can effectively be thought of as the volume. The volume of either occurs as a melody versus the loud noise possible in unhealthy states. Unhealthy states are consistent with loud noise. Excessive amounts of the steroids are as destructive as the wrong steroids directing a cells DNA. It is also true that in some owners the melody is great, but the pressure is low because their gonads and/or adrenals are failing to make adequate steroid pressure.

The owners' adrenals and gonads create the 'pressure head' for steroids. For vitamin A, the liver is usually determines this hormones release. Vitamin A is stored and released from the liver as needed. The processed food diet is typically deficient in vitamin A. Thyroid pressure is generated from the thyroid gland. The steroid-like hormones produced here behave like a gas defusing from a high concentration to the far periphery of the tissues. When the skin no longer receives adequate steroid tone and/or pressure, its cells behave like other cells when there is sub-optimal informational direction. Like other cells, skin cells need direction on how to spend cellular energy. This is largely determined by which DNA programs are turned off or on in a cell.

Gonad and/or adrenal insufficiency first appears in the peripheral tissues of skin, joints, and bone. This is obvious when studying the chemical behavior of molecules like steroids. Anatomically, the skin is the outward periphery of tissues and is last in line with the receiving of hormones and nutrients. Pressure gradients for oxygen and steroids are lowest when they travel to the periphery. The outer living layer of skin is more vulnerable because it has no direct blood supply. The skin relies on the slower process of diffusion of nutrients and hormones down their concentration gradient.

Excess fat can hide the earlier stages of gonad and/ or adrenal insufficiency by stretching the dermal layer of skin in a misleading way. This shows up in subtle ways to the trained eye. These owners often have a bloated look that coincides with how the dermal layer feels. Owners are often fooled into thinking things are great when the bad is hiding amongst the fat. Missing the earliest clues of falling steroid pressure and tone leads to prolonged recovery.

Skin is the outward expression of the peripheral tissues. Deficiencies of steroid output or quality show up here first. The facial skin begins to lose taught ness, fine wrinkles appear, and puffiness follows. The general process makes the face less recognizable compared to the face of their youth. Processes that increase steroid pressure and tone slow this development.

Close in onset of facial changes are the first signs that the joints are less capable. They begin to creak and ache. Later in the process, the upper back begins to hunch over. As the steroid deficiency progresses, the internal organs begin to shrink and falter. This happens when organs no longer receive sufficient message content directing the cell types in the wise use of cellular energy.

Each owner's body has its own subtle unique order in which different cell types respond to insufficient message content. No one will deteriorate in the same sequence as another. As steroid imbalance progresses this syndrome becomes more predictable. These owners have a look of someone who is beaten down by life. It is at this stage the joints become widely involved with degenerative osteoarthritic changes. This causes deformity, pain, and loss of usefulness. Other processes contribute to cellular age. In the peripheral tissues there seems to be a particular predilection for the ravages of diminished message content leading these cells to aging.

Skin – Taking Out the Garbage

The skin is well supplied with sweat glands that operate on the same principle as the kidneys. The sweat glands depend on aldosterone to determine the final mineral composition of sweat. When aldosterone levels are high, the sweat contains high amounts of potassium and the body conserves sodium. When aldosterone levels are low the sweat becomes high in sodium and the body conserves potassium. Many other toxins are eliminated by the sweat glands and provide aid to the kidneys.

Taking out the garbage that piles up in the peripheral tissues of the skin domain is accomplished in two ways. Drink water. Skin cells are anatomically on the periphery and will be most vulnerable to dehydrating forces. Extremes of environmental drying situations will only exacerbate an ongoing deficiency of the most powerful medicine of all. Adequate water promotes adequate water content in the skin. The skin dries out first when body water content decreases.

The second method of taking out the skin garbage involves perspiration. Traditional medicine men living in the northwest illustrate the power of this for taking out the skin garbage. These people have nice skin because they sweat in their lodges regularly and flush the garbage out of the peripheral tissues. It also facilitates hydration of wrinkled skin. People who exercise to the point of breaking a healthy sweat will notice the improved skin appearance following a work out. With increased pollution from all sources, it makes sense to include effort in the regular flushing of the peripheral tissues through breaking a sweat.

Skin and Nutrition

Many skin conditions are the result of nutritional deficiencies. One group of nutritional deficiencies is the inappropriate hormonal fats precursors that line the dermal layer of skin cells. These fats produce inflammatory conditions like psoriasis, seborrhea, and dermatitis conditions. Optimizing hormonal fats (ecosanoids) will go along way toward healing skin conditions. The right hormonal fats are only possible when attending to diets that encourage the right hormones (level 2 hormones). The right essential fatty acids are also essential in the diet.

Summary of the inflammatory conditions of the skin as they relate to nutritional fat

1. Avoid inappropriate hormonal fats (polyunsaturated and partially hydrogenated fats)
2. Optimize the level two hormones ratios between insulin and glucagon, by consuming a diet that encourages this.
3. Consume the best hormonal fat precursor sources (olive oil, fish oil, borage oil, and primrose oil).

Flax seed oil is missing from the list for sources of essential fatty acids. Flax seed oil does contain large amounts of the essential fatty acids. Flax seed contains other oils that require it to be refrigerated, protected from air, and protected from light. Once flax seed oil gains entry in the tissues, it is exposed

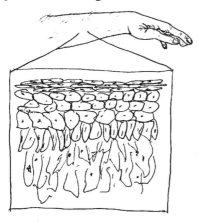

to heat and oxygen. This reactive combination allows the other oils in flax seeds to oxidize. The oxidation propensity of flax seed is well documented in the house painting industry. Oil based paints of yesteryear were formed from flax seed oil. Flax seed oil is also known as linseed oil. Linseed oil was chosen because of the speed at which it oxidizes when exposed to air. Once oils become oxidized they harden and this is not consistent with body health.

Vitamin C is also important for the support layer of the outer lying epidermis. The internal layer of support tissue is called the dermis and contains a blood and nervous supply. The integrity of the dermal layer determines the elastic quality of the skin. Sufficient skin elasticity occurs when this layer contains optimal amounts of the connective tissue proteins of collagen and elastin. Vitamin C is a critical ingredient needed for the manufacture of this connective tissue layer because it serves as a cofactor in its synthesis. Without adequate vitamin C there is insufficient manufacture of this layer. Deficiency of the dermis layer creates another way for the skin to deteriorate.

A and B vitamin deficiencies are also possibilities in skin disease. Live food sources for these vitamins are emerging as superior in their ability to be utilized by the body. Processed food diets lead owners to become deficient in either or both vitamin A complex and B vitamins. Vitamin A deficiency dramatically increases the likelihood of skin cancer because it instructs the skin cell DNA program on how to differentiate (mature). Skin cells stay immature without adequate vitamin A message content. Immaturity is a central property of cancer cells. Conventionally trained physician should be encouraged to inquire into the vitamin A status of skin cancer patients.

Chapter 19

The Liver

The liver serves multiple roles in the body. The tasks of the liver can be arranged into five main groups.[19]

1. Disarm and remove toxins
2. Controls the availability of fuel in the blood stream
3. Facilitates the assimilation of fat into the body
4. Storing and releasing minerals, vitamins and hormones
5. Manufacture and release transport proteins in the blood serum.

Each of these five main liver tasks is fundamental to health. The assessment on how the liver performs in these five main areas is often superficially addressed. Longevity requires that all five of these liver tasks perform at efficient rates.

Disarm and Remove Toxins

The liver needs certain molecular parts to disarm many different types of toxins that are encountered when the owner creates or ingests them.

Toxins made by every day processes:

Natural body waste	Drugs
Ingested toxins	Cookware
Food additives	Food pollutants
Air pollutants	Water pollutants
Herbicides	Heavy metals
Toxins absorbed from an unhealthy colon	

The liver has a choice on how it will disarm any toxin. There are five common mechanisms for the initial inactivation of toxins. In general, all five of these processes facilitate the next phase of liver detoxification. It is in the initial stage that the liver machinery creates a molecular appendage which the body can attach the final removal compounds to. This allows the toxin to become water soluble or inactive. The final removal compounds cannot attach until one of five initial reactions occur. The five initial liver deactivation methods are:

1. Oxidation
2. Hydrogen addition
3. Hydration (addition of water)

4. Cleavage through hydrolysis (removal of water)
5. Removal of chloride, fluoride, bromide or iodide

The trouble with these processes is that they each tend to create reactive intermediates. The liver needs protection from these intermediates. The protective molecules needed by the liver are commonly called anti-oxidants or 'rust retardants'. The better the supply of these substances the liver has, the more protection one has from liver injury. The greater the load of toxins, the more anti-oxidants is needed. More anti-oxidants become necessary because they will be used up quickly.

The basic list of liver anti-oxidants is:

Vitamin A	Vitamin E
Vitamin C	Bioflavonoids (berries)
Selenium	Zinc
Coenzyme Q10	Pycnogenol (grape seeds)
Lipoic acid (real foods only)	

Thiols that are found in garlic, onions, and cruciferous vegetables

These anti-oxidants are the basic protectors of the liver tissue. The liver cells need the protection of anti-oxidants because of the reactive intermediates created when the liver begins the first phase of deactivating and/or removing a body toxin. There are also certain vitamins and nutrients that are needed to power the molecular machinery that performs the task of disarmament.

The basic list of these vitamins is:

Vitamin B1	Vitamin B1
Vitamin B2	2Lipoic acid Co enzyme Q10
Vitamin B3	Pantothenic acid Folic acid
Vitamin B6	Phospholipids like lecithin

The liver must begin the initial attachment of molecular appendages without releasing reactive molecules that can oxidize liver cells. It is the anti-oxidants that prevent the oxidants from causing liver rust. These initial deactivation steps require specific vitamins to power the enzymatic machinery needed for these activities. Once the liver cell has created the various appendages on a toxin, it needs to proceed on to deactivation.

The basic choices for the final reaction in toxin removal are the addition of:
Sulfate
Glucuronic acid
Glutathione or n-acetyl cysteine
Acetate
Methyl
Certain amino acids: glycine, taurine, glutamine, ornithine, and arginine

Depending on the final solubility characteristics, the deactivated toxin will either be excreted in the bile or blood stream. When excreted in the bile it will be removed in the feces. However, poor bacteria content in the colon can prevent this and the toxin can be absorbed back into the body. Some toxins are reabsorbed because the wrong bacteria rip apart the deactivation appendage that the liver attached.

When the toxin is excreted into the blood stream, it is destined for the kidneys that can remove large amounts of toxins. Many toxins and hormone excesses that the kidney removes must first be made water-soluble by the liver. This includes ammonia, steroids, small chains of amino acids, and heavy metal complexes.

The liver is one tissue that possesses remarkable capabilities for regenerating new cells until its underlying architecture becomes disrupted. Disruption of the architecture state of the liver is cirrhosis. Healing is compromised because cell regeneration is disorganized. At the level of cirrhosis the energy template of where cells belong has been disrupted. When the energy template is disrupted a progressive cellular disorganization ensues.

The liver is responsible for the up take of ammonia. Ammonia is generated by amino acid breakdown when protein is converted to sugar (gluconeogenesis). The ammonia formed in the breakdown process is converted to urea in the liver and removed in the urine. The kidney has the ability to excrete a limited amount of ammonia. However, it is the liver that neutralizes the majority of this toxin. The liver through the use of bile or the kidney detoxifies many environmental toxins and prescription drugs. The liver requires numerous nutritional factors to effectively remove toxins and is greatly diminished without sufficient nutrition.

A rich system of blood vessels (liver sinusoids) exists in the liver. These are arranged to allow immune system scavenger cells room to grab unwanted material out of the blood stream. They are fed directly from the portal vein that is the drain for all the blood in the intestines and colon.

The Liver Determines Fuel Availability

Inappropriate fuel types in the blood stream is the primary cause of diseases like diabetes, heart disease, strokes, and peripheral vascular disease. These diseases can have their origins in the liver. When it treats fuel types inappropriately, the blood vessels begin to break down. Inappropriate fuel types released by the liver with consequent blood vessel injury are the high blood sugar of diabetes and the high rate of release into the blood stream of LDL cholesterol. In both cases the blood vessel walls are injured by excess of these fuels. In both cases the liver creating and releasing these fuels inappropriately causes the excess. The source of the release results from the liver receiving the wrong hormones.

Healing involves attention to lifestyles, nutritional nutrient intake, and hormone balance at the level of the liver. Owners are told the hopeless mantra about the cruel hand that genetics has dealt them. The typical approach sells drugs and procedures. Healing involves improving the hormone types and amounts that instruct the liver on whether to store or release fuel.

Like other organs, the liver follows the message content it receives. Healing involves an assessment of the proportions of the hormones that deliver message content at the level of the liver cell. Only when the proper amounts of hormones instruct the liver will these diseases begin to heal.

The hormone message delivered to the liver determines whether the liver takes fuel out or puts fuel into the blood stream. Five main hormones determine how the liver directs fuel - insulin, glucagon, growth hormone, cortisol, and epinephrine. The message content arriving at the liver determines whether the liver will manufacture fuel in storage forms (glycogen and LDL cholesterol) or release them as readily combustible types for use in the cellular power plants (mitochondria). If the fuel is in storage form, it does this by removing fuel in the blood stream. The liver synthesizes LDL cholesterol particles with storage in mind. Even though the liver eventually releases them, their design is such that they head for the storage destinations of the macrophages that line the arteries and the fat cells.

The opposite situation occurs when the liver releases sugar and fatty acids into the blood stream. These types of fuel are immediately accessible to the cells when adequate IGF-1 is present in the blood stream. Once inside the cells these fuels are either combusted in their power plants or utilized for structural components in the cell. The other four hormones encourage this type of fuel release, as well.

It is helpful to arrange the hormones interacting with the liver in the antique weight scale analogy. This arrangement reveals that only insulin is on the side of the scale tipping it in the direction of storing fuels (glycogen and LDL cholesterol). The other four hormones (at the level of the liver) counter storage and encourage the power plant accessible types of fuel release by the liver into the blood stream.

The insulin predominant hormone situation allows a tremendous increase in fat because insulin behaves like the body's fuel nozzle. It desires to fill the cellular fuel tanks for cellular build up purposes and not fuel burning purposes. When the cell fuel tanks are full for carbohydrate, insulin instructs the liver to make the extra sugar into fat and cholesterol. This is why insulin is necessary for fat cell growth and in the storage of muscle and liver glycogen.

Counter regulatory hormones can overpower insulin's ability to direct carbohydrate storage and fat in the liver (each to varying degrees). Counter regulatory hormones direct the liver to dump stored fuel into the blood stream for usage in cell power plants.

When between meals or physically stressed the counter regulatory hormones become elevated. The fat stores are needed during intense and prolonged exercise. Exercising muscles and heart prefer fat as their fuel source. Carbohydrate storage is limited to about 1500 calories in the liver and about 500 calories in the muscles. When the glycogen stores are burned, as in the case of prolonged exercise, the body needs other fuel sources for energy. A 150 pound athlete with 15% body fat has access to 22.5 pounds of fat times 3500 calories per pound of fat. The proper counter regulatory hormones allow access to the tremendous fat fuel storehouses.

Nerves and red blood cells need exclusively sugar for all their energy needs. This fact explains the desirability of adequate counter hormones that direct the additional release of fat. Processes that conserve glycogen for the nerve and red blood cells enhance endurance because nerve and red blood cell optimal function are preserved when their sugar supply remains available. This happens when the muscles and heart have access to more fat for their energy needs. Conversely, exercising owners that insist on promoting high insulin states compromise their red blood cells and nerves due to sugar stores being consumed more quickly. When insulin excess occurs in the liver, it competes with the ability of liver to dump fat into the blood stream and create more sugar from amino acids. The sugar stores dry up with the same level of activity because less fat is available. Exhausted sugar stores in the exercising athlete are commonly known as the 'wall'. The wall will arrive more quickly when insulin levels are high.

Longevity and exercise performance are critically related to the balance of hormones that instruct the liver. When these hormones are improved not only exercise ability but also heart disease, blood vessel disease and diabetes risk and complications are reduced.

Insulin Causes Fuel Storage as Fat or Glycogen

The counter hormones, glucagon, growth hormone, cortisol, and epinephrine all cause the liver to release and synthesize readily accessible fuels into the blood stream.

Initially, insulin will only direct the liver to remove sugar from the blood stream for storage as glycogen. It can store about four hundred grams of sugar in this manner. Sedentary owners have livers that are almost always full of stored sugar. In this case, insulin directs the liver to make the excess sugar into fat and cholesterol that are packaged for the fat depots. These depots are in the fat cells and in the macrophages that line the arteries. At the level of the liver, insulin is the only hormone that promotes storage of fuel. The other four hormones oppose the message content of insulin at the level of the liver.

Glucagon counters insulin in four ways in the liver. It stimulates the liver to change available amino acids into sugar (gluconeogenesis). Second, it stimulates the release of stored sugar (glycogen) from the liver into the blood stream. Third, it stimulates the release of stored fat into the blood stream. Glucagon message content makes body fuel available. Fourth, the glucagon message content decreases cholesterol and fat synthesis from carbohydrate. When cholesterol and fat are manufactured at slower rates, LDL cholesterol levels in the blood stream will go down.

Growth hormone has the same effect as glucogon on the liver. There are two important exceptions. It inhibits the conversion of amino acids into fuel. This is known as a protein sparring effect. When growth hormone levels are high, it counters the ability of glucagon to convert protein into sugar. The advantage of having high growth hormone levels relative to the other counter regulatory hormones is that it conserves protein. In contrast, all other counter regulatory hormones to insulin are catabolic toward protein stores.

The second unique affect of growth hormone's message is its ability to direct the liver to release insulin-like growth factor (IGF). When this hormone is outside the liver, it acts like insulin by facilitating the muscle cells to take up fuel (sugar). In healthy owners insulin-like growth factor (IGF) is found at levels one hundred times that of insulin in the blood stream. This liver secreted hormone reduces the need for insulin and does not stimulate the liver to make fat and cholesterol. A longevity advantage occurs when IGF levels are high. High IGF levels depend on three things, an adequate release of growth hormone, a healthy liver capable of high rates of IGF manufacture, and adequate DHEA levels to stimulate the liver cell DNA programs to direct the manufacture of IGF.

Growth hormone effects on the body need to be understood in a tandem-like fashion. Once the tandem of growth hormone release followed by IGF release is recognized one can avoid the confusion discussed in the scientific literature. Medical physiology textbooks describe growth hormone as a diabetogenic hormone. This is a half-truth except when the liver is diseased or growth hormone production becomes abnormally high. In this case, increased growth hormone levels can occur with the disease acromegaly and with high dose growth hormone replacement therapy.

Growth hormone will counter a diabetes tendency by its message directing the release of IGF. IGF behaves like insulin in the circulation. This happens because of the tandem effects of growth hormone release followed by IGF release. Medical physiology textbooks focus on the fact that growth hormone initially causes the release of sugar into the blood stream. However, the tandem of IGF release that follows causes the peripheral uptake of sugar out of the blood stream. It is the tandem of growth hormone release followed by IGF release that prevents the overall rise of blood sugar. The insulin-like effect of IGF explains why growth hormone in normal amounts lowers insulin requirements in patients who have a normal liver. IGF is released when growth hormone is elevated. The insulin-like growth factor released acts like insulin in the cells outside of the liver (the periphery). In the periphery, insulin-like growth factor directs many cells to take sugar out of the blood stream. When adequate insulin-like growth factor is secreted, the insulin needed to normalize the blood sugar decreases. Some physicians believe that insulin, outside of the liver in the healthful state, is unnecessary beyond very low levels.

IGF has the additional benefit of facilitating the uptake of cell nutrition and minerals. IGF occurs at one hundred times the amount of insulin in the circulation when an owner is healthy. High levels of IGF prevent the need for insulin in the cells outside the liver. Conversely, low levels of IGF require an increased insulin secretion because a sugar load will require more insulin to return the blood sugar to normal following a carbohydrate meal. However, healthy owners have one hundred times more IGF in the blood stream as compared to insulin. Unhealthy owners have liver strain because more insulin forces the liver into sucking excessive sugar out of the blood stream. This also increases the amount of LDL cholesterol synthesis. Therefore the imbalance between insulin levels and IGF levels creates a situation that favors increased body fat.

Cortisol is the next counter hormone to insulin message content. Cortisol is powerful in preventing insulin from removing sugar molecules from the blood stream. Cortisol directs the liver to release stored liver sugar and fat into the blood stream and the fat cells to release fatty acid fuels into the blood stream. In addition, it acts on the protein stores of the body to release amino acids into the blood stream. The liver then sucks up the released amino acids for processing into sugar. The process of gluconeogenesis denotes the conversion of liver sequestered amino acids into sugar. Extremely high cortisol release tends to deplete body protein content. High cortisol release occurs with stress.

Cortisol instructs the liver cell DNA. The liver cell DNA when instructed by cortisol leads to the formation of certain cell receptors. The cell receptors are needed to recognize hormones that are not as powerful as level one hormones. Only level one hormones, like cortisol, can instruct the DNA programs. The cortisol directed receptors are necessary to recognize adrenalin (epinephrine) and glucagon. These are level three and two hormones respectively (hierarchy of hormones). The liver will be unable to recognize the message content of epinephrine and glucagon without sufficient cortisol. Cortisol deficiency therefore, sets up a situation of the 'lesser hormones' not being able to deliver their message content (elevate the blood sugar in this case). The only other counter regulatory hormone to insulin, growth hormone, will cause the release of IGF that exacerbates low blood sugars. Here lies the under recognized mechanism for low blood sugar between meals.

Low blood sugars (hypoglycemia) are the hallmark of diminished adrenal reserve (section two). The adrenal gland manufactures all body cortisol. Deficient cortisol in the setting of high insulin will lead to diminished blood sugar levels. Unfortunately, many of these hypoglycemic prone owners are prescribed frequent feedings. This approach leads to weight gain and a compounding of problems with the passage of time.

However, a twenty-four hour urine test will document diminished adrenal cortisol production. Occasionally, the additional test of cortrosyn challenge of the adrenal reserve function will be needed to elucidate borderline cortisol reserve. There are several considerations for healing from diminished adrenal function. First, dietary changes for carbohydrate and mineral imbalances are a strong start. Second, the results of the twenty-four hour urine test document the scope of the steroid imbalance that includes cortisol deficiency. In some cases replacement with real steroid hormones is necessary. In others, diet and life style changes are all that will be necessary. Customizing replacements to actual needs prevents side effects from cortisol replacement. In addition, changing the carbohydrate and mineral content of the diet prevents side effects. The replacement program often includes other adrenal steroids as indicated by the twenty-four hour urine test. When these factors are considered together, side effects are reduced or eliminated.

Epinephrine is one other counter regulatory hormone that opposes insulin. The other counter regulatory hormone, growth hormone acts mostly in the liver in its opposition to insulin. Epinephrine acts like cortisol in its ability to free fatty acids from the fat stores.

The Liver Controls Fat Content

Diabetes and heart disease are often diseases that are secondary to the liver receiving poor informational direction. Ninety percent of all diabetics have an excess of total body insulin. Most heart disease owners also have an excess message content from insulin. These diseases, when insulin is the cause, begin with poor message content at the level of the liver. The poor message content arises from excess insulin. The liver cell follows the message content it receives. Insulin in the liver is opposed by growth hormone, epinephrine, cortisol, and glucagon message content. The balance of message content between the hormone insulin and the other four counter hormones is a major determinant in the risk of an owner for developing these diseases.

The complete cholesterol profile that is typically performed on an annual basis provides clues as to the summation of message content in one's liver. Some owners may have a normal blood cholesterol profile, but an obese body. Only fifty percent of heart disease victims have abnormal cholesterol. The fact that they are obese says they have too much insulin because it is always a pre-requisite for body fat. With more insulin there is more fat for the body to hang on to. High insulin fills the macrophages that line the inside of arteries. Fat laden macrophages eventually plug an artery even if the cholesterol is normal.

Whenever the lab results are sub-optimal or the owner is obese, several things need to be considered and investigated. With this and some life style changes are adopted diseases are often effectively curtailed. Altering the message content that the liver receives is critical. When these primary factors are ignored symptom control medicine is all that is possible.

Healing from heart disease or diabetes involves alleviating these abnormalities.
1. Insulin and glucagon ratio of message content in the liver
2. Potassium deficiency leads to insulin resistance connection
3. Growth hormone connection
    a) Excess
    b) Deficiency
4. Cortisol excess
    a) Normal pancreas
    b) Wounded pancreas
5. Thyroid status
6. Growth hormone when the liver is unhealthy
7. Insulin pro-hormone levels and body fat
8. Excessively high estrogen levels lead to higher insulin levels

There is a common factor between the disease processes of diabetes and heart disease. Although ninety percent of diabetics have elevated insulin levels almost all heart disease involves elevated insulin levels. In diabetics, their body fat has finally elevated to the point (genetically determined) where their pancreas can no longer handle the insulin need. Insulin need rises when body mass goes up or carbohydrate consumption increases. When a pancreas cannot meet the insulin demanded by either body mass or carbohydrate consumption blood sugar will rise. By definition, when blood sugar rises beyond one hundred and forty diabetes is diagnosed. However, the same process of elevated insulin plugs up the heart diseased owner. However, the pure heart diseased owner, and not diabetic, can still make enough insulin to keep his blood sugar normal.

Many heart disease patients start out with normal blood sugars and only after many years the pancreas becomes exhausted. This commonality between these two diseases explains why mainstream medicine is finally acknowledging that at diagnosis of adult onset diabetes, heart disease is presumed to already exist. Ninety percent of diabetes and almost all heart diseases owners have elevated blood insulin levels. High insulin levels that occur in both diseases leads to increased blood fat abnormalities. However, in the case of the adult onset diabetic, the amount of insulin needed exceeds the ability of the pancreas. When body mass and carbohydrate consumption exceed the pancreas ability to excrete enough insulin, adult onset diabetes results. In both cases, high insulin is required. High insulin levels direct the liver to make excess LDL cholesterol. The excess LDL cholesterol released into the blood stream then causes the vessel walls to collect LDL cholesterol in the macrophages. The elevated blood sugar of diabetics is an additional mechanism that injures the blood vessel.

Mainstream medicine tends to focus on normalizing the blood sugar at the price of increasing insulin message content. Conventional physicians are then taught to peripherally address the increased insulin fat making side effect with cholesterol lowering drugs. Healing requires that insulin levels come down rather than pummel the liver with poison.

This common denominator is particularly disturbing when realizing how mainstream medicine treats these disease types. They sidestep the central determinant, insulin excess. Ninety percent of diabetics are treated by methodologies that raise insulin. This may normalize blood sugars, but it will only make the fat coating the arteries worse. In the case of heart disease, the common class of liver poison, the statin drugs, is given to inhibit cholesterol making enzymes, HMG CoA reductase. However, in biochemistry textbooks it is known that if insulin message content is decreased, this enzyme turns down its activity level naturally. All of these eight factors affect the message content at the level of the liver by an effect on insulin message content.

Insulin and Glucagon Message Content in the Liver

It is more accurate to say the activity of the cholesterol- manufacturing enzyme in the liver is determined by the ratio, in amount, between glucagon and insulin. A high protein and low carbohydrate diet will tend to increase glucagon levels relative to insulin. Owners who eat steak and eggs while simultaneously decreasing carbohydrates will tend to see a drop in their cholesterol. There are other factors that influence blood cholesterol level, but this ratio is all-important in most owners. Without attention appropriately placed on an improved insulin and glucagon ratio healing a blood cholesterol problem is difficult.

Diminished Potassium leads to an Increased Insulin Level Requirement

Potassium deficiency causes an increased insulin message in the liver. Diminished body potassium has detrimental effects to the insulin and glucagon ratio. This mechanism of altered blood fat creation from the liver is rarely recognized in America today. This basic defect arises because owners who subsist on a processed food diet stuff their cells chronically with the wrong mineral ratios. The body was designed to intake three times as much potassium as sodium. Processed foods contain a reversal of this natural mineral requirement. Around middle age the kidney begins to falter in its ability to conserve potassium and excrete excess sodium.

The potassium deficiency of middle age means less of this mineral becomes available to bring the blood sugar down following a carbohydrate meal. One potassium is necessary to bring one sugar molecule inside a liver cell for sugar storage purposes. This is also true for all cells except in the brain and red blood cells. When there is inadequate potassium the pancreas will secrete extra insulin eventually because it senses the delay in the blood sugar fall after eating. This will be met with resistance because the basic defect is not enough potassium to uptake the sugar into the liver cells. It is slightly more complicated than this because of the IGF that is released between meals. Potassium deficiency impedes the storage of sugar as glycogen because potassium is needed in a fixed amount per gram of glycogen in the liver. The liver manufacture of fat and cholesterol is not dependent on potassium levels.

The extra insulin that occurs in these situations will activate the fat making machinery in the liver. This happens whenever it receives a excess in the insulin message. In contrast, the healthy body has ample potassium to facilitate the rapid liver uptake of sugar out of the blood stream following a meal. Between meals or with exercise the liver stored potassium and IGF are secreted together. IGF with adequate potassium can promote the uptake of nutrients. The potassium and other nutrients are needed for cell energy and rejuvenation (i.e. strong, large muscles). When there is not enough potassium, the blood sugar is normalized more by the liver than by the peripheral cells.

The dependency of insulin on adequate body potassium exposes a defect in the high protein diet proponents. It clarifies how the fruit and vegetable proponents have a piece of the puzzle that pertains to diets that work. When both of these pieces are correctly re-united a superior diet and cholesterol profile will be possible.

The high protein diet premise improves when adding in the optimal ratio of potassium to sodium mineral content. This drastically lowers the insulin message content needed in their bodies. A lower message content of insulin will improve the ratio between it and glucagon. This will allow less cholesterol and fat synthesis in the liver. Diminished cholesterol and fat synthesis leads to improved blood cholesterol. When less insulin is needed the pancreas strain is reduced. In the case of diabetes the need for extra insulin becomes less likely.

Growth Hormone Connection - What Message the Liver Receives and the Effects on Diabetes and Heart Disease

Growth Hormone Excess

Excessive growth hormone tends to promote diabetes when the ability of the liver to secrete the consequent insulin-like growth factor (IGF) is exceeded. Within the liver it promotes the release of sugar and fat into the blood stream. The second effect concerns the simultaneous release of insulin-like growth factor (IGF-1). IGF-1 acts like insulin out in the periphery, muscle, and organ cells, in directing of sugar uptake from the blood stream. When the liver is diseased the second effect fails to occur to varying degrees. Elevated GH with a diminished IGF-1 release will cause the blood sugar to rise. When blood sugar rises beyond the pancreas ability to manufacture the insulin necessary to counter act the excess growth hormone, diabetes results. Growth hormone excess can occur either in acromegaly or with high dose growth hormone replacement protocols. It is the increased insulin, in the above scenario that leads to altered blood cholesterol profiles. When this occurs heart disease and diabetes are more likely.

Growth Hormone Deficiency

Problems with blood sugar control occur in this situation, but for different reasons. Blood sugar will tend to rise because there is less liver direction to release insulin like growth factor (IGF). IGF levels occur at levels greater than one hundred times those of insulin in the blood stream in a healthy owner. With less IGF, more insulin must be secreted for the sugar load. The increased demand for insulin can exhaust the pancreas of some owners and diabetes develops. Sedentary lifestyles promote a decline in growth hormone secretion. Conversely owners that exercise have higher growth hormone levels. That means less insulin will be required because of the increased liver stimulation to secrete IGF. Less insulin creates less message content in the liver to make fat and cholesterol. Athletic training will decrease cholesterol levels.

Excess Cortisol Levels - The Message the Liver Receives Depends on the Health of the Pancreas

Excess Cortisol

Excess cortisol creates obesity or borderline diabetes. In either case the blood vessels are damaged. The phenotype distinguishes which process is occurring. The twenty-four hour urine test confirms the physical exam and blood findings. When owners have a normal pancreas with increased cortisol they tend to become obese. With the passage of time they will tend to appear cushingoid (moon face, buffalo hump, stria on the abdomen, panus formation on the abdomen, muscle loss). If the cortisol level is high enough they can reach the upper limit of the pancreas for insulin production. Diabetes results. It is the insulin that makes them fat. It is the cortisol that elevates their blood sugar and sucks down their body protein content (catabolic effect).

Mainstream physicians are generally groomed into thinking that cortisol directly makes these owners fat. This is not true. First, the elevated cortisol directs the liver to begin creating and dumping blood sugar into the blood stream. This result is from the fact that when cortisol levels are increased the body thinks there is an emergency. When modern stress creates increased cortisol, no physical challenge ever comes and the body eventually recognizes the increased blood sugar as inappropriate. When the body recognizes that an increase in blood sugar is inappropriate, insulin levels rise. When insulin is secreted in these higher amounts, the liver receives a higher message content to make fat. Increased fat synthesis leads to weight gain.

The second group of increased cortisol producers is often missed because the lack of body fat fools the physician. Any owner who has heart disease and appears on the emaciated side of physical body habitués deserves a deeper inquiry. Although they have increased cortisol output, they have a 'wounded' pancreas. Wounded pancreas cannot increase insulin production to match the increased sugar output of high cortisol. Increased blood sugar is only transient. The normal fasting sugars are almost always normal, but the glucose challenge tests are not. These owners acquire blood vessel injury from the episodic elevations of sugar following the cortisol surges or carbohydrate binges. Increased blood vessel injury occurs from the rust processes that high sugar causes to the vessel walls.

Thyroid Levels

Thyroid levels are a determinate of how fast the cell power plants can utilize blood fat. Owners with low thyroid levels have a diminished ability to utilize fuel in their power plants (mitochondria). Their livers are feeble because of the diminished thyroid message content at the level of the liver cell DNA program. Scientific experiments on dogs that had their thyroids partially or totally destroyed clearly showed the pathologic changes at the level of the liver. Without adequate thyroid, the liver becomes pathologic because it lacks appropriate instruction at the level the DNA programs.

Growth Hormone and the Unhealthy Liver

Unhealthy livers are unable to release adequate insulin-like growth factor (IGF) when growth hormone instructs them to do so. The growth hormone can be diabetogenic in these situations. Injured liver cells still make fuel available when directed to do so long after their ability to make proteins is curtailed. Insulin-like growth hormone is a liver manufactured protein. There are many different reasons for the liver to become defective. Some of them include poor nutrition, excessive liver toxin exposure (alcohol, prescription drugs, putrefaction of colon with liver reabsorption, and poor trophic hormone levels (cortisol, thyroid, androgens, etc.).

Insulin - Pro-hormone Levels

Insulin is first made within a 'package', the pro-hormone, that is converted to insulin before release into the blood stream. There are certain situations that create an increased release of the pro-hormone form of insulin (in the package). This is when the pancreas is forced to increase insulin production in response to some other body condition (obesity, high carbohydrate diets, insulin resistance). When this occurs the effectiveness to remove sugar from the blood stream is diminished per amount of pancreas secretion. The pro-hormone seems to retain some of its message content in the ability to make the liver create fat from sugar. This also happened in the growth of fat cells.

High Estrogen Levels and Increased Insulin

There has been a flurry of media attention toward supposed new evidence about increased estrogen levels and the increased risk for heart disease. All along the evidence for this predictable association has been buried in the medical textbooks.

This chain of events is high estrogen leads to increased growth hormone release and simultaneously curtails the liver's release of insulin like-growth hormone. The decrease of insulin-like growth hormone and the increased growth hormone message causes the sugar release to be uncompensated because there is a diminished release of insulin-like growth hormone. In this situation, the blood sugar will rise higher than it does when excess estrogen is not present. The body eventually senses that the blood sugar is elevated and insulin is secreted. When this happens, the liver receives increased message content to manufacture sugar into fat and cholesterol. Fat and cholesterol are released as LDL cholesterol. The blood has more LDL cholesterol and the triglyceride levels will be higher when measured. Triglyceride levels are only the summation of all the fat in the blood stream (the fat content of HDL, LDL, and VLDL cholesterol). Both high triglycerides and LDL cholesterol are associated with an increased risk of heart disease.

Liver Facilitates the Assimilation of Fat from the Digestive Tube

There is a system in the liver for breaking down spent hemoglobin molecules by utilizing certain parts of these aged hemoglobin molecules, bilirubin, for the manufacture of bile. Bile facilitates the ability of the digestive tracts to absorb dietary fat and the excretion of certain body wastes that are processed in the liver. The bile system is anatomically like a 'tree' in the liver. The smaller branches of bile containing the fluid coalesce into larger bile containing branches until they all converge in the common hepatic duct. The bile system tree has its root in the gall bladder that lies outside the liver. Salts of cholesterol are also used in the chemical concoction called bile (digestion chapter). All the constituents that make up the bile facilitate the assimilation of dietary fat. When the liver is sick the bile can back up into the blood stream. Jaundice is the result of certain components backing up in the blood stream. It is the hemoglobin breakdown product, bilirubin, being too high, which causes the skin color changes of jaundice.

The message content that the liver receives can help or hinder the fat content in the blood vessels and body. Equally important to overall body health is the molecular parts needed by the liver to deactivate numerous toxins.

The Liver Stores and Manufactures Vitamins, Minerals, and Hormones

The liver stores many vitamins such as vitamin D, A, and B12. In the case of vitamin A, the liver also manufactures the transport protein, retinol-binding protein. When carotene is absorbed from the diet, it requires a capable liver to split carotene in half. Two vitamins A are formed from one carotene. Some owners begin to turn yellow when their liver is unable to split this. Vitamin A is best thought of as a hormone. The vitamin A 'hormone' belongs to the most powerful class the level one hormones. All level one hormones share the unique ability to regulate the DNA programs. Healthy owners have ample vitamin A stored in the liver.

Part of the ability to intake nutrition at the cellular level depends on the liver storing adequate potassium. A high potassium diet facilitates this ability. One potassium is used to move one sugar molecule out of the blood stream. Cells need adequate potassium to stabilize the proteins in the cell. The size of muscle cells serves as an example of the importance of adequate potassium.

IGF levels also determine the ability of muscle cells to intake nutrients out of the blood stream. Once nutrients are inside a cell, they can be incorporated into power plant generation activities or regeneration projects. IGF activity also depends on adequate potassium release from the liver. Normally potassium and IGF are released from the liver at the same time. Owners who possess high potassium and IGF stores in their liver have a health advantage. The rate of IGF manufacture in the liver is determined by the amount of DHEA that reaches the liver DNA programs. The amount of IGF released by the liver is determined by the amount of growth hormone released from the pituitary. Common factors that encourage the release of growth hormone from the pituitary are exercise, fasting between meals, high dopamine levels, and low blood sugar. Conversely, high estrogen depresses the ability of growth hormone to cause IGF release.

Here lies the mechanism for how estrogen causes insulin resistance (higher insulin need). Insulin resistance occurs because more insulin is needed when IGF secretion is diminished. This happens when estrogen, at high levels inhibits IGF-1's release from the liver. The diminished IGF-1 released despite the GH directed dumping of sugar into the blood stream leads to the need for more insulin than normal. IGF-1 is essentially ineffective in the liver and fat cells for directing these types of cells in the taking of nutrition out of the blood stream. In contrast insulin is less effective for directing the uptake of sugar in cells like muscle but many times more effective in directing the liver and fat cells to remove sugar for storage. A fat making consequence of increased insulin regards the fact that it is most effective in the liver and fat cells for taking nutrition out of the blood stream). In contrast, IGF-1 is more effective for facilitating cells like organs and muscles in their up-taking of nutrition. Increased estrogen then promotes the need for increased insulin to make up the deficit of IGF-1 in the peripheral cells.

The Liver Manufactures Most Transport Proteins in the Serum of the Blood Stream

The liver makes most of the many proteins circulating in the blood other than the immune proteins. Many liver manufactured proteins are needed for diverse reasons. The liver manufactured proteins include transport proteins for the different steroids and minerals (iron and calcium). The liver also makes the clotting protein that prevents bleeding when a blood vessel tears. Lastly, the liver makes stress survival type proteins.

Common examples of liver manufactured proteins by type

1. Transport proteins   molecules transported

   Sex hormone binding globulin   estrogen, testosterone and
                                                            some progesterone
   Albumin   calcium and some progesterone

   Thyroid binding globulin   thyroid hormones
   Retinol binding protein   vitamin A
   Cortisol binding protein   cortisol
   Transferrin   iron
   Ceruloplasmin   copper
   Insulin-like growth factor binding proteins   insulin like growth factor

2. Blood clotting proteins

        Factors 1-12

3. Acute phase reactant proteins that are secreted during stress

        Complement proteins
        Fibrinogen
        C reactive protein
        Interferon

        This concludes the taking out the trash section. In the next section the
ability of the one hundred trillion or so cell batteries to charge up is explained.
The immune system, joints and bones all lend themselves to understanding this
important body feature. In addition, the above three organ systems themselves
are explained and what they each need to stay healthy.

SECTION V

CELLULAR CHARGE

Principle 6

While alive, the cells must maintain an electrical charge that is contained in various membranes. These membranes are the cell membrane, mitochondria membrane, nucleus membrane, lysosomal membrane, and endoplasmic reticulum membrane. The outside cell membrane selectively controls which molecules move in or out of a cell (the force field). This electrical charge is also the basis for providing the energy to accomplish cellular work. In general, all membranes in the cells and around the cells are electrically charged. The quality of these electrically charged barriers determines how much work is possible and the ability to defend the cell from harmful ions.

Brand new car batteries are similar to healthy cells. When the battery or cell is charged and activated, it can perform and discharge electrical energy. In the case of batteries, the post begins to oxidize inside and out in a few years. As time passes the electrical gradient between the positive and negative posts possess less energy to perform. As batteries age the metal posts oxidize and form corroded terminals that are less capable of performing energetic work. The oxidation process is similar to the process that occurs in the cells. Oxidation of the components decreases the production capacity of the cell.

In the battery and the cell less productive capacity is secondary to the process of oxidation and decreased minerals in the fluids. These two effects result in a decreased electrical charge with the consequence of there being less energy output from a battery or a cell. When the battery is unable to deliver adequate charge it is replaced. Corroded, depleted cells are best repaired or diminished function manifests.

During the life of the battery the clues to its decreased energetic capacity are subtle, until one day it fails. The analogy between car batteries and the cells is similar for why cells lose electrical vitality. Cells are different in regards to the ease of repair and replacement once oxidation or altered minerals damages a cell. Healing here involves repair of the damage to the cell charge systems. One of the ways to comprehend how to heal is to appreciate the similarities between cells and car batteries. Later, their differences will be explained.

The various cells are like different sized car batteries. The size of the charge varies with the different cell types. Each cell type has an optimal charge that is necessary for efficiency in the life of the cell. Efficient living cells have achieved the right proportions of minerals around their membranes. All cells maintain an optimal charge by maintaining high intracellular concentrations of potassium and magnesium. These two electrolytes (minerals) are electrically opposed by high concentrations outside the cell of sodium and calcium.

Batteries, including the cell, charge by moving minerals against the concentration gradient around the membrane. It is the membrane difference between the various mineral concentrations that determines the strength of any battery. As the difference decreases, the energy in the membrane decreases. Cells charge their membranes by moving opposing minerals against their concentration gradient. When they move into their gradient through specific channels, energy is released. It is the mitochondria (power plant) that constantly supply the ATP energy packets that are used to concentrate the minerals against their concentration gradient. When the minerals have a increased concentration differences around the membrane, it contains more energy. This process creates a living little battery.

The living cell battery serves two basic purposes. It is the electrical charge of the cell membrane that keeps out unwanted molecules. When a cell membrane is fully charged there is maximal protection for the contents inside the cell from outside hostile ions. When the membrane charge is depleted below a critical threshold, these ions harm the cell. The life of the cell depends on the membrane charge to protect it from external, harmful molecules. Second, the cells, in order to perform biochemical reactions, must discharges the energy contained in their membranes. This process is much like a car battery that performs electrical work by discharging the energy contained by the difference of mineral concentrations between the two different battery posts.

There are processes that diminish cellular batteries. When these processes occur they each cause two immediate consequences to any cell. First, if cellular charge is too low, the cell becomes vulnerable to a massive influx of damaging charged ions. Among these ions calcium and sodium are in high concentrations outside of the cell. When a cell is vulnerable due to low cellular charge, ions like calcium rush in and irreversibly harm numerous structures. The cellular charge is a force field that needs adequate electrical energy to be maintained. These harmful processes occur with decreased oxygen delivery, decreased fuel availability, or an increased stimulus to membrane excitability (discharge) beyond the cells energetic ability to recharge. All of these processes can be permanently destructive to cellular contents within minutes to the metabolically active tissues (brain).

The second consequence resulting from membrane energy depletion is that there will be less energy available within the cell to perform the job of living. This job is powered by the electrical energy contained within the cell membrane. When the electrical energy contained in the cell membrane diminishes, life-sustaining work is not possible. Aging results when cells head toward a diminished energetic capacity.

This section concerns how the principle of cellular charge must be optimized in order for health to continue. Like the other principles of health, a failure to satisfy the requirements will subdue the body's performance despite the other six being in full operation. The satisfaction of the principle of cellular charge is interdependent on the other principles to come to fruition.

This section will explain the different organ systems that best exemplify the principle of cellular charge. Basic explanations will be given as to how the organs function in regard to this principle. The other six principles will be touched upon where they are pertinent.

Cellular Batteries are like Car Batteries

The entry of charged metal ions, like calcium and sodium, into cells is carefully regulated (gated). This process occurs simultaneously with potassium and magnesium flowing outside the cell. Cellular function is possible only when calcium and sodium flow into the cells and potassium and magnesium flow outside the cell. There is a price for this function. The ions that are flowing deplete the electronic energy contained in the cell membrane. The cell power plants, mitochondria, must continuously provide energy packets for recharging the cell membranes (force field).

Adequate cellular charge energy determines the ability of the cell to obtain the proper proportions of molecular supplies and these supplies need to be constantly available. This consists of fuels (carbohydrate, fat, and protein), correctly proportioned minerals, specific vitamins, and oxygen to burn them.

All cells need proper informational direction on how to spend available cellular energy contained in the molecular supplies. A cell in possession of all the correct molecular supplies needs informational direction. The energy availability in the mitochondria is dependent on which hormones are directing the operation of this facility. Mitochondria function depends on ample thyroid hormone. When adequate thyroid message content instructs cells mitochondria these power plants burn fuel more efficiently (section two).

Cells age when either or both of these processes begin to occur. All cells need adequate molecular replacement parts and proper informational direction on what to do with these parts. This section combines these two processes and explains cell charge and the consequences to cells when the cell charge system fails.

When cell charge systems fail they are like old car batteries with the oxidized posts. In living cells, there is an occasional ion (fluoride, lead, calcium etc.) that slips inside and reacts with intracellular structures (an oxidation process). Their mechanisms of destruction are the same as when unsupervised, these charged ions irreversibly bind delicate intracellular support structures and machinery (enzymes). This binding often times causes deformation because shape and size matter in the molecular world. Incapacitation of enzymatic machines and structural support systems follow and can block breakdown and removal of the molecular junk that results. Junk contributes to the intracellular landfill of useless protein structures and oxidized fat. Dysfunctional proteins and oxidized fat can't participate in the chemical reactions of life.

The body's systems of chemical reactions that sustain life are dependent on a proper gradient between opposing minerals. They create an electrical force field that can be discharged to perform cellular work. The high concentration of magnesium and potassium inside the cell are opposed by the high concentration sodium and calcium outside the cell. This allows an electrical gradient that the cell can harness. Electrical energy contained in the membrane is constantly used and therefore requires recharging. The electrical energy of the cell battery is maintained by the gradient between calcium and magnesium and sodium and potassium, as well.

This is similar to a car battery that continuously needs to be recharged while the car burns fuel. In the body the combustion of protein, fat, and sugar can only occur after all three are processed into a common combustible derivative called acetate. Acetate is only combusted when exposed to oxygen in the cell's power plant. The acetate requirement for the power plants is analogous to the fact that different power plants require specific fuels inherent to their design. Some require coal and others require natural gas. The body's power plants are designed to only combust the fuel called acetate. Processing protein, carbohydrate, or fat creates acetate. Numerous and specific vitamins are necessary to convert these different three fuel groups to acetate. Owners who are deficient in vitamins have a diminished ability to burn fuel in their power plants.

The power plants allow the recharging of cellular batteries. Healthy cells avoid unnecessary oxidation. Adequate cell charge (the force field) prevents oxidation by preventing the inappropriate penetration of un-channeled ions inside the cell. The prevention of inappropriate calcium entry into the cell requires an adequate force field (cell charge) at all times.

There are appropriate and inappropriate ways for calcium to enter a cell. When calcium enters through appropriate cell channels the energy liberated allows for useful cell function. The cell has many reasons to keep calcium in these appropriate channels. Calcium within the appropriate channels allows it to be pumped back outside. In order for this to happen energy packets, created in the mitochondria, are used up and the membrane receives a slight recharge from having less calcium inside the cell. This is the basis for how the cell charges the membrane energy content.

Any cells must power up energetically against the influx of calcium through inappropriate channels. When calcium slips inside a cell inappropriately it is analogous to an intracellular missile. Calcium outside of appropriate channels will damage inside the cell structures. It is the strength of the electrical charge in the membrane that protects the cell from harmful penetration of ions. Examples of cellular energetic depletion are where blood or oxygen supply is compromised (drowning or cardiac arrest) or if vulnerable tissue is excited beyond its energetic capacity to maintain adequate cellular energy (seizure). All of these mechanisms injure cells by allowing depletion of the cellular membrane electrical charge (the force field) with a resultant massive influx of inappropriate calcium. These inappropriate ions flood inward when the membrane energy is depleted. Once inside the depleted membrane energy cell these ions readily react detrimentally with intracellular contents.

Cell batteries must maintain a full charge to maintain health. Fully charged cell membranes have mineral balance. Mineral imbalance results from a diet of processed food. America is a land of diseases caused by deficiencies. Many owners are unaware of the sickening consequences when arriving at middle age after eating a processed food diet. They stuff their body cells year after year with the wrong ratio of minerals contained in processed food.

Middle-aged owners are often not aware of the need for optimal hormonal direction that determines how their cells are directed to spend energy. Only good hormonal directions allow appropriate use of available energy. Conversely, poor hormonal directions lead to the inappropriate use of energy and diminished cellular charge.

The typical middle age American can be typified as an owner who has diminished cellular charge. These cells cannot maintain their charge without adequate molecular parts and proper hormone direction. The depletion of cellular charge shows up clinically as fatigue, high blood pressure, more fat, less muscle, bone weakening, memory loss, depression, and irregular heart rate. From this menu of ailments there is common denominator of the perfect American way to become weak and fatigued. The loss of cellular charge is another determinant of how youth is lost.

The American Method of Becoming Weak and Fatigued

The mineral content of processed food has been significantly altered from the natural state. Real food is high in magnesium and potassium. The body was designed to eat food in the natural state for cell charge to remain strong (table of mineral values section 1).

Processed food, among other depletions, is low in these nutrients. The other mineral aberration contained in processed food is unnaturally high sodium content. The food industry adds sodium to prolong the shelf life of these processed products. Sometimes processed food is only relatively low in regard to the magnesium and potassium content because of all the sodium that has been added. The mineral content of processed food has been significantly diminished from the natural state. When an owner eats these processed foods and experiences chronic stress health is further compromised. Stress hormones alter the ability to remove extra salt from the body causing fluid retention. Stress hormones increase the loss of magnesium and potassium from the tissues creating further health consequences.

As a general rule, 4,000 mg of potassium day, 1000 mg sodium, 300 mg of magnesium, and 500 mg of calcium are needed every day. Most Americans consume the reverse ratio between sodium and potassium. The ideal mineral ratio occurs when there are normal kidneys and adrenals. Extremes of environmental heat or exercise habits increase sodium requirements. There is individual variation on the optimal amounts of minerals needed. This reference will put the owner back on the path to adequate cellular charge.

When food is consumed that confers these mineral ratios, the body can effectively charge the cell batteries. This is true even when an owner is under stress. If the kidneys have not been damaged from the processed food diet, then blood pressure should drop. This is especially true when there is a concomitant effort to diminish insulin production and obtain optimal vitamin status.

Seven Reasons the Potassium Deficient Diet Leads to Old Cells

The importance of ample potassium in the diet has been over looked as a determinant of health. The half-truth about the desirability for a low sodium diet has been substituted for an appropriate emphasis on potassium. There is also the preoccupation about the importance of calcium for the bones while the need for magnesium is ignored. The truth would include a balanced discussion of all four important minerals. A real food diet is the only way these four minerals are correctly proportioned in consumption relative to need. The focus here will be on potassium only to allow clarity on how mineral balance is fundamental to health. Potassium is an excellent example of the importance of achieving appropriate ratios of mineral intake.

Optimal potassium facilitates:

1. Stability and conservation of protein
2. Protection of the kidney
3. Insulin efficiency and function
4. Red blood cell flexibility and health
5. Choice of normal testosterone with normal blood pressure versus normal blood pressure from medication with a consequent decreased testosterone production
6. Electrical charge of the cellular force field
7. Optimal cellular function

Potassium and Protein

Potassium is a crucial determinant of the cellular ability to hold onto protein. Adequate potassium content within a cell is necessary to stabilize protein content. For every gram of protein, 2.6 milliequivalents of potassium are needed. Those who consistently eat low potassium diets begin to notice an increase in body fat and a decrease in muscle mass around middle age. Often the loss of muscle is largely the result of inadequate potassium and/or excess sodium intake. In addition, chronic stress accelerates potassium loss, which contributes to muscle loss.

Muscle wasting is often the result of the body compensating for a potassium deficiency. The body will raid the cells for potassium if it is not provided in the diet. The price of raiding the inside the cell storehouse of potassium is the loss of cellular protein. When cells give up protein they lose structural and functional integrity.

Potassium and the Kidney

It has been known for many years that low potassium diets carry the risk of kidney damage. A processed food diet and stress increased the risk of hypokalemic nephropathy. The kidney damage will increase when the potassium deficiency persists. This type of kidney damage can lead to high blood pressure

There is a correlation between kidney damage and high blood pressure caused by the potassium deficiency. Many owners in America are not informed about this simple consideration. The longer the time that the owner spends with symptom control, the longer the potassium deficiency will exist to do further damage.

The Function and Efficiency of Insulin

The effectiveness of insulin to lower blood sugar requires potassium. One potassium ion is required for each glucose molecule that enters a cell. The more carbohydrates in the diet, the more need there is to increase potassium consumption. Owners who fail to consume potassium in their diet will have insulin caused health consequences.

They will become insulin resistant meaning for a certain sugar intake more insulin is required to bring the blood sugar back to normal. The increased insulin level that is required will tend to stimulate the liver to uptake more sugar. When this occurs the liver will increase the manufacture of sticky fat and cholesterol particles (LDL). The higher blood sugar stimulates the secondary liver sugar removal pathway that does not require potassium. Only the brain, red blood cells, and liver can take up blood sugar without potassium. All other cells need adequate potassium to feed on the sugar in the blood stream.

Potassium in the cells is sacrificed to the blood stream. Cells donate potassium when more carbohydrates are consumed than there is potassium available. Over time the body begins to become depleted in cellular potassium. With greater potassium deficiency the ability of the cells to donate potassium for sugar uptake is slowed. There is less potassium in the cells so they are more reluctant to part with it. When an owner is healthy, potassium donation occurs quickly to allow the blood sugar to return to normal because there is an optimal supply of potassium relative to sodium in the diet. In contrast, when the potassium deficiency becomes chronic many cells are depleted in optimal potassium content. This process accelerates when an owner is under stress. Stress increases potassium loss.

All seven principles must be applied in life. An owner could be practicing all other six principles of health and fail only because they have not been counseled to turn off the desire of the liver to make more sticky fat. They need to know this important mechanism of how a potassium deficiency will increase insulin's fat maker role in the body.

Red Blood Cell Flexibility

The red cells have the feeblest electrical charges of any cells. These cells are often the first to sacrifice potassium content to keep the serum potassium level normal. A mild potassium deficiency can be missed when the doctor only checks a serum potassium level.

When red cells lose potassium content their ability to charge their force field diminishes and they weaken. Weak red cells are less effective at squeezing out their contents of nutrients, oxygen, and hormones at the capillary level. Red blood cells with diminished flexibility raise blood pressure.

Testosterone and Blood Pressure

Normal testosterone synthesis with a normal blood pressure is not possible in certain owners that eat a processed food diet. The combination of high salt with low potassium and magnesium commonly lead to high blood pressure. These situations are often treated in the mainstream medical paradigm with ACE inhibitors that lower aldosterone production. The aldosterone level is the rate limiting step for testosterone production as well as other steroids. Conventionally trained physicians are trained to reduce aldosterone levels. The fundamental role aldosterone plays in all the steroids biosynthesis is largely down played or ignored.

A real food diet allows for normal aldosterone levels and normal blood pressure. It contains high potassium and magnesium plus low sodium. In some owners, only when these electrolytes are properly proportioned are blood pressure problems avoided. The body was designed to consume the mineral proportions that are provided by the real food diet. Conversely, the processed food diet violates the basic body design theme in that the mineral proportions are drastically altered. There is individual variation in how long a body can tolerate an aberrant mineral intake.

The analogy to understand how a processed food diet will eventually harm owner's cells is similar to purposely violating the composition of battery fluid. Just like batteries, human batteries were designed for specific mineral intake. There is remarkable resilience to chronically reversed mineral consumption, but there is a tolerance limit. Cells that reach their tolerance limit behave in electrically aberrant ways. Electrical aberrancy is the culprit, but aldosterone is blamed.

Western trained physicians are taught to decrease aldosterone levels when blood pressure is elevated. Aldosterone will only elevate blood pressure when the minerals within are imbalanced. The elevated aldosterone effect is further exacerbated when stress is also present by increasing potassium and magnesium losses while retaining sodium. With sodium retention comes fluid retention. The fluid retained is the second contribution of stress to blood pressure.

Owners who are stressed, but consume the proper mineral ratio are less vulnerable to fluid retention induced high blood pressure. They will tend to tolerate a higher aldosterone level that allows a proper stimulus for the production of other steroids. Proper mineral consumption is a determinant of the rate of steroid synthesis.

Most physicians are schooled in the vague principle of a low sodium diet only. Very few doctors are aware of food types that are low in sodium such as real food. There are even fewer physicians that understand the importance of increasing the potassium and magnesium containing foods in the diet. Real food is high in magnesium and potassium. Processed food has less magnesium and potassium content. Only when physicians understand the facts about the different natural mineral proportions can they begin to counsel on diets that will heal. Owners heal from correcting cellular charge related health problems.

The Cellular Force Field

The amount of potassium is a central determinant of the cellular ability to keep unwanted molecules out. The potassium level permits the membrane to maintain a protective electrical charge. When a potassium deficiency exists there is less protection. This leads to the destruction of the cell. Elevated sodium levels decrease cellular potassium levels. Sodium is over abundant in America and potassium deficiency is prevalent. To maintain cellular health, there must be proper proportions between sodium and potassium within the body.

Potassium Availability and Cell Charge

Cell charge is directly proportional to the amount of potassium available in the cell. Adequate potassium levels are necessary for optimal cellular function. Owners with diminished potassium content have weak cells that cannot accomplish the same function as properly nourished cells. The availability and proportions of potassium, sodium, calcium, and magnesium determine how much work a cell can perform.

Owners that understand the importance of this mineral ratio take the time to create a diet that reflects this. A real food diet will naturally provide these ratios and amounts (food ratio and amounts list). When this consideration becomes habit another principle is better satisfied of the seven.

These first four minerals help introduce the idea of cellular charge. Certain organ systems exemplify this process when they charge themselves. There are other minerals that the body uses to charge different anatomical areas. Some of these additional minerals will be explained in the chapters that follow. Although these organ systems may use different minerals the principle is the same. The joint tissue of the body is the first illustrative example.

The Concept of the Electrical Extraction Architecture That Keeps the Cells Inflated

Consistently present among the cells, but beyond the view of the electron microscope, there exists an important anti-aging architectural framework. This sub-microscopic architecture solves the problem of internal cell pressure. Inside the cell, neighboring cells that are stacked on top of and around every cell create pressure. Healthy owners have a high integrity framework operating inside and around each cell. The architectural framework of the body is also electrically charged. This prevents the gravitational forces from expressing cellular fluid.

One of the reasons owners age is that this sub-microscopic framework becomes compromised under certain conditions. When the framework of a cell crumbles, cellular collapse appears clinically as the shrinkage of old age. As the water is squeezed out, the framework of the cell begins to collapse and everything becomes smaller. The architectural framework attracts sufficient water by the amount of its electrical charge. When a sufficient electrical charge exists, in the framework, water is sucked in to further inflate this framework creating wrinkle free cells.

Processes that accelerate this sub-microscopic framework deterioration also accelerate the shrinkage into old age. Conversely, processes that re-enforce this framework's continued rejuvenation maintain a prolonged youthful vitality. The cartilage cells serve as an excellent example of how this electrically charged architecture keeps itself in repair. The ongoing repair process exemplifies the importance of an adequate electrically charged architectural framework.

Chapter 20

The Cartilage in the Joints

Many things can go wrong when the integrity of the sub-microscopic framework becomes compromised and cellular collapse begins. Once the framework begins to give way, re-inflating the cell becomes difficult. Understanding ways to slow down deflationary cellular forces is most effective early in the aging process.

The same electrically charged architecture that is responsible for keeping the majority of the cells inflated also applies to the joint cells. The difference concerns the amount of reinforcement-architecture needed because of the environmental variations that the different cell types experience.

Healthy joints need a few basic molecular building parts supplied on a regular basis. Joint cells also need adequately equipped cellular factories. Cellular factories must be able to manufacture new framework structures during the entire life of the cell. Cell factories need informational direction that can only be given by contact with high quality hormones. Joints are on a path to deterioration unless these three elements are present.

Facilitating the Health of Joints

Joint Cells Need Molecular Building Materials to Make Cartilage

Joint cartilage has three basic components, collagen (a structural protein), modified simple sugars that contain varying added amounts of nitrogen and sulfate groups, and ample water to inflate the structure into a hard rubber consistency. These raw material components are capable electrical charge generators in the body. Electrically charged molecules are able to attract water when the opposing gravitational forces want to extract water from a cell. Before a owner can have enough of these electrically charged molecules there needs to be an adequate supply of the necessary building blocks.

Cell Factories are Vulnerable

In general, cartilage cells are affixed to the end of the bones. They are usually on the ends of two bones to form a joint. Cartilage serves to cushion the trauma of gravitational forces. Each cartilage cell contains many factories that produce the structural framework and the cells are spaced far apart. In between the cartilage producing cells lies the elaborate framework that is in need of constant repair and maintenance. Healthy cartilage cells are capable of producing adequate new framework structure. Healthy framework contains a sufficient electrical charge.

The cartilage cell factories produce the electrically charged framework. The wide spacing between the cartilage cells, with the intervening support framework, makes sense functionally. Cartilage cells are given more gravitational stress than other types of cells. This occurs because of the added structural support role that they play.

Each cartilage cell needs to be re-enforced by more surrounding support framework due to added gravitational pressure created by its weight-bearing role. The other extreme is the red blood cell that needs almost no outside supporting framework. Less support framework is necessary because they are floating inside the blood stream where the imploding force is less. Different body cells need unique amounts of electrically charged support framework to defend from being crushed. Cartilage cell factories produce an extreme amount of this protective framework because of the role they play.

Joint Cell Factories and Message Content

The third element required for healthy joints is a high quality message content contained in the hormones. Many different organs and glands provide these messages to the joint cells. Like other cells, cartilage cells are dependent on receiving quality message content do to direct the use of cellular energy appropriately.

Three Ommisions Perpetuating Joint Destruction

The biochemistry of joint health is not discussed in a straightforward way. This leads to erroneous thinking that comes from three main areas. There is a failure to remember that the human body cannot digest wood. Second, there is confusion regarding which hormones are centrally responsible for directing the joint cartilage cell. Third, owners are not counseled regarding the importance of facilitating the removal of joint trash water. Avoiding these pitfalls allows healing.

Chondroitin is a Wood-like Molecule

When clinicians prescribe chondroitin to be taken orally, they are asking their patients to digest a wood-like molecule. If human bodies digestive tracts were equipped to digest wood, these endorsements would be valid. Human bodies cannot digest wood.

Wood (cellulose) is made of glucose molecules strung together in a beta linkage. Beta denotes the angle of the repeating sugar molecules linkage that humans cannot split. Human's digestive systems can digest (split) alpha linkages. The human digestive tract machinery is ill equipped to dismantle beta linkage into glucose building blocks.

Dietary fiber is cellulose or plant wood. Cellulose has water-conserving properties in the colon because the indigestible beta linked sugar molecules remains osmotically active. This linkage is the reason lettuce and grass provides so few calories to the digestive tracts of humans. Life forms like rabbits, horses, cows, and termites have the ability to digest this beta linkage. They derive caloric benefit from the liberated simple glucose contained in the fiber.

Human digestive tracts can only break down the alpha linked glucose molecules that are found in complex carbohydrates. Members of this group include potatoes, grains, pasta, breads, and corn. Human bodies also store sugar fuel (glycogen) in the alpha linked arrangement.

A problem arises when clinicians endorse the consumption of chondroitin by mouth in the hopes of helping joint tissue regenerate. The building blocks making up chondroitin are in fact useful for part of the renewal reactions in cartilage synthesis. However, consuming chondroitin by mouth is futile because the building blocks making up its structure are linked together in a beta like arrangement. Oral chondroitin supplementation is nothing more than an expensive form of dietary fiber. Human bodies digestive tracts machinery cannot access and split the building blocks making up the chondroitin molecule. Hence, it is not absorbed out of the digestive tract as molecular building blocks (chapter three).

The other part of the endorsement usually involves glucosamine sulfate. This is a simple molecule and is readily absorbed when taken orally. Glucosamine sulfate is a necessary building block molecular component, but it is only part of the crucial molecules that are needed for new cartilage synthesis. If glucosamine is accompanied by the building blocks that make up chondroitin (galactosamine and glucosamine), the combination is much more powerful in contributing to healing. The other critical building block molecular component contained in chondroitin is galactosamine. The other part of chondroitin is made from simple sugar. Ideally supplementation protocols for healthier joints would include both glucosamine and galactosamine because healthy joint cartilage is composed of these building blocks.

Until someone takes the initiative to bring about a reliable source of galactosamine supplementation with commercially available glucosamine and gelatin will help because it is composed of partially digested cartilage. Complete digestion would increase the effect, but it is currently unavailable.

Building Blocks and the Hormones that Order Them to Be Built

A mental picture of these structural building blocks after processing in the joint (cartilage) cell is helpful. Galactosamine and glucosamine are derived from galactose and glucose by the addition of varying amounts of sulfate, short carbon chains, and nitrogen containing groups (amino groups). Synthesis of these compounds under youthful circumstances is routine and not complicated. The manufacture of these modified sugar building blocks can only occur when there is adequate message content from a hormone, insulin-like growth factor type 1 (IGF-1). When owners are young, there are ample amounts of this hormone being produced and delivered to the chondrocytes (cartilage producing cells). As owners age, total body production of this hormone decreases. Supplementing with glucosamine and galactosamine makes sense as age progresses because providing these building blocks gets around the obstacle of the falling IGF-1 message content. When message content falls, there is less direction for the manufacture of more of these components. Synergism is achieved when methods that increase insulin-like growth factor production are included. Lifestyle choices that promote high hormone tone will raise the hormones necessary for joint rejuvenation (chapter 2).

The material that makes up the supporting framework occurring inside and outside the cells is similar. At the molecular level, the same molecular material produced in excess outside of cartilage cells is also around most other body cells. The supporting framework occurring outside the cell is called the extra-cellular matrix. The supporting framework that expands the cell from inside is called the cyto-skeleton. Throughout the body the adequacy of the cellular support framework preventing the flattened look of old age is dependent on the same three criteria as are necessary for cartilage health.

Visualize the different cells as different types of fruit. The different cells and different cell membranes become analogous to the different skins of different fruits. The cytoskeleton becomes analogous to the different fruits internally. When fruit is ripe they have a firm consistency and resist pressure forces. As fruit ripens they begin to lose water and become mushy. Eventually they begin to wrinkle. Mushy fruit occurs for the same reasons as mushy and wrinkled cells. They have a common loss in the integrity of the supporting electrically charged framework that expands them and holds in the water content.

All these galactosamine or glucosamine derived products are composed with an alternating sequence of one of the simple sugars (either glucose or galactose). These molecular associations extend into chains that are made from thousands of simpler molecules. These long chains are precisely crisscrossed and reinforced generously with the protein collagen. The resulting sub-molecular structure is like the steel support structures contained in the skyscrapers. These molecular 'sky scrapers' have the additional property of being electrically charged. It is the strength of this electrical charge that is a powerful determinant of how much water remains in a cell.

Building Block Properties and Joint Health

The presence of galactosamine and glucosamine type molecules is critical to joint health. This is one of the pivotal points to achieving prolonged joint health. They possess the right electrical charge properties and are able to powerfully suck water into the framework. This framework is created by their formation into long chains of electrically activated building blocks. These molecules are elaborately crisscrossed to make up the overall structure. The electrically charged chains result in a mesh net configuration. The higher the electrical charge, the more powerfully water is drawn into the meshwork.

Joints are a sophisticated combination of shock absorbers and a hinge. The shock absorber feature works best when adequate water is lubricating into and out of the cartilage. Old age begins to occur when the flow of water into and out of the shock absorber diminishes. Cartilage (shock absorber) possesses enough crisscrossed (electrically charged) chains made up of electrically charged building blocks, glucosamine and galactosamine, to be healthy. Healthy joints are only possible when these repeating units occur in optimal amounts and are associated with adequate water. The molecular meshwork allows water to be electrically sucked into the joint space whenever joint pressure is released. The water is then squeezed out when pressure is re-applied. The ebb and flow of water moving back and forth serves two important functions. It creates a cushion (shock absorber) for the traumas inflicted by resisting gravity. Secondly, it is the way joint cells eliminate waste and take in the nutrition they need.

Cartilage cells (chondrocytes) have no direct blood supply making them critically dependent on adequate water flowing back and forth. This flushes waste and brings nutrients in.

Processes that contribute to the degeneration of the cartilage architecture are ones that create the presence of less elaborately crisscrossed chains derived from galactosamine, glucosamine, and collagen. The degree of diminution of the electrically active meshwork that results parallels the decreased function in the joint tissue.

Joint Deterioration – Part of the Solution

Whenever there is a process that decreases the performance of the electrical meshwork abilities, a vicious cycle of continued joint deterioration is normal. With decreasing electrical power to suck in water, there becomes also an ever-increasing defect in the ability to achieve adequate waste removal and nutrient delivery.

Part of the solution is in providing adequate, preformed building blocks necessary to jump-start the synthesis of new framework material. If the other joint cell needs are satisfied there will be an optimal response toward regenerative healing.

Joint Deterioration - the Rest of the Solution

Cartilage cells are dependent on reliable message content delivered to them via the informational substances (hormones) directing them on how to spend energy. Cartilage cells are no different from other cells throughout the body in regards to the need for informational direction. They are different in that they are more vulnerable because they have no direct blood supply. These isolated cells are critically dependent on the functional power of the electrical sucking grid (healthy cartilage) for waste removal and nutrients intake. In addition, as the electrical power of the meshwork begins to fail there is a corresponding decreased ability to attract informational substances. When there is less power to suck in water, there is a corresponding drop in the amount of informational substance arriving at the cartilage-producing cell. Less message content directing cartilage production leads to less work performed.

Owners on an accelerated path to old age have poor hormone tone (section 2). Poor message content results from sub-optimal hormone types and amounts being the norm in these owners. Some nutritional supplementation programs are without the desired benefit in these owners. Nutritional supplements for joint health can only benefit those owners that have some message content from the informational substances (hormones) directing the joint cells to utilize it. This is the second failure occurring in clinical medicine. Clinicians have good intent when they instruct their patients in the need to take nutritional supplements, but fail in assessing whether the patient has adequate hormone tone to derive the intended benefit.

Hormones direct the cells in energy expenditure. Healthy owners have optimal message content from the right amount of each hormone occurring at the proper times and for the proper duration. Conversely, unhealthy owners have diminished quality in their message content leading to the inefficient usage of energy. Over time inefficient use of energy results in a breakdown of tissue. This result occurs from the cells not receiving the message to invest appropriately in cellular rejuvenation.

When clinicians ignore an inquiry into the status of the patient's hormone tone, they often observe diminished clinical results, if hormone tone is the problem. The science exists to measure many of the body's hormone levels. Healing becomes facilitated when an assessment is made where an owner's message content lies. It can be between the extremes of healthy joints and the deteriorating processes that result from poor hormone tone.

Ensuring that adequate growth hormone, androgens, and thyroid hormones are reaching the joint cell is a fundamental consideration in the management of improving joint health. Opposing these hormones effects by inhibition are the counter-regulatory hormones estrogen and cortisol. There are inhibitory effects of the estrogen hormone class on the regeneration abilities of joint cells. Patentable estrogens and cortisol derivatives are big business and therefore, a disincentive exists to advertise the well-documented downside of excessive usage.

Cortisol Injections - The Other Side of the Story

Many owners by age forty have received at least one cortisol injection into a painful joint. Most often it is a finger, shoulder, or knee. Most people remember the dramatic improvement that followed these injections. Some are lucky and no further problems arise. The upside of these injections is the power of cortisol's message to diminish inflammatory activity within an injured joint. This rosy outcome is unusual because of the often-unmentioned side effect. This type of injection inhibits the message of rejuvenation in the injected joint. The lack of rejuvenation increases the likelihood of further degeneration. The cortisol message is amplified from the injection and the rejuvenation message is dwarfed.

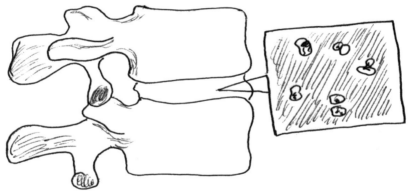

The majority of these cortisol injectable formulations are designed to remain localized and active for about six weeks meaning the injected joint will receive decreased message content for rejuvenation and repair during this time. The usual consequence when the medication wears off is that further joint deterioration occurs. Joints deteriorate when there is a lack of message content directing rejuvenation.

One example of suppressing joint rejuvenation is the spinal disc injection. This procedure involves using patentable cortisol derivatives and is a favorite practice of many specialists. Too often the injured disc, after initially seeming less painful (appearing better clinically), succumbs to the biochemical forces that result when cellular energy is directed away from rejuvenation. The consequence of ignoring this detail is often the need for a surgical procedure.

This does not mean that there is never an indication for cortisol injections, but rather patients should be included in the risk versus benefits analysis.

Estrogen Inhibits the Joints Rejuvenation

The second major counter-regulatory hormone that directs energy away from ongoing joint rejuvenation is the estrogen group of hormones. There are different estrogens occurring in nature. Basic medical textbooks counsel on this fact. There is a discrepancy in regards to what science has revealed contrasted to what is being practiced in the clinical setting. Too much estrogen message content has a direct inhibitory effect on rejuvenation in joint cells. This can occur with the environmental estrogen mimics (chapter 2) in both men and women. It can also result from taking inappropriate amounts of estrogen replacement therapy.

Whenever estrogen's message content is too high, at the cartilage cell level, there needs to be an increase in the counter weights (increased IGF-1, androgens, thyroid). Without an effective counter hormone response these cells do not direct energy into cellular rejuvenation (estrogen effects in the liver chapter). If this situation becomes chronic joint deterioration begins.

Androgens – Messengers of Cartilage Rejuvenation

On the opposite extreme of informational content are the androgen hormones that are manufactured mostly in the gonads (ovaries and testes) and the adrenal glands that rest on top of the kidneys. There is a small amount of these steroids manufactured in the brain itself. Men tend to make more androgen and therefore initially have a joint longevity advantage. Women's tendency for joint deterioration is exacerbated by the medical custom of ovary removal and then failing to supplement them with adequate androgen replacement therapy. Some women without their ovaries have strong enough adrenals to manufacture adequate androgen. Adequate androgen allows enough message content to direct the joints to both repair and rejuvenate. The adrenals of many women are not up to the task of increased androgen manufacture. A consequence of this is an increased likelihood of joint problems. The joints of many males have the disadvantage of joint insults acquired early in life that exceed the ability of the body to repair the damage.

The Cartilage Cell's Dilemma

There is a cartilage cell dilemma. While awake there is constant compression and decompression as an owner goes about the activities of living. Rest provides opportunity for rejuvenation when the right informational content reaches the cartilage cells. Remembering the analogy of the antique weight scale helps. Often disease states are reflected in this loss of balance between the opposing hormonal forces. When energy is allowed to move too far in any one direction in the body imbalance occurs and is detrimental to continued health.

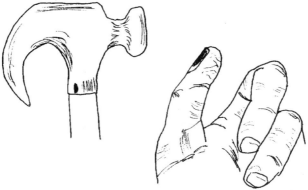

Cortisol's message content is involved in joint health as a counter-regulatory hormone. Any hormone will convey different message content that is dependent on the tissue with which it interacts. This subtle point is often missed when trying to understand the effects that a simple molecule like cortisol can have on different tissues.

Cortisol is a powerful and important hormone that counter-regulates many other hormones. For example, there is the tug of war of cortisol opposing the actions of insulin. Cortisol has another counter-regulatory role in a different body tissue, cartilage cells. These joint cells are caught between the 'weight' and the 'counterweight' of opposing hormones. Understanding balance facilitates the problem of the continued existence of a cartilage-producing cell. One extreme is the tendency to swell as physical traumas are inflicted on these cells. If one were to take any other tissue outside the musculoskeletal system and compress and decompress it for any length of time, it would become inflamed (swollen). The process of swelling when tissue is overused is mediated by the release of informational substances that give the cells permission to begin swelling. Swelling of tissue is perceived consciously as pain.

Within the musculoskeletal system the body eludes this problem by secreting small amounts of anti-inflammatory cortisol into these tissues just before the owner wakes up each morning. Cortisol is a powerful inhibitor of inflammation. The risk of this process comes in the form that there is an operating deficit of the counter hormones to cortisol. Too much cortisol message content leads a cell into disrepair. The anti-inflammatory message content has the side affect of inhibiting ongoing cellular rejuvenation.

Ideally, when healthy owners are resting their counter response to cortisol is optimal in the form of released androgens and growth hormone. The net effect that occurs is appropriate cycles of cellular rejuvenation that are balanced with cellular rest. The counterweights to cortisol's message content are the androgens and growth hormone. These hormones stimulate joint cells to invest in cellular infrastructure investment activities and encourage factory synthesis of new meshwork (cartilage, the extra-cellular matrix). Without adequate cortisol secretion into the musculoskeletal tissues each morning, an owner would soon become stiff and swollen. Conversely, inadequate counter response from both the androgen class of hormones and growth hormone will lead to painful and stiff musculoskeletal tissues from the disrepair that follows when there is an inadequate message to these cells to invest in rejuvenation. The practical operational principle is the awareness that balance between opposing hormones allows health to continue.

Joint Health - Taking Out the Trash Water

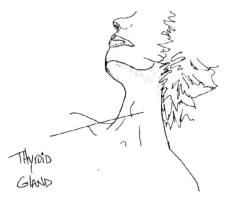

Adequate elimination of toxins and waste is the third requirement for the facilitation of joint healing. Overlooking the need for the most powerful medicine of all, water, is behind many joint ailments. The joint cells produce waste on a regular basis. Adequate free water intake removes the waste generated in the cells. The cartilage cells, within the joints, are more vulnerable to toxins and waste buildup because they have no direct blood supply. Sufficient water squishing back and forth is necessary to remove the waste and toxins. When the joint cells do not receive adequate water between the joint spaces, the tissues begin the process of sequestering (taking out the garbage chapter).

The effect of an inadequate water supply is exacerbated by diminished thyroid system function. This affects all six garbage removal organ systems (section four). Further obstructing this discovery is the lack of appropriate clinical attention into the physical signs of low thyroid function at the tissue level (seven links of the thyroid health chain). Instead mainstream doctors are found dutifully checking owner's thyroid function superficially by obtaining often only a TSH (Thyroid Stimulating Hormone). This is despite the medical physiological textbook fact that events like stress will depress TSH. Over reliance here misleads clinicians into thinking that the thyroid health, in their patient is good when in fact it is not. Accumulating evidence suggests that at the very least patients should be instructed to take an armpit temperature before getting out of bed. If the temperature is more than one degree below 98.6 degrees then thyroid hormone replacement should be a consideration.

When the thyroid message is inadequate at the level of the joint the cell trash water begins to accumulate and the afflicted owner's joints hurt. Sometimes healing the hurt is only an accurate thyroid test away. Sometimes the afflicted owner only needs to realize the potential contained in the most powerful medicine of all, water.

Chapter 21

The Immune System

Most owners have been supplied with a standard equipped immune system. The different powers contained in this standard equipment have far reaching longevity potential. Scientist like big words and often make matters worse by having numerous examples of non-communicating duplicity among the many different competing ways to say the same thing. The end result is usually a powerless owner. This means that an owner has less ability to choose intelligently in regard to discernment between 'hype' and 'helpful'.

Less obvious is the confusion that disjointed scientific writings has on a physician's ability to offer their patients the best advice. Duplicity of scientific vocabulary and information overload are effective methods for the suppression of how healing takes place. One way around this is going back to basic medical textbooks and reviewing what is known about a subject.

A presentation of the big picture has the power to facilitate healing many immune imbalances through insight. Insight allows for seeing cause and effect relationships. At this level, symptom control medicine begins to look less attractive.

The sixth principle is that of cellular charge adequacy. This principle is exemplified in the immune system because these cells require a highly functional 'power grid' to supply the energy needs that arise when the weapons of destruction (immune system) are activated.

The Standard Equipment of the Immune System

The different elements (soldiers) in the standard equipment immune system can be divided into the army, navy, air force, and Special Forces conceptually. This will serve as the analogy for this system. Each service has a weapon of destruction. The effectiveness of these forces is constrained by the military budget of the body. The budget is composed of the energy available to power these various defenses. The types and amounts of hormones available to the cells control the use and distribution of this budget. The level one (section two) hormone quality is the congress. They are either wise or foolish in their appropriations.

The types and amounts of more powerful hormones (level one hormones) determine the immune cell energy budget. Once the energy budget is decided, the communication system carries out the directives. One of these systems can be thought of as the E-mail system of the immune cells. The E-mail system communicates among the different types of soldiers and weapons. The quality of the message content (immune system E-mail) in this lesser communication system orchestrates where and when different immune system soldiers are going. It gives them their individual orders. Technically, this communication system is still a hormone system because it contains message content carried in the blood stream. There are many basic types of soldiers available to defend the homeland.

All immune cells (soldiers) arise from one of three main areas: the thymus, the lymph, or the bone marrow. The basic immune cell types are leukocytes, lymphocytes, macrophages, eosinophils, basophils, and mast cells. There are general requirements to keep these different immune cells (soldiers) well populated in total number and in proportion to the other forces. They must be well equipped with their unique weapons, have properly constructed components that make up the different immune cells, and operate with the different communication systems that can either help or harm the defense systems.

The Immune System Communication

Communication systems (hormones) differ with the different soldiers while they are out in the field. The E-mail system is known as cytokines among the various soldier types. The E-mail system is capable of sending many types of messages that can become complicated by the use of big words and duplicity of expression. Some scientific descriptors are words like interleukin, tumor necrosis factor, and interferon. These names are unnecessary if thought of as different E-mail message types. The E-mail is a type of hormone that the immune system cells use for communication. The different types of immune system cells secrete different types of E-mails that contain unique message content intended for other immune cell types. The immune cells receive these E-mails via the blood stream or lymphatics. Occasionally they can be delivered out into the tissues.

The E-mail choices that each cell type is capable of carrying into the blood stream are limited to short cryptic communiqués. These communiqués are the way that the different soldiers and weapons in the immune system communicate to one another. The type of E-mail secreted into the blood stream is one of the determinants of immune system readiness for defending the homeland. As a general rule, the more all seven principles of health are actualized, the higher the quality of E-mail message that will predominate.

The immune system is composed of various types of armed forces and each is equipped with weapons of destruction. When this system is well numbered and equipped there is a formidable obstacle against potential enemies that want to invade the homeland. There are also potential enemies created from the rebel cells within. The military budget directors determine the strength and size of each of these forces and the weapons they use. The budget directors are made up of powerful hormones that determine the amount of body energy available for defense purposes. The qualities that the collective budget directors impart determine the overall maintenance schedule, number of new recruits, and repair activities that are allowed from total body resources.

There are four basic determinants of the overall readiness of the immune system:

1. The size of each type of soldier population (army, navy, air force, and special forces)
2. The amount of weapons that each soldier type is allotted (each type of immune system cell has a special way to destroy the enemy)
3. The nutritional integrity available for the construction of the various components that create the operating system of the immune cell
4. The overall tone of the message content that the immune cells receive

E-mail is only one type of message content within the larger system. The other message content occurs in the blood stream, as well, and originates from a large number of different body locations. Healing the immune system is best understood by explaining the overall design.

Processes that organize message content in E-mail confer a performance advantage for the owner. Conversely, processes that impair the quality of the message content in the E-mail system weaken the performance. E-mail is just a construct to help lump together one class of hormones, which are secreted by the immune system cells. Immune system cells secrete other types of hormones. All hormones contain message content designed to be understood by other cell types. In the case of immune system cells these hormone messages are designed to communicate almost exclusively with other immune cells. One of the immune system cells hormone types is best conceptualized into a general group by the construct of E-mail.

Sometimes the quality of E-mail communiqués can be rebellious in nature and contradict the desires of the budget directors (powerful hormones that act like a congress). In these situations increasing the forceful presence of the budget directors (level one hormone amount) is required to subjugate the rebellious E-mails sent by the various soldiers. When different soldier types are sending out rebellious message content disease can eventually result such as allergies, autoimmune disease, asthma, and various skin conditions.

Each immune cell 'soldier type' comes equipped with another communication system. This standard equipment is most analogous to each soldier having voice of its own. This type of message content can communicate with other soldiers in the vicinity of the cell that sends the message. The length of time that the message lasts is only one to two seconds. This is similar to the voice being only heard as it is articulated and only as far as the voice will carry.

This voice equipment feature of the standard immune system is the ecosanoids. Molecular reality of this concept is more complicated. This is another hormone class. The different hormone classes all contain message content. All hormones deliver their message content in the blood stream initially. The ecosanoids are locally heard and short lived messages that are analogous to the voice message in many ways.

The ecosanoid class of substances contains the prostaglandins, leukotrienes, and the lipoxins and is made from essential fatty acids. Depending on the types of ecosanoid precursors produced (determined by diet) this determines the quality of the various voice communication possibilities in an owner. If an owner indulges in processed food consistently for essential fatty acids, he will be more inclined to make the pro-inflammatory types of voice messages. The problem with loading the immune system cells with the pro-inflammatory essential fatty acids is that certain diseases are created when these messages predominate. Examples are some asthma, some allergies, some autoimmune disease, and some skin problems.

This is in contrast with owners who obtain regular high quality essential fatty acids from cold-water fish, fresh vegetables, borage oil, evening primrose oil, and olive oil. These foods supply the non-inflammatory essential fatty acids to the immune system cells. Many inflammatory aches and pains that begin in middle age can be resolved by a simple change in these 'voice messages' that are communicated by the different soldiers. Choosing real foods in place of the processed foods will increase these hormone precursors on the immune cells. When the hormone precursors contained on immune system cells are of the non-inflammatory variety, there will be a diminished ability to propagate diseases. Taking this step before committing to a symptom control approach with all the side effects will improve the immune system.

Healing doesn't require controlled double blind studies although it would be a nice validation. These studies are rare when profit is at stake. Healing has no side effects and some argue this should always be tried first.

The 'voice' system that delivers inflammatory message content is a cause for owner suffering. The complex largely ignores this fact. A bigger mental picture develops the ways to heal. Healing from the inflammatory diseases that result from poor message content in the immune system is possible. Understanding the interplay between the different message systems within the immune system plays a significant roll.

In the world of humans, the lifespan of spoken language is only during the moment of articulation. It is only operational over the distance that it can be heard. The louder the voice the farther it will carry. There is contrast between the 'voice' system (ecosanoids) of communication and the more powerful and far reaching E-mail system (cytokines). E-mail communiqués are capable of traveling throughout the homeland whereas vocal (ecosanoids) are only heard locally.

Nutritional fat choices determine the type of 'speaking manners' that these local vocal messages communicate and also depend on other factors. Some of these general factors are whether a soldier is properly equipped, properly fed with quality rations, and the quality of the energy in the soldier's environment. Traditional medicine doesn't give much attention to the environment in which these soldiers operate.

Environment is the emotional state of the owner. Environmental energies are in part determined by the qualities of the emotions that an owner experiences. These energies range from those that heal to those that maim cells. The quality of emotional energy circulating is a concept quite foreign to many western owners. Opening to the possibility that the western view of the universe contains inconsistencies is to open to more possibilities of healing. Science has revealed the importance of the emotional environment and the energy it contains. Emotions are another determinant of how well the immune cells function (section VI).

Immune Performance and Longevity

The different performance parameters of the immune system are dependent on certain nutritional building blocks. Nutritional imbalances lead immune cells to disease risk possibilities. The quality of the essential fatty acids in the diet is only the first determinant of maximizing immune cell performance. There are necessary vitamins for the immune cell power plants to generate maximal energy to power the weapons of destruction. Weapon performance is tied directly to the energy that powers them.

The ability to deliver oxygen and fuel to the immune cell furnaces is one determinant of the energy available for living. The trapping of energy from this combustion process, which occurs in the cellular mitochondria, is part of a cell's energy requirement. When immune cells cannot sufficiently power up their force fields they lack the energy to defend the homeland. The owner's immune cells have the ability to trap the heat energy only when there are sufficient molecular building blocks available. When the heat energy of combustion is trapped it can be converted to useable energy packets. The trapping of the heat energy of combustion requires numerous vitamins and cofactors. The energy packets are used for cellular work (body defense).

The ability of the cell to function is analogous to the ability of a car engine to move the vehicle down the highway. Superior automobile engines have more energy (gas combustion) transfer to the drive train. There is less gas wasted and more (efficient combustion of energy) moves the vehicle. Inferior automobiles waste energy (gas) and there is less efficient combustion that equals fewer miles per gallon. This situation can exists in body cells. These cells lack one or more of the nutritionally derived molecular parts that are necessary to trap cell furnace heat energy to power cellular electronics (force fields).

The immune system describes the general process of electronic charge that is contained in the cell membrane. The membrane's charge directly affects the energy contained in a cell. The immune system cells activate the weapons that defend the body. It takes adequate membrane energy for these weapon systems to function properly.

The immune system cells need adequate supply lines of certain key molecular parts or immune cell energy becomes compromised. A deficiency of critically needed molecular components (vitamins and cofactors) causes the power plant to generate heat instead of supplying defensive energy. Over time the furnace flame diminishes despite the presence of adequate hormone direction. Appropriate molecular parts are required to process fuel (sugar, protein, fats) into acceptable shapes to keep the combustion chamber full. Think of a gasoline engine that requires gas instead of unrefined oil. Cell furnaces are engines that have precise fuel groups that they can combust. Like oil that must be refined into gasoline before a car engine can utilize it, the cells need to refine raw fuels into refined fuel (acetate). Many owners get infections, feel overwhelming fatigue, or even get cancer because certain types of their cells are nutritionally deficient. The immune cells cannot protect them.

> The science that discusses these basic principles has existed for years. It often lies buried in confusing descriptors. Owner empowerment is bolstered when some of these basic (but less profitable) understandings are brought back into the discussion that concerns this complex subject.

The immune system has a ravenous need for a continuous supply of nutritional components. This is one of the first places that malfunctions when vitamin supply lines are compromised. Deficient molecular replacement parts often leads to diminished cellular force fields. In the immune system this can manifest as frequent infections, chronic fatigue, and eventually as cancer. The ways the cells charge themselves becomes relevant to longevity. Immune dysfunction often has at its roots the overlooked nutritional molecular components that are necessary to power weapons of destruction. Vitamins and proportioned minerals allow for superior cell performance. They often accomplish this feat by virtue of the cellular charge that becomes possible when the right supply of these ions and building blocks occurs.

Hormones direct the use of energy in the immune system. The relationship between hormone tone and the nutritional adequacy available to power cellular charge is critical. Vitamins and other nutrients allow the hormonal directions to be followed. This will not happen appropriately if the owner is deficient in certain vitamin-like substances. An owner with a vitamin deficiency, in a setting of high hormone tone, is analogous to a fine tuned engine that has had its transmission and drive train progressively degraded by improper lubrication.

Appropriate nutritional components must occur in the presence of effective hormonal direction. When the body contains nutritional components, but doesn't have good hormone tone, use of available energy is improperly directed (chapter 2). The relationship between the directors (the hormones) and the adequacy of available molecular building parts and minerals is critical. It makes possible the sixth principle of optimal cellular charge. The quality of the hormones within is a determinant of the sixth principle.

Proper nutritional building blocks are needed to maximize the immune cells force field generation ability. Only when the immune cells have both of these determinants in operation can the owner defend himself with optimal cellular charge.

The Immune System and the Hierarchy of Hormones

Level 1 Hormones

The powerful Level 1 hormones are the generals and the only hormones that directly instruct the immune cell DNA programs (genes) to turn off and on. This group of hormones contains the steroids, thyroid hormone, and vitamin A. The quality of this mixture is a central determinant of the competency of an immune cell. This group of hormones can access all tissues and move freely into the nucleus of the cell to instruct the DNA to put the cell in an active or resting state.

The cortisol message content directs the white blood cells known as lymphocytes into cellular rest and decreased new cell production. With insufficient cortisol message content inappropriate activity of immune system cells occur causing allergies, some asthma, some autoimmune disease and various other diseases. When thyroid hormone direction diminishes the immune cellular furnace (mitochondria) decreases in burning capabilities (section 2). Vitamin A deficiency leads to a lack of DNA direction for immune system cells to grow up (differentiate).

This class of hormones powerfully sets the stage for what the other 'lesser' hormones must confront before their influence can be felt. All other hormones are limited by the body tissues they can penetrate and by not being allowed to directly influence DNA programs.

Level 2 Hormones

In the hierarchy of hormones, level 2 includes insulin, glucagon, growth hormone, cytokines, and prolactin. These are made from sequences of amino acids that confer precise messages to different cell receptors throughout the body. The effectiveness of theses hormones is dependent on the presence of their unique cell receptors. The level 1 hormones need to 'set a stage' that directs the manufacture for the level 2 hormone receptor that fit on a specific immune cell. Only when this occurs can a level two hormone have an effect in directing how that cell spends its energy content (storing energy versus combustion).

Once these amino acid chain type hormones deliver their message, the cellular digestion machinery disassembles them. Before disassembling, they leave a directive that instructs the cell in available energy options. These options are only available for few seconds (level four hormones). In the case of immune cells, this directive affects how reactive they become to immune stimulants (appropriate and inappropriate). This is accomplished by affecting which hormone fat precursors are allowed to form on the immune cell surface (level four hormones).[20]

This directive is accomplished through level two hormones having an influence on which level four hormones will be possible. Level 2 hormones have an extensive roll in the domination of level 4 hormones. The ratios of insulin versus glucagon levels will powerfully affect, which level four hormone precursors are possible.

In the case of immune cells this directive affects how reactive they become to immune stimulants (appropriate and inappropriate). The type of predominant level two hormones instructing the immune cell largely determines this reactivity. The level 2 hormones accomplish this by affecting which level four hormone precursors are allowed to form on the immune cell surface.

The level two hormones, glucagon and insulin, are largely determined by an owner's diet preferences. The relative levels between these opposing hormones determine what level four hormones are possible. When wise choices are made in food consumption good level 4-hormone precursors form. Poor nutritional choices affect the types of level 2 hormones released. Too much insulin prevents the good level four hormone precursors from forming. Dietary indiscretion produces immune dysfunction. The immune problems that occur from hormonal mismatch include allergies, painful joints, painful tissues, immune compromise, etc. Extreme cases can lead to the inability to destroy cancer cells that are made daily.

Level 3 Hormones

Level 3 hormones direct blood flow. The ability to perform this function is established by level 1 and 2 hormones. Level 3 hormones include epinephrine, serotonin, histamine, dopamine, nor-epinephrine, and acetylcholine. This level of hormones is critically dependent on adequate intake and absorption of amino acid precursors in the diet. Nutritional deficiencies lead to impaired blood flow in afflicted owners because the manufacture of these types of hormones requires many different vitamins. Manufacture of level 3 hormones requires the nutritional cofactors and vitamins B1, B2, B3, B5, B6, B12, SAMe, folate, magnesium, vitamin C, and tetrahydrobiopterin. These have proven biochemical validity.

> There is an advantage for the physician inquiring into the nutritional status of those patients that suffer from blood flow problems, like high blood pressure. Many physicians are not appropriately schooled in how nutrition effects blood pressure and blood flow. The power of the pharmaceutically influenced education is truly amazing. This fact is not meant to criticize the many devoted and conventionally trained physicians, but rather to point out the missing educational guidance that their training involves. Matters are made worse by the ways text books are worded and organized that steers many curious physicians down erroneous thinking paths that perpetuate the complex's interest.)

The immune system is only as good as what is absorbed nutritionally. Many owners have disease processes caused by unrecognized mal-absorption. This is particularly relevant with level 3 because these hormones need many nutritional factors that must be present for their manufacture. Immune system diseases are made worse from deficiencies in level 3-hormone production. Failure to recognize this factor increases the need for the symptom control approaches.

Both nor-epinephrine and serotonin tend to raise blood pressure and histamine tends to lower it. Histamine also increases blood vessel wall permeability, which allows certain immune system cells to penetrate the tissues and reach their destination more quickly. Epinephrine raises blood pressure slightly but has the immune advantage of keeping allergy and asthma tendencies inactive. For this reason appropriate attention to ones methyl donor system makes sense with these two diseases because epinephrine synthesis requires methyl. In addition, epinephrine's presence avoids the leaky capillary side effect which histamine causes.

Level 4 Hormones

Level 4 hormones are part of the weapons of destruction employed by a functional immune system and the 'voice' system of the hormonal fats.[21] This level of hormones has a local effect and is only active for a few seconds. There are limitations of the voice because it can only be heard while speaking and only over the distance it can travel. Level 4 'voices' are short-lived hormones that can only be heard by neighboring cells for an instant. There are two examples of level four type hormones that are relevant to the immune system.

The ecosanoids are made from the essential fatty acids and are absorbed from the diet. The types of level 2 hormones, which predominate, determine the hormonal fat precursors formed from the essential fatty acids ingested. Though all hormones contain message content, the level 4 hormones are short-lived and cannot travel very far from their point of origin.

Even if an owner manages to consume adequate essential fatty acids, they can still receive immune system diseases from the wrong level 2 hormones. The main level 2-hormone opposition for the immune system occurs between insulin and glucagon. Insulin promoting diets increase production of the wrong hormonal fat precursors on the cells and alter immune function with time. In contrast, diets that promote more glucagon promote creation of the desired hormonal fat precursors that line cells. When the good hormonal fat precursors dominate, immune cell's can respond appropriately.

A Level 4 Hormone - An Immune Cell Weapon

The second type of level 4 hormone is made from oxidizing nitrogen to nitric oxide. The cells that line the arteries, the endothelium, manufacture the hormone nitric oxide that produces local vasodilatation. In other cells, nitric oxide is released in much lower concentrations and has hormonal properties. Nitric oxide that occurs at low levels is one of the ways local blood vessels are directed to relax, a hormonal effect.

In the immune system it is generated in concentrations many times greater than needed for hormonal effects and becomes a weapon of destruction when it is released. It is only at high production levels in the macrophage cells that it is toxic to targeted recipient cells. Macrophages roam the body in search of an enemy. Sufficient nitric oxide production capabilities depend on key nutritional components. These nutritional components are thiols, tetrahydrobiopterin, niacin, riboflavin, and adequate arginine.

Macrophages need sufficient nutritional factors to generate sufficient 'killing gas' (nitric oxide). These are adequate thiols (found in garlic and onions), tetrahydrobiopterin, niacin, and riboflavin. All of these chemicals must be present to produce nitric oxide. If any one of these is deficient then nitric oxide production becomes impossible. Any deficiency in these cofactors gives the advantage to foreign bacteria, virus, yeast, and cancer cells. This gas lasts only a few seconds before it is deactivated.

Nitric oxide is poisonous to foreign organisms and cancer cells only when high enough concentrations are generated by a functional macrophage. This is analogous to automobile exhaust fumes that kill when a high concentration is generated. When the immune system is healthy, it can generate sufficient nitric oxide to become a toxic gas when released upon the enemy.

A methodical approach assesses where an owner is in the different levels of energy directors (hormones). Focus on the hormone 'generals' (level one hormones). Then consider successive steps down through the level 4 hormones. Concurrently, an assessment of the nutritional needs of the immune system should occur. These two insights lead to healing.

The Immune Cellular Charge and Nutrition

The nutritional needs of the immune system are no different than that of other energized cells in the body. The magnitude of body dysfunction makes their needs paramount. Nutritional deficiencies often show up in immune cell performance long before a serious disease manifests. To avoid symptom control paradigms, the owner needs to be empowered to 'think outside the official box' when thinking in terms of nutritional vitamin needs.

The science is present to expose the fallacies of the inconsistencies and detrimental practices of the profit driven approaches to immune dysfunction. One of the most extreme and tragic outcomes of ignoring the central role of the immune system that regards health versus disease is found in the way main stream medicine treats cancer. The role that specific vitamin-like nutrients play in the immune cell ability to power weapons and their cellular force fields is critical to healing.

The different immune cell types need to have adequate supplies of 'energy packets' in order to power the systems. All the proper hormones instructing the immune cells to defend does little good if the energy force to power the system is missing molecular components. The opposite is also true. Poor hormone instruction can be equally destructive to defenses against disease. It usually is a mixture of these two interrelated processes that leads to disease. Healing involves a cognizance of interrelating health principles.

Nutrients are needed to burn fat and carbohydrate in the immune cell power plants. The ability of an immune cell type to destroy unwanted cells is directly proportional to the amount of energy contained in the cell membrane force field (cellular charge). The ability of the cell to function is directly related to the amount of cellular energy available. Fully charged immune cellular batteries are capable of powering their weapons of destruction.

A major impairment operates in the immune system of many owners because of their chronic decision to eat dead foods in place of live food. This fact is effectively down played by arbitrarily low official daily values of key vitamins. Exacerbating this involves the practice of minimizing the importance of certain nutrients chemical instability. Nutrient instability secrets are the result of not educating the public. The public is not educated in the loss of vitamin content once food has been processed, fortified, or cooked. Even official publications that the public rarely reads acknowledge that most Americans are deficient in multiple vitamins and minerals. Many of these deficiencies are caused by processed foods that have little nutritional value. This fact receives little press.

A startling reality arises out of the American preference for dead food (processed food) in place of live food (nutrients are intact). There is healing power contained in live foods and changing the diet can change the owner's health for the better. The role that optimal nutrients play in healing from diseases like cancer arises from the way the complex has groomed (neuro-linguistic programming) the thinking patterns of doctors and patients. When adding the holism of what nutritional science has revealed, which includes the needs of the immune system and its performance capabilities, there is an underutilized way to heal. This can be accomplished in some instances without the cut, burn, and poison approaches pandered by the complex. At the very least, even if cut, burn and poison approaches were utilized, it makes good scientific sense to inform owners about maximizing their immune system performance. The holistic approach is routinely done in countries like Germany that do not operate within a profit driven health care system.

It is critical to increase the energetic advantage of the immune system cells. Enemies want to harm the body and immune cell weapons need ample energy to power them with increased cellular charge. Nutritional deficiencies lower the amount of energy packets created in an immune cell. Ample energy packet formation is necessary to allow body defenses to function properly.

There are critical nutrients necessary for trapping energy from fat combustion and there are specific things carbohydrates need to be maximally utilized in the formation of these energy packets. Most of these nutrients allow the immune system cells to trap fat and carbohydrate combustion energy. In turn, the usable packets created can be used to power the defensive weapons. When any of these critical nutrients is deficient the immune cellular power plants (mitochondria) make more heat. More heat equals less ability to trap energy for cellular function.

Carnitine, pantothenic acid, vitamins B1, B2, B3, B6, and coenzyme Q10 are the molecular components needed to trap energy packets from fat combustion. If a deficiency exists in any of these nutrients the immune cell is compromised in its ability to create energy packets. When this happens two different detrimental processes occur that depend on which nutrient becomes deficient. First, the severity of certain deficiencies directly limits how much of the fat can get processed into acetate. Without acetate formation, combustion cannot occur within the immune cell power plant. The second detriment concerns the fact that some of these deficiencies make the combustion process more wasteful. When this happens there becomes less energy packets formed, but an increase in heat production occurs.

Several factors influence why Americans today are deficient in one or more nutrients. Most of these vital nutrients are extremely heat and light sensitive. Owners who subsist on processed foods are likely to be deficient. A highly functional digestive tract is critical for proper absorption. Around middle age owners develop mineral imbalances because of poor absorption in the digestive tract cells. Owners are only as good as what they absorb.

Nutrients are crucial for immune cells to form energy packets from fat. Carnitine moves fatty acids into the outer furnace compartment. This is the first layer of 'armor' in the mitochondria. Carnitine is the shuttle carrier of the body for common sized fatty acids destined for combustion. Deficiencies manifest clinically as rising blood fat, fatty liver deterioration, heart failure, and bleeding kidneys.

SAMe, vitamin B6, vitamin B12, lysine, and vitamin C are required in tremendous amounts for the manufacture of carnitine. This nutrient is also available by consuming meat that has not been over cooked though some people have known for quite some time that cellular carnitine levels are a determinant of how fast the cell can suck fat into the cellular power plant. Supplementation is worth considering for these individuals.

Immune cells need ample pantothenic acid to manufacture coenzyme A. Pantothenic acids role concerns the strict fuel requirements of the cell power plant in that power plants can only combust one size of 'brickete' (acetate). This requirement is similar to power plants in the physical world that can only burn a specific fuel. The raw materials of fats, proteins, and carbohydrate must be processed into acetate 'bricketes' before they can be combusted in the cellular power plant. Fatty acids always contain even numbers of carbon in their chains. Coenzyme A is necessary to accept the two carbon fragments (acetate) that are broken off sequentially in the mitochondria. Once this acceptance occurs Coenzyme A derived from panothenic acid is a carrier of these bricketts. A deficiency of pantothenic acid reduces the amount of Coenzyme A. Less Coenzyme A means less available bricketts to stoke the cellular power plant flame. Pantothenic acid is contained in diminished amounts within B complex vitamin formulations. Owners are advised that this could be a weak link in their nutrient supplementation strategies.

Availability of vitamins B1, B2, B3, B6, and coenzyme Q10 in the immune cell determines how much of the power plant flame energy can be trapped into energy packets or cellular function is impossible. A failure to trap the power plant flame energy creates only heat.

This situation becomes analogous to power plants in the physical world. They only create heat if they cannot trap some of the combustion energy and convert into to the energy packets of electricity. Power plants in the physical world require specific functional components that facilitate the conversion of raw energy into electricity. In the cell power plants, a deficiency of any nutrient diminishes the ability of the mitochondria machinery to trap combustion energy packets (ATP). In deficiency situations, the more heat energy formed, the less energy packet formation is possible. Each of these vitamins becomes a facilitator for trapping some of the combustion energy in the cell power plant.

A coenzyme Q10 deficiency is possible in owners who consume the class of cholesterol lowering drugs known as the statins because the same enzyme, HMG Co A reductase, that begins the manufacture of cholesterol also begins the manufacture of coenzyme Q10. The statin drugs lower cholesterol by poisoning this common enzyme in the liver. Heart cells and immune system cells require tremendous amounts of Co enzyme Q10 to power their function. Their health is dependent on the liver manufacturing adequate amounts of this molecule.

This fact will probably eventually explain the suspected increased cancer rate and increased incidence of heart failure in some of those owners who chronically take this medication. In the case of cancer it has to do with the decreased energy that the immune cell has available to power the weapons of destruction against the daily occurrence of cancer in the body. Most owners on these prescriptions could avoid them entirely if they became committed to a low carbohydrate diet, optimized the hormones (section 2), ate mineral balanced foods, and absorbed nutrients (section 3). For those that have a rare form of dyslipidemia or lack motivation to change, they could be taking high quality coenzyme Q10 supplementation.

Carbohydrates as a raw fuel source in the immune system cell have additional vitamin requirements for its conversion to acetate. Only acetate can be burned in the immune cell power plants. So the immune cell has a similar dilemma, as it has with the other raw fuels (fat and amino acids), with the need for key nutrients. Key nutrients need to be present to receive carbohydrate derived (brickets) acetate. Deficiency in these cofactors forces the cell to burn sugar anaerobically (like cancer cells). Without these five nutritional cofactors sugar cannot be processed inside the mitochondria and the anaerobic metabolism limitation occurs. Without these five factors there is no way to cut the head off of the three-carbon intermediate of sugar breakdown into two-carbon (acetate).

Metastatic cancer cells initially lack the ability to burn fuel aerobically. This occurs even with all the nutritional factors because they usually possess deficient cellular machinery and initially have a poor blood supply. An owner who wants to survive cancer would insure the availability of these nutrients to their body.[22]

Burning sugar is inefficient and wasteful when anaerobic metabolism is involved due to the obligatory creation of lactic acid. Lactic acid build up manifests clinically as sore and painful tissues. There are many sufferers of fibromyalgia whose main problem arises from the decreased ability to handle listed nutritional deficiencies. Adrenal deficiency is often in operation in fibromyalgia syndrome. When receiving appropriate treatment for adrenal function, fibromyalgia improves (adrenal chapter). These patients also have stiff red blood cells that need to be addressed (section one). In addition, many fibromyalgia patients suffer from undiagnosed thyroid insufficiency although any defect in the seven links of the thyroid chain can do this (thyroid chapter).

Diseases like chronic fatigue often have an immune dysfunction component resulting from nutritional deficiencies regarding the combustion of carbohydrate. In order to convert from the three-carbon intermediate of sugar breakdown to the two-carbon brickett (acetate) adequate amounts of five nutritional molecules are needed. Lipoic acid, vitamin B1, panothenic acid, vitamin B2, and B3 must be available or the process will not occur.

In contrast, fat combustion deficiencies tend to decrease cell energy as the amount of deficiency increases. In the case of sugar combustion preparation, all five of these factors need to be present in the cellular machine complex called pyruvate dehydrogenase complex. This enzyme cleaves the three-carbon fragment, pyruvate, to form the two-carbon molecule acetate. Only acetate forms the perfect bricket for the cellular power plant.

When any of these five vitamins is deficient in the breakdown of carbohydrate it leads to lactic acid formation or sore muscles clinically. This enzyme, pyruvate dehydrogenase, needs all five vitamins.

Owners that have this type of deficiency when carbohydrate is the fuel source have diminished energy in afflicted immune cells. Lower energy occurs in early cancer cells, because anaerobic combustion of carbohydrate is their only fuel source. The immune system advantage over cancer cells concerns the increased energy in the immune cell when all nutritional factors are present. This advantage is lost when deficiencies occur. High levels of lactic acid that form daily hurt the ability of the liver to detoxify other problem molecules and cause a increased inflammation in the body.

Owners who are ill can consider intra-muscular or intra-venous vitamin replacement therapy to revitalize their cellular situation. Thiamine injections need to be done cautiously because of occasional anaphylactic reactions. Intra-muscular reactions tend to be less severe.

An additional consideration involves the fact that lipoic acid is a common vitamin missing from most multivitamins. This is another mechanism for disease development. Taking supplements doesn't necessarily prevent nutritional deficiencies. Lipoic acid prevents this above mechanism from manifesting as lactic acid excess. Lipoic acid is not common in multivitamins and B complex vitamins do little good until it is available. Cells need sufficient lipoic acid or the combustion of carbohydrate in the power plants is impossible.

All five vitamins are necessary for processing pyruvate to acetate or the cell power plant cannot combust it to carbon dioxide and water. When the cell cannot combust sugar to carbon dioxide and water anaerobic metabolism occurs and creates lactic acid. Lactic acid leads to a higher liver toxin load and sore tissues.

Oral therapy with a combined effort of both more live foods in one's diet and high quality supplements makes sense in the absence of overt disease. The owner needs to be cautioned to remain mindful of only deriving benefit from that which he/she absorbs.

The above nutritional discussion has proven biochemical validity within the mainstream biochemistry and medical physiology textbooks. When the above nutritionally dependent processes are running smoothly an owners immune system cells can charge themselves up fully. Conversely, when the above nutritionally dependent processes are enfeebled the immune cell charge is also weakened. Paradoxically these biochemical requirements of cellular charge have yet to become incorporated within most clinical settings. When owners are fighting for their lives it seems rather cruel to with hold this knowledge in favor of more lucrative ways of treating a given illness.

Nutrients that DNA Needs to Behave Itself

The methyl donor system is a process in the context of the immune system that gains particular importance when trying to understand another way to lower the risk of cancer. Removal of the abstractions contained in scientific literature becomes the challenge. The owner is prevented from identifying the power of the methyl donor system to heal or deteriorate their physical form with abstract information.

There is a central problem for cells when the methyl donor system is depleted. A depleted methyl donor system allows an increase in the number of cells that want to misbehave. Some of these cells become cancer cells with properties that disregard total body protocol. One way the body stabilizes cellular DNA programs is the methyl donor system. Cancer cells uniformly have turned on the DNA programs inappropriately.

There are many functions of the methyl donor system such as epinephrine biosynthesis, estrogen metabolism, hormone deactivation, and specialized brain fats manufacture. Stabilizing the DNA in the cells with the addition of methyl groups is important here.

The addition of a methyl group to many biologically active molecules confers either activity or silence depending on which biological molecule receives this molecular addition. In regards to the immune system, adequate methylation rates on the DNA do much to stabilize cellular rebellion. Effective methylation rates occurring on the DNA lowers the 'police force' role of the immune system. There is a reduction in anarchy among the cells. The cells behave when they contain adequate methylation of the DNA programs and the job of the immune cells becomes easier in regards to the surveillance of rogue cells.

Methyl is a very simple, small molecule in comparison to most biologically active molecular components in the body. It contains one carbon and three hydrogen atoms. Often times it becomes proportional to a biological molecule wearing a 'crown'. The crown analogy proportions the methyl group for how it changes the size and shape of an average body molecule. Despite its simplicity, it confers powerful abilities to activate and silence some of the most important molecular players such as DNA programs, steroid hormone types, level three hormone types, quality of brain fats, and blood vessel health.

What directs the quality of cellular DNA methylation rate and occurrence is determined by which steroids reach the DNA program of the cell. There is a bridge in the relationship between hormone tone and nutritional adequacy. Cellular activation or deactivation of DNA programs (genes) is directly determined by the amount and type of level 1 hormones presence. Only level 1 hormones instruct the DNA directly. These steroid-like hormones can accomplish silencing DNA programs by the action of methylation. Other level 1 hormones can activate these same programs by the process of de-methylation of a cellular DNA. Each level 1 hormone contains message content inherent in its precise shape and that determines how the DNA is instructed to behave. Different level 1 messages effect the DNA program in opposing ways. One of the main on and off switches is whether DNA programs are methylated or un-methylated.

In order to minimize the risk of cancer both optimal amounts of level 1 hormone instruction and a nutritionally supplied methyl donor system must be available. This is a powerful measure that can be taken toward controlling rebellious DNA total body load.

Craig Cooney, Ph.D. in Biochemistry, wrote an insightful book *Methyl Magic*, 1999. His career long research into many body processes that rely on an operational methyl donor system has lead him to estimate that methyl groups are changing places at one billion times per second. That is the rate at which an owner runs the risk of their genetic program rebelling. Genetic program rebellion is a centrally observed feature of cancer cells behavior.

One billion times a second the body needs to supply methyl groups somewhere in the body. Dr. Cooney and other medical texts provide a short list of documented roles for the production of methylation; melatonin, epinephrine, acetylcholine, carnitine, creatine, lecithin, deactivate histamine and dopamine, estrogen metabolism, DNA methylation, myelin sheath integrity, and in repair of damaged proteins.

These processes are central to lasting or regaining health. The methyl donor system critically needs to be nutritionally supplemented. A healthy methyl donor system occurs when SAMe (S-Adenosyl methionine) levels are high and homocysteine levels are low. The cell must possess the nutritional components to continuously recharge SAMe. Simplistically, one billion times a second the body uses SAMe when it donates a methyl group and becomes homocysteine. The ability to recharge SAMe is the yardstick for how well the methyl donor system is performing. Owners who are methyl donor deficient tend to have elevated blood homocysteine levels.

One billion times a second the body needs to have adequate supplies of SAMe. Deficiency to recharge to SAMe leads to rationing among methyl donor vital processes. In some owners the DNA begins to become unstable in rebellious cells. In others the adrenals supply of methyl becomes deficient causing epinephrine synthesis to suffer. This leads to elevated blood pressure (heart chapter) and/or asthma. In still others the methyl donor deficiency manifests as a delay in the elimination of histamine. This decreased ability to eliminate histamine leads to worse allergy symptoms. Conventionally trained physician usually prescribe symptom control methods before suggesting correction of nutritional deficiency possibilities. This is not meant as a criticism, but a red flag that something is missing from the educational emphasis of conventionally trained physicians.

Basic medical biochemistry textbooks contain methyl donor reactions. They are rarely applied in the clinical setting. All the molecules in the methyl donor system are concerned with keeping SAMe levels sufficient. In order for SAMe to recharge, there has to be adequate serine, vitamin B6, Vitamin B12, and folate in the tissues. Some authorities feel that the official government recognized minimum daily requirements for these nutrients are too low. These nutrients are necessary for the prevention of methyl donor deficiency.

There is a concern regarding the confusion in the addition versus avoidance of methionine in the methyl donor supplementation programs. Methionine is an essential amino acid (the body cannot manufacture it). SAMe contains methionine that degrades to homocysteine each time it donates a methyl group to another biological molecule. In the absence of a highly functioning methyl donor system, blood levels of homocysteine rise as available SAMe is consumed.

When SAMe degrades to homocysteine without other adequate molecular components of the methyl donor system, homocysteine levels rise. Elevated homocysteine levels are a well-recognized risk factor for blood vessel disease. In most owners the homocysteine level will only rise when one or more of the other members of the methyl donor system are deficient. All the hype about limiting the intake of methionine in the diet seems ludicrous because the real problem results from some other component of the methyl donor system being deficient. The curtailment of the essential amino acid methionine is unwise in most cases. Correction of the methyl donor supply team deficiency is the recommended course of action.

Some clinicians endorse the consumption of SAMe. This has been shown to be of great benefit in treating some forms of depression and insomnia. Biochemically, SAMe is necessary for the manufacture of epinephrine (a mood elevator in the central nervous system) and for melatonin synthesis (necessary for a good nights sleep).

SAMe contains methionine. This means that without an adequately recharging methyl donor system, the supplementation of either one of these will lead to a rise in the blood homocysteine levels. In extreme cases this will occur at the rate of one billion new homocysteine molecules a second. Without attending to maximizing the methyl donor system nutrients, the supplementation with either one of these will lead to elevated blood homocysteine levels.

This means that there are many owners with elevated blood homocysteine levels who are at major risk for heart disease. In most cases elevated homocysteine levels result solely from inattention to vitamin status.

Rarely are there genetic defects in one or more enzyme machines that facilitate the transfer of methyl groups in the methyl system. The most famous of these genetic diseases is known as homocystinuria that results from the enzyme absence of cystathionine synthase. Normal owners use this enzyme to transfer the methyl group from serine to reform methionine from homocysteine. Folate, vitamins B6, and B12 are required to complete this series of reactions. Even in cases of this rare genetic condition, the consumption of methyl donor nutrients is beneficial.

Some prominent researchers like Dr. Cooney, Dr. Sears, Dr. McCully, and Dr. Bolan feel that the methylation rate on immune cell DNA gone awry leads to some of the autoimmune diseases including systemic lupus erythromatosis, multiple sclerosis, and fibromyalgia. Other research would add equal attention to restoring adrenal health in these autoimmune diseases. The importance of methylation in the prevention of autoimmune diseases is that drugs that tend to cause lupus (hydralazine, quinidine, and procainamide) all have the ability to decrease certain immune cells DNA methylation rates.[23] Methylation is important in the prevention of diseases concerning the cerebral spinal fluid. The cerebral spinal fluid of multiple sclerosis and fibromyalgia patients has elevated homocysteine levels. Both of these diseases seem to have an immune system malfunction component.

Sufferers of these diseases should be advised in healing their methyl donor system and inquiring into their adrenal derived steroid tone (section two). Steroid-like content should involve adequate attention on evaluating the adrenal status of these owners. This is particularly important for multiple sclerosis sufferers because of the remission that occurs while these patients are pregnant. Pregnancy produces high progesterone and cortisol levels. Multiple sclerosis patients have a disease process where there is progressive injury to the nerve sheath (myelin sheath) surrounding the nerve. Most clinicians feel that this disease involves an autoimmune component.

Progesterone is known to be a factor in allowing the continued health of the brain cell type layer, the Schwann cell. Most patients with multiple sclerosis, under the care of conventionally trained physicians, do not have their progesterone status evaluated. They do not have the benefit of a state of the art twenty-four hour urine test for analysis of the steroids. Many multiple sclerosis patients have toxic levels of heavy metals in their bodies. A hair screening analysis and heavy metal provocation test can evaluate the heavy metal factor.

There are other ways to acquire a methyl donor in the recharging of SAMe. When pressed, the body can rip methyl groups off of other molecules. This desperate approach comes with the price of a deficiency in the type of molecule from which the methyl group was taken. The conversion of testosterone into estrogen by the enzyme aromatase is an example. When this occurs one methyl group is free for use somewhere else in the body. This desperate method for obtaining methyl groups has the powerful side effect of decreasing testosterone and increasing the estrogen message content.

The body is forced to sacrifice many active biological molecules that contain methyl groups when the supply of methyl donors becomes deficient. This variability between how individual owners prioritize the rationing of methyl groups helps explain individual clinical variation. There is individual variation in the possible diseases that can result when abnormal adrenal steroids occur. In some, the DNA programs become unstable. In others the DNA molecules that require methylation are preferentially given the little methyl that is available. In others hormone manufacture like epinephrine in the adrenals is dramatically reduced leading to asthma and/or high blood pressure (lung and heart sections). It is possible that the breakdown of allergy producing histamine is curtailed. The protective specialized fat coating around nerves can become deficient in its molecular supply. A major component of this coating comes from lecithin. When adequate lecithin is not obtained in the diet it can only be made from an adequate functioning methyl donor system. Each molecule of lecithin requires three SAMe's to form. Owners that subsist on low fat diets and have a methyl donor deficiency are at risk for brain fat deficiencies.

This reveals an additional role that diets play in helping or exacerbating the methyl deficiency. Certain fats are needed in such large amounts in the nervous system that diets lacking these fats put a tremendous strain on the methyl donor system. This is in addition to having all the right vitamins because diets deficient in certain fats require these bodies to manufacture this by using large amounts of methyl. The need for methyl increases tremendously because some diets are deficient in preformed nutrients like choline, lecithin, and carnitine. Owners who consume adequate amounts of these nutrients help their bodies have ample methyl donors available for the other reactions to life

Methyl donors are needed one billion times a second. In some owners the deficient methyl donor state forces their immune system to police the increased numbers of rebellious cells. Methyl donor deficient owners have increased rebellious cell numbers because the DNA is inappropriately active. Inappropriate DNA program activity puts extra strain on the need for policing cells. Cancer cells are the most extreme example of this process.

Inappropriate immune cell activation can also be attributed to other problems. The autoimmune problem can also occur when the level 1 hormones are of poor quality and amount. Autoimmune problems can occur when the poor integrity of the digestive tract allows foreign shaped molecules into the body. Foreign molecules activate the immune system. Trouble begins when tissues cross react. For example, when joint tissue is mistaken for foreign material, the owner's own immune system attacks inappropriately and injury occurs.

Chapter 22

The Immune System and the Joints

Sometimes the immune system and joint disease are interrelated. This relationship stems from the fact that bacteria, fungi, and virus' have a cell wall that is supposedly absent from human cells outer coating. Human cells have an under developed outer coating that is derived from various combinations of glucosamine and galactosamine. The same building blocks are used in the outer cell coating of these other organisms. The difference lies in how much of this support framework surrounds a certain type of body cell. Cartilage cells have more of this molecular material around them than any body cell type.

This architectural framework lies outside the cartilage cells. Scientist long ago declared that by definition mammalian cells lack sufficient framework to call it a cell wall. This confuses and limits the way people think. There are structural similarities between human cells and those of the bacteria, virus, and fungi. For all practical purposes, the human cell wall is just under developed. If the immune system isn't functioning within normal parameters, it can inappropriately think joint tissue is a foreign invader (bacteria, fungus, or virus). This misguided activation is analogous to microscopic missiles launching into joint tissue.

There is some technical truth in the delineation between the difference in the cell wall material in bacteria, fungus and virus' versus the human cells outer coating. This centers on the ability of this framework to protect these single cell life forms from environmental extremes of temperature, humidity, and salinazation. Human cells could never survive these environmental conditions.

Similar molecular building materials surround both human cells and pathogens. In all cases, these materials are constructed into a support architecture that keeps the outside of the cell from collapsing. Human cells differ in the tightness of the weave that denotes the interlocking chains of these molecules crisscrossed and woven together. The human cell is unprotected from extremes because of the loose molecular weave.

This is how the immune artillery can make mistakes between human cells and invader organisms. These mistakes are more likely under altered circumstances. Joint tissues are potentially one of the most vulnerable to these mistaken attacks by the immune system. They have the most abundant amount of these substances surrounding each cell. These building blocks when altered and arranged in unique sequence under normal circumstances alert the immune system that an invader cell is present. Under normal conditions the immune system can tell the difference in the outside architecture of human cells by sequence and type of the building block components.

The immune system is poised to recognize the material making up the cell walls of invading organisms. The molecular material (glucosamine and galactosamine-like building blocks) is also found in, and surrounds cells (most prominently in cartilage cells). There is always the potential for an inappropriate immune system attack on the joint tissues.

Under normal circumstances the immune system cells are able to differentiate the sequencing of the invading organism cell wall and human cell coatings. These sequence differences are so slight that cross reactivity occur against some owners own cartilage cells under certain conditions. This explains one of the causes of rheumatoid arthritis. Once the immune system has been activated against a specific sequence, massive joint tissue destruction ensues.

When the digestive tract leaks, dysfunction occurs in the immune system affecting the joints. This can allow seepage of partially digested substances made from the building blocks. The immune system is designed to activate against any sequence of these that is longer than three. When this occurs there is the possibility that this sequence exists in the joint tissue. A healthy digestive tract poses an impenetrable barrier to large molecules like chondroitin once the immune system has been activated. If the foreign sequence of chondroitin were to slip inside the blood stream even partially intact, it would activate the immune system. When the immune system activates against foreign sequences, there is a chance that these same sequences are in the joint tissue. This would start the process of joint destruction and is one possible mechanism for rheumatoid arthritis.

The sequences that make up cartilage are unique in each owner. Joint cartilage is made up of varying amounts of glucosamine, galactosamine, glucose, and galactose. Building block molecules are arranged in chains of thousands, crisscrossed with other chains, and then wrapped together on a bed of the protein, collagen. These individual building blocks are further customized by the addition of varying amounts of sulfate, amide, and acetate groups.

When these molecular building blocks occur individually in the blood stream, they are too small to activate the immune system. This is a reoccurring theme. The body is able to place new molecular building parts inside the blood stream and transport them to their building sites. These individual molecules are too small to activate the immune system. A similar process occurs when the digestive track first breaks down the proteins into individual amino acids and they are transported in the blood stream to building sites (digestion chapter). Like the undigested cartilage, undigested protein will also activate an immune response.

The danger of leaky gut syndrome allows larger than normal (partially digested molecules) to be absorbed into the blood stream. There is grave danger of immune activation against these larger molecules. Some researchers feel this explains one of the reasons infants fed solids too early in life develop food allergies. Other research suggests an association with leaky gut and other more harmful autoimmune system diseases such as systemic lupus erythematosus.

Leaky gut situations are encouraged wherever the bacteria in the digestive tract are sub-optimal. This can occur with candida over growth, chronic chlorine poisoning, excessive iron intake, excessive fluoride intake, recurrent antibiotic usage, poor nutrition, and inflammatory bowel. Many holistic physicians take an active role in counseling their patients to prevent these situations. Imbibing in clean water and taking steps to optimize the bacteria growing in the colon are good first steps in preventing a leaky gut situation. Immune cell function is sometimes tied to the health of the digestive tract. When leaky gut causes the immune destruction of the joints, improvement will not be possible until the leaky gut resolves (digestion chapter).

Some forms of arthritis are activated when certain bacteria or virus' get inside a particular joint space. When pathogens begin to multiply in the joint space, the resulting attack from the immune system cells leads to joint damage. Streptococcus, staphylococcus, Lyme disease bacteria, and chlamydia are common microscopic organisms known to invade the joint spaces and activate joint destruction. Attack by these organisms is one of the times that early and aggressive antibiotic treatment is warranted over alternative treatment strategies.

Some owners have an unprovoked attack on their joint tissues. These owners defy explanation even after a diligent searching. Research suggests that these patients are suffering from damaged adrenal glands and that this would cause an inappropriate balance of message content to be directed at the immune system cells. The adrenals are a prime site of immune regulation by proportioning and timing cortisol and DHEA (counterweight) release. There are others like androstenedione and progesterone as well.

The common approach to immune dysfunction involves routine prescriptions of the synthetic versions of cortisol derivatives. The detrimental consequences can be understood by loading one side of an antique weight scale. Loading one side of the scale without considering the counter weight side has health consequences. This approach always has side effects. With cortisol-like prescriptions the inaproriate immune response is suppressed.

Commonly, cortisol-like derivatives are prescribed to suppress either inflammation or immune response, in diseases like rheumatoid arthritis and systemic lupus. Synthetic cortisol derivatives contain an altered message content through altered shape and amount. The price for this approach is energy directed away from other immune processes and a substantial decrease in cellular rejuvenation.

Cellular rejuvenation is suppressed by two mechanisms when cortisol substitutes are taken. Cortisol substitutes do not contain real cortisol and therefore do not contain true message content. Changed message content causes side effects. By increasing cortisol substitutes the other counter weight hormones like DHEA are not released. The presence of the substitute fools the body into to thinking the other adrenal steroids are available.[24]

One promising new understanding in promoting a balanced approach in the treatment of systemic lupus comes out of Japanese research. Here they correctly posited that in some autoimmune diseases the problem is the counter hormone DHEA is too low. Dramatic improvement was noted when DHEA was given.

The effectiveness of DHEA makes sense in the holism of autoimmune diseases like lupus because there is a glandular defect operating in the adrenal tissue. Treating only one side of the weight scale (cortisol) exacerbates the deficiency in other adrenal counter regulatory hormones like DHEA (i.e. DHEA and cortisol are operationally deficient in the disease process). Basically, cortisol needs to be counter balanced by DHEA or health consequences occur. Supplementing with one side of the hormone balance equation leads to unnecessary complications that can be avoided if the holism of what science has revealed comes into practice.

Healing is possible when healthy adrenal glands secrete DHEA and cortisol (also progesterone and androstenedione) at the same time. The adrenal secretion of these two hormones occurs when the pituitary directs it by releasing ACTH. Medical textbooks fail to unite the simultaneous releases that occur in predetermined ratios whenever the adrenal gland is activated. This relationship has been ignored for a long time. The inclusion of this scientific fact is profound in healing from diseases like systemic lupus erythematosus, rheumatoid arthritis, asthma, allergies, and chronic fatigue.

Supplementing only one component of a multi component system compromises the balance/counter balance relationship. This practice occurs when diseases are treated with cortisol substitutes only. The pharmaceutical dosing of cortisol suppresses the adrenals from further DHEA, and other adrenal steroid, production. Here lies a major cause of cortisol replacement associated toxicity. The antique weight scale is totally out of balance. Knowledge of this gives a better way to approximate the health of the adrenal glands. This method includes both DHEA and cortisol replacement (possibly progesterone and androstenedione as well).

The final dose between these powerful hormones is individually determined. Unbalanced, these hormones are usually the true culprits of diseases. The nature of the unbalanced ratio is decided after the results of a twenty-four hour urine test. Sometimes an adrenal challenge test is required as well.

The failure to consider the status of other adrenal steroids causes many fears about cortisol. If mainstream physicians were trained in the need to assess adrenal status before they began symptom control medical treatments for disease, many owners would be saved from countless complications. The side effects from cortisone-like drugs are often traced back to a lack of this initial consideration. A 24-hour urine test, which evaluates for steroid output, would help assess what doses are needed for DHEA, cortisol and other adrenal steroids. Performing an adrenal challenge test provides added information in marginal cases. When these approaches are utilized there will be fewer side effects because much of the guesswork has been eliminated.

Autoimmune diseases like lupus are related to androgen deficiency. This is shown in the rate of occurrence of lupus based on gender differences. DHEA is an androgen steroid that stimulates investment in cellular rejuvenation. Lupus occurs in females nine times more often than in men. This fact alone warrants a detailed, scientifically valid hormone assessment for any patient suffering from these diseases. In most cases this will require a twenty-four hour urine sample to accurately measure a patients steroid hormone profile. Blood analysis fails to address all six links in the adrenal health chain and is therefore and inferior test. All six links in the adrenal system need to be diligently investigated (adrenal glands). This is in contrast to with the moment of the blood draw where this value could be high or low depending on the time of day. The other links in the adrenal health chain can fool the physician who only checks one link, the blood stream. Blood draws, although most doctors use this method, do not make scientific sense.

The association of estrogen usage and blood clot formation can cause an overlooked risk for adrenal injury occurring in females. The risks increase with higher dosages, prolonged sitting, cigarette smoking and obesity. The adrenal gland is particularly vulnerable to clot formation because of its unique venous drainage anatomy. The adrenal gland has four arteries leading into it, but only one vein heading out making it susceptible to venous clot induced damage. Females who suffer clot formation here would notice a subtle decrease in their ability to participate in a quality life experience. These changes are confused with other imbalances. This misdiagnosis causes needless suffering. Autoimmune disease, thyroid disease, hypoglycemia, depression, and, in some, hypochondria are attributable to diminished adrenal function. These errors in primary diagnosis are best avoided by employing the best scientific methods available to assess the true hormone status. Steroid breakdown chemistry is complex and often confuses physicians who want to help.

Several laboratories now offer 24-hour urine assessment steroid profile. Now that there are several good laboratories performing these steroid assessments, there needs to be an increase in the understanding among physicians regarding the interpretation of the results. The importance of steroid status has been chronically ignored by all but the most superficial inquiries.

This fact is disturbing. The steroid class of hormones is the only hormones other than vitamin A and thyroid that directly activate or suppress the DNA program in cells. The quality of the types and amounts of steroids circulating determines the quality of DNA programs that are being expressed or repressed. All other hormones act on the periphery in their ability to influence

DNA programs. It is the steroid class of hormones that plays the central role in youth versus' old age. The time has come that this basic central consideration in health versus' disease comes to the forefront. Adrenal evaluation needs to be clinically considered for those whose immune system begins to malfunction in middle of their earthing experience.

The upright position is another important part of the earthling experience. Since the upright position defies the laws of gravity the skeletal integrity is not possible without bone cell health.

Chapter 23

Bones

Like other cell types the bones that make up the skeleton are dependent on the seven principles of longevity. Above all other principles two of these are exemplified in the bones. These are cell charge and the fact that the hormones giveth and the hormones taketh away. The knowledge of these principles is only partially acknowledged in their relationship to the bones. In the first part of this chapter, the hormones and bone health will be reviewed. The cellular charge principle as it involves bone health will be discussed along with the other principles where appropriate.

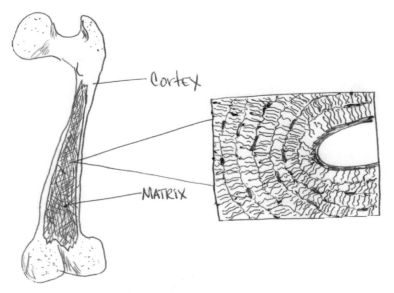

Message quality is the 'bulls eye' for optimal cellular performance. Almost weekly media sound bytes or newspaper articles discuss the 'latest information' on the prevention of the disease osteoporosis. Press coverage has been occupied with peripheral considerations while central scientific facts are disregarded about preventing skeletal deterioration.

The growing body of evidence linking the mainstream cornerstone of osteoporosis prevention, estrogen replacement therapy, to accelerated heart disease risk, breast cancer, and uterine cancer makes matters worse. Most authorities go on about the difficult decisions women face in the light of this 'new data'.

Looking into what is known about the role of estrogen in tissues it is no surprise about its role in cancer. Estrogen can increase the overall tendency to develop cancer. It comes down to a failure to understand balance. Estrogen when unopposed by its counter regulatory hormone is a potent stimulus for cancer growth in estrogen responsive tissues in the breast, ovaries, uterus, and prostates in men. The central message content property of estrogen in these tissues promotes cell division. One of the central features of cancer cells regards their ability to divide and multiply.

When an owner is healthy and free of environmental estrogens (chapter two) estrogen is unopposed in the first half of the female menstrual cycle. In optimum health, in the second half of the cycle estrogen is counter regulated by adequate progesterone. Progesterone serves as the counter response (counter weight in the antique weight scale analogy) putting the biological breaks on estrogens message to stimulate cell division. Progesterone in many tissues behaves in an androgen fashion by directing cells to invest energy in cellular rejuvenation. This property of progesterone in the bones is one of the central prerequisites for continued bone health. Situations arise that lead to a deficient progesterone output, which allows the estrogen message to be amplified to dangerous levels. Clinically these states show up as fibrocystic breast growths, uterine fibroids, cyclical migraine headaches, thyroid dysfunction, and weight gain in the hips and thighs, and in extreme cases as cancer. The more severe the progesterone deficiency, the greater the tendency will be to develop osteoporosis especially if other androgens are deficient (testosterone, DHEA, androstenedione, etc.).

Bone rejuvenation should optimally occur in the monthly cycle when progesterone is the highest. Rejuvenation is only possible when the bones receive proper message content at the DNA level. Around middle age the slow decrease of progesterone message content in the monthly cycles affects the bones by decreasing instruction to rejuvenate.

The other problem in the bones of some women as they approach middle age regards their decreased adrenal performance. The adrenal abnormalities can be quite variable (section two), but the main effect results from a decreased output of androgens (DHEA and androstenedione). There can also be an increase in the relative amount of cortisol message content. Cortisol message content at the level of the bone channels energy into survival and away from rejuvenation.

Many times both their adrenal and ovaries are less capable in the manufacture of sufficient androgen message content. This deficit effects how fast women lose bone mass. Androgen deficiency increases bone mass loss because it contains message content that directs bone restoration.

Bones Need Real Progesterone

There is only one true progesterone molecule found in nature. Forgetting this fact confuses many physicians into prescribing synthetic substitutes in pill form. Natural progesterone helps in owners who are unable to manufacture adequate progesterone on their own. It is a natural substance and therefore not as profitable (chapter two). Synthetic progesterone substitutes cannot be used in the manufacture of the other steroids. When synthetic progesterone penetrates adrenal and gonad tissues there is the risk of impeding these glands ability to manufacture other steroids.

Bone health is more dependent on progesterone and androgens (testosterone, DHEA, etc.) than the numerous peripheral solutions pandered by the medical industrial complex. Realize the reoccurring body design theme of the androgen hormone class telling the different cells that it is important to invest energy in cellular rejuvenation reactions. Body tissues only differ in which type of androgen steroid they prefer to be stimulated by. The bone cells are no different than other cell types in regards to the need for high quality message content that directs the wise use of cellular energy.

There is some feeble truth in the consideration of estrogen in the prevention of bone loss. There is a weakness of the ability of estrogen to impede bone loss. Bone occurs as a living dynamic tissue that constantly replaces its old electrically charged matrix with new matrix (minerals). In broad general terms, at any time approximately eight percent of the bone mass is in the remodeling stage. The average skeleton completely replaces itself every twelve years. This remodeling creates a tug of war between the cells that must eat bone matrix and the cells that make bone matrix. Bone matrix describes the mineral part of bone that occurs outside the widely spaced bone cells. This is the only thread of scientific evidence for the role estrogen plays in bone health. The peripheral bone support that estrogen imparts concerns its message content. The estrogen message will impede the bone eating cells for up to five whole years after the menopause. What isn't being said regards the additional hormones responsible for new bone formation. The hormones that direct bone formation are all in the androgen class (progesterone, testosterone, DHEA, etc.). When androgens are included in the healing program the bones begin to strengthen. This approach lessens the estrogen related side effects.

Other hormones direct the manufacture and maintenance of healthy bones. This is found in the different rates of occurrence for developing osteoporosis between men and women. Men with healthy gonads do not develop osteoporosis even though their total body estrogen content is less than women. If estrogen were the central hormone directing new bone formation, osteoporosis would be higher in men. Consistency among reoccurring hormone themes bears out that androgen message content as being central to healthy bone formation.

Many a good scientist has suffered over the last few years by pointing out which hormone class is truly responsible for maintaining bone health in men and women. Osteoporosis prevention medications and the technology to detect and follow its course make big money for the complex. Though there is some doubt about a true conspiracy, there is the suspicion that this process occurs one decision at a time protecting the profitable ways of treating a disease process. Therefore profitable decisions receive the advertising dollar. There is no incentive and in some cases even a disincentive for advertising the holism of what science has revealed. Owners should be aware of the reasons they have not heard of this more contrary approach.

Adequate progesterone message content is a necessary prerequisite for continued bone health. The relationship of the relative potencies of the other androgens and their contribution to healthy bone formation is less understood. Perhaps members in the androgen class of steroids contribute significantly to the total message content telling the bone cells to invest in rejuvenation. There are ways to ensure adequate progesterone content in women's bodies, which provide adequate stimulus for new bone formation in most cases. However, other androgens play substantial roles in bone health.

There are two caveats women deal with, in the androgen class of steroids, other than natural progesterone. Androgens-like testosterone and dihydro-testosterone have marked physical masculine message content in female bodies. Exceeding the natural optimum will have unwanted side effects. Second, female owners have a remarkable process at work to protect them from presenting physically masculine traits and still deliver androgen steroid message content to the target cells (bone, muscle, organ and nerve cells etc.). This process involves the action of peripheral conversion whereby weaker androgens initially formed and released into the blood stream. Later they are converted into more powerful androgens. This conversion takes place when the relatively weaker androgens changes to the more potent androgens once inside the target cells. This is a way of getting powerful rejuvenation message content in a female cell type, but not getting unwanted male characteristics (hair growth, clitoral enlargement, increased aggressiveness, and acne). There is erroneous thinking when clinicians counsel patients about androgens like DHEA, androstenedione, and progesterone being relatively weak and unimportant. They are forgetting the powerful concept of peripheral conversion operating in the healthy female body. This conversion allows female cells to convert the weaker androgens into the more powerful androgens. This process occurs after the blood stream phase and thus the male characteristic side effects are prevented. There is no increased testosterone in areas like facial hair, clitoris, or chest hair.

Natural progesterone levels begin to decline in the mid-thirties creating an ineffective counter balance to estrogens message content. Ineffective progesterone message content results in increased complications. In the bone the deficiency allows accelerated bone loss.

Progesterone is generally thought of as a female hormone. Scientific inquiries, in regards the properties of progesterone, fail to bear this out. Progesterone behaves in a sex neutral fashion. If men have abnormally high estrogen content progesterone contributes to breast duct cell enlargement. When progesterone behaves in a strictly androgen fashion, it facilitates the infrastructure rejuvenation cell message in the myelin nerve sheath in the central nervous system, in bone cells strengthening activity, and the enlargement of uterus lining cells.

The power of having adequate progesterone in men and women is due to progesterone serving as the precursor molecule for making many other steroids. Processes that harm the ability to manufacture progesterone have far reaching health consequences. Steroid hormone synthesis begins with the steroid building block, cholesterol. As gonads and adrenals age, these tissues decrease in their ability to obtain cholesterol. This initial step is necessary to start the process of making the precursor steroids leading eventually to progesterone (the chassis for multiple other models of steroids). Bone cells are no different from other cells. They need continuous, quality cellular direction provided by hormones. The most powerful hormones are level 1 hormones because they instruct the DNA program directly. The bone cell expends energy according to the DNA programs that are activated.

The DNA program activity primarily depends on certain level 1 hormones that are made in the adrenals and gonads. The first few steps in the conversion process towards making progesterone from cholesterol occur in the mitochondria. As aldosterone output diminishes with age, gonads and adrenals have a decreased ability to send cholesterol into the mitochondria (the adrenal chapter). Functionally these structures can be thought of as the armored power plant of a cell. When real progesterone is supplemented to aging gonads and adrenals there is little difficulty converting this steroid to other biologically active steroids. These reactions of biosynthesis occur in the cytoplasm of the cell and are not as susceptible to the ravages of old age. The initial conversion of cholesterol depends on adequate aldosterone message content. The remaining manufacture activities occur in the cell cytoplasm and continue when real progesterone is available.

Adequate progesterone plays a significant role in bone health, especially females. Effective plants preparations exist that can jump-start aging adrenals and gonads into producing the hormones that lag with age. This works by getting the aging gonad and adrenal around the hurdle of the decreased ability of the mitochondria to begin steroid biosynthesis. Evidence has emerged that progesterone replacement (standardized and pharmaceutical grade only) can reliably enhance the aging gonad and adrenal to increase production of the anti-aging steroids. With sufficient anti-aging steroids there will be adequate direction on bone strengthening activities.

There is a consistent and important theme emphasized throughout the body in the need for specific instruction from level 1 hormones on how to expend cellular energy. A little knowledge can be dangerous when considering the importance of the power contained in the level 1 hormones.

Pregnenolone is a prototypical example of how partial knowledge applied to lagging hormone production can have deleterious and unwanted consequences. Pregnenolone is a steroid precursor that occurs on the path to DHEA and progesterone biosynthesis. It is the intermediary between cholesterol and the biosynthetic pathway to making all steroids including progesterone, testosterone, and DHEA.

Some clinicians routinely prescribe this steroid precursor in the belief that it will simply jumpstart the aging gonads and adrenals in their ability to manufacture the anti-aging steroids. There are better and safer ways to bring about the desired results. The side effects are not worth the price. The side effects occur because pregnenolone contains a message content that is very similar to that of the cortisol message content. If the cortisol message is higher than necessary, the cells are directed to take energy away from cellular rejuvenation and into survival pathways (chapter 2).

This cautions owners to consult a physician who has competency and a complete understanding of steroids. An increased cortisol-like message content in the bone cell will behave as cortisol does. This becomes an unacceptable side effect in the case where bone rejuvenation are concerned.   The effect of pregnenolone creates opposite to the desired effect that is strengthening weak bones.

> The official stand is to demand double blind studies. When pursuing official policies, it is very apparent that there is significant control in what is studied and what the public receives about the results of these studies through mainstream media. It is a cozy arrangement.

Supplementation with progesterone under the guidance of a competent and hormone knowledgeable physician is the safest approach to health. This allows for a trial in usage for several months to document objective benefits. Proving the ability of progesterone to reverse osteoporosis involves the obtaining of a bone density scan as a baseline before treatment. At the end of a six month trial period the bone density scan can be repeated and compared to the before treatment scan.

Progesterone cream leads to wonderful facial skin. For this reason some progesterone should be given as a cream. The cream can also be applied to the breast to help protect them from estrogen dominance.   Use only pharmaceutical grade true progesterone. Without adequate potency the desired benefits will go unrecognized.

There are other methods of progesterone replacement that may be relevant for certain owners. Reputable sources for these progesterone products are obtained through a prescription to the compounding pharmacist. A physician can best advise a patient on how to time, which time of the month, will be best for cream application and when to abstain. Hormone holidays allow for the recognition of the natural ebb and flow of the cycle between estrogen and progesterone.

An excellent summary of natural hormone replacement for women was written by Uzzi Reis, M.D., in his book, *Natural Hormone Balance for Women*, Pocket Books, 2001. He explains the benefits of real hormone replacement instead of patentable hormone replacement. Overall this book is written and informative for women past thirty-five years of age.

When viewing the disease osteoporosis holistically, scientific evidence is more accurately described as gonad and/or adrenal insufficiency. Lagging gonad or adrenal function leads bones down the path of deterioration from the lack of hormone message content. The androgen steroid message content directs the bone cells in ongoing rejuvenation. There are more peripheral considerations that have potential to contribute to the overall severity of the disease process. It is the more peripheral considerations that are receiving the advertising dollar. These peripheral approaches occur without the benefit of implementing the central role that the anabolic steroids play in creating a lessened consumer demand for the services of the complex.

A caution as to why progesterone is being endorsed over other anabolic steroids. Competent advice is needed when considering steroid supplementation to invigorate aging cells. Steroids with the additions of vitamin A, and thyroid hormones are the only hormones that directly interact with DNA. The quality and amounts of the different types of steroids interacting with cells determine direction of expenditure of available cellular energy. The power of steroid message content to switch off or on DNA programs is critical. All other hormones that effect the cell DNA act more peripherally and indirectly if at all. The steroids are extremely powerful and deserve respect, much like being taught respect for a loaded gun.

Progesterone, for one's bones, has a known safety profile that the other steroids fall short of in one way of another. Under certain circumstances other anabolic steroids may be warranted. However, one really needs to be followed by a knowledgeable physician in these cases because of the risks versus benefits considerations. Risks are always lurking with these ever more powerful hormones.

The need to supplement with powerful steroids does occur. Females who have had their ovaries surgically removed may be at increased risk for developing osteoporosis. Owners suffering from autoimmune disease and owners who have diminished adrenal reserve could benefit from stronger forms of therapy. A complete twenty-four hour urine test is the basic starting point to assess for steroids. This tests an important part of the overall hormone report card that helps guide the physician toward healing.

Another caution is in order when considering steroid supplementation for a patient that has a history of a hormone responsive malignancy. These cases often occur in breast, uterine, ovarian, and prostate cancers. Counsel from a knowledgeable physician is essential. Progesterone that arrives at capable gonads and adrenals is easily converted to other steroids. This is an important, but subtle clinical point that is often overlooked. This approach relies on the body possessing an intelligence to do the wise thing when given the chance.

The Chinese have recognized this fact for millennia in their routine supplementation with high quality ginseng to combat the lagging hormones. As a general rule, at the age of forty, it is a common practice to begin supplementing with ginseng. When inquiring into why this practice is reverently adhered, interesting biochemical support emerges. The complex creates smoke and mirrors tactics to discount this information that has been successful through the ages.

Ginseng is progesterone in a package. Before the package is ripped off, the intact ginseng molecule is a type of surfactant (lung chapter). This revered quality facilitates an optimal breathing function resulting from regular use. The body is intelligent. The intact ginseng molecule will go where needed. If there more is needed in the aging gonads and adrenals, that is where it will go. This property will also make the androgen message content available to the increase of bone structure.

When the progesterone precursor package is ripped off, natural progesterone is made available to jumpstart the aging hormone glands into renewed production of lagging steroids. Life style choices in exercise and nutritional adequacy will influence this ability.

The use of ginseng to strengthen bones includes the need to realize that quality ginseng is the most difficult medicinal herb to find in this country. There are over 2 billion Asians and a good proportion of them are over forty years old. Good medicinal ginseng takes a minimum of seven years to grow before there is sufficient bioactive ingredient present (source guide).

There are two cautions in the use of ginseng. Regular ginseng usage may raise blood pressure. Monitoring this should be a safety measure. Raising the androgen content can result in hair thinning in genetically predisposed males after forty. Around this age testosterone production decreases enough in males to slow down their hair loss and increase the tendency to get a beer gut. Insulin levels become less opposed to the fat burning effects that testosterone creates. The tough decision becomes which facet of youth the owner wishes to maintain. A knowledgeable physician should monitor these decisions.

Some owners supplement with progesterone and high quality ginseng for increasing bone mass. A report card can be obtained through a twenty-four hour urine test for steroid content before beginning any supplement program. Follow this up in ninety 90 days with a repeat test.

Ginseng builds stronger bones by stimulating steroid synthesis in the adrenals and gonads. Men usually notice a discernable increase in the size of their testicles in about seven days. Some owners do not absorb ginseng like the normal population. In these cases it is worth experimenting with taking it on an empty stomach versus a meal containing eggs or cheese. Without certain vitamins, ginseng can be taken for a long time without any benefit because these vitamins are needed for the body to process it into more active forms.

Halatorrhea floribunda, suma (Brazilian ginseng), macca, pomegranates, European mistletoe berries, and possibly Mexican wild yams are a few of the plants that contain progesterone or a similar precursor. None of these have the thousands of years of safety and efficiency that ginseng possesses. People will continue to gather information and compare notes and eventually more will be known about these other medicinal plants. Until then, it is wise to proceed cautiously and stay in the areas where common safety guidelines are established.

There are cases where stronger anabolic steroid creams and potions are warranted. The ability of testosterone creams applied over the fracture site to speed bone healing is one of them. Another effect is in the ability of testosterone injections to facilitate ligament and joint injury healing. These are all predictable when considering the stimulatory message content that anabolic steroids play in healing these tissues. There are other hormones to consider (growth hormone and insulin), but they have obstacles because of potential side effects.

A case in point involved a naturopathic physician who broke his knee. He also has an 18-year history of insulin dependent diabetes. This was a concern to the orthopedic surgeon who reconstructed the joint and tibia fracture fragments with pins and plates. The concern was founded on the general knowledge that long-time, severe diabetic patients heal poorly and very slowly. Unbeknownst to this talented surgeon was the fact that his patient had two things in his base of knowledge that powerfully enhanced his ability to heal. He was a faithful adherent to the pioneering work of Richard Bernstein, M.D., in the solutions to diabetes mastery (***Diabetes Solutions***, 1998, Little Brown Co.) and was entirely free of the usual diabetic complications. Second, he applied a mixture of testosterone and progesterone cream over the fracture site daily, at this authors suggestion. This resulted in an acceleration of fracture healing time. At the time of his 4½-week exam x ray there was 9 weeks of healing when compared to healing in the normal population.

The quality of the homones and their direct relationship to anabolic steroids greatly influences the healing processes of the bones and how cellular energy is expended. Throughout the cell types, health requires optimum message content or aging results. Clinical assessment is critical to rejuvenation and should be applied skillfully and holistically. Today's knowledge about different hormone's ability to preserve youthful properties should be fully applied in the office setting.

Other hormones play a less central role in the health or deterioration of bone mass. These along with different lifestyle choices, nutritional adequacy, and emotional energy impact bone health and the youthful state of cells.

Bones and Exercise

Exercise is a powerful stimulant for strong bone formation when an owner has capable gonads and adrenals. Unhealthy gonads and adrenals when faced with the physiological demands of exercise are analogous to making a cash withdrawal when the safe is empty. Without previous deposits, no withdrawals can be made. The inability of some owners to maintain an adequate fitness program stems from this.

Exercise proficiency is limited by the quality of the steroids being secreted in the months before starting to exercise and by current ability. Exercise encourages the gonads and adrenals to function efficiently. If they are capable, there are far reaching performance and longevity advantages. Some exercise can be harmful if the gonad and adrenals ability to produce adequate anabolic steroids is chronically exceeded. Exercise increases the need for message content to direct the appropriate investment into muscular-skeletal strengthening.

Simply, exceeding gonad and adrenal ability to generate sufficient message content (anabolic steroids) causes soreness and potential injury. Normal training can also produce some soreness. Injury verses exercise training soreness can be differentiated. Exceeding the level of current gonad and adrenal ability creates sore joints or ligaments after exercising. Regular exercise with cautious increases in intensity will stimulate the adrenals and gonads to increase output of anabolic steroids.

Increased demand of anabolic steroid production goes unrecognized in owners who lack adequate response of gonad and adrenal ability. Signs of aging elicit unnecessary counseling to slow down. With an appropriate inquiry into balancing lagging hormones, slowing down may not be the answer.

Once the hormones have been attended to an exercise program will have remarkable restorative affects. The interrelationship between exercise and hormone quality and the bones is obvious. Weak bones can come from either a sedentary lifestyle or poor hormone production ability in the adrenals and gonads. Healing is possible when there is awareness of both possibilities.

The Bones and Calcium

The importance of calcium plays a significant role in bone health. The press on a regular basis covers adequate calcium intake. The average adult contains about 2½ pounds of calcium in their body. 99% of this amount is in the bones. Increasing dietary calcium has little effect on increasing overall absorption. That is determined by which hormones are present. The hormone quality also further determines where calcium ends up in the body. Eating meals rich in phosphates and oxalates causes calcium to bind and exit in the formation of microscopic gravel in the stool.

1% of calcium that is not in the bones needs to be carefully channeled and regulated. Organism havoc ensues when this pool of calcium is altered minutely. This concept is often lost in trying to make sense of the complex medical phraseology that is in print. Making informed choices regarding adequate calcium requires the need for the body to keep 1% of the calcium constant. This calcium influences whether the owner lives from one moment to the next. If free calcium falls 10% below normal, tetany promptly ensues and the next step is fatal laryngospasm. The body has an elaborate system of hormones that regulate and counter regulate the 1% calcium content on multiple levels. These hormones ensure that an adequate and constant supply of calcium is maintained.

There are two classes of hormones operating that concern calcium. The first group includes vitamin D, parathyroid hormone, and calcitonin. These hormones ensure that calcium in the free form is kept constant to maintain life. This must occur in a wide variety of metabolic circumstances.

Parathyroid hormone is secreted from six little glands behind the thyroid. These glands promptly respond to calcium content falling in the blood stream by secreting sufficient parathyroid hormone. That increases active vitamin D formation in the kidneys and tells bone tissue to release calcium.

Increasing active vitamin D content increases absorption of dietary calcium, puts it into the accessible bone pool of calcium, and increases the ability of the kidney to retain calcium from excretion in the urine.

The role of thyroid-derived calcitonin seems to speed the uptake of calcium increase in the blood stream that may occur following a meal. Deficient calcium encourages the release of parathyroid hormone, which in turn promotes the absorption sequence. This calcium is destined to the readily accessible bone calcium that is separated from true mineralized bone structure.

The second group of hormones determines how adequately bone quality is being addressed at any given time. It is these and not the first group that needs sufficient quality and amount occurring with proper timing to maintain bone health. This is contrasted conceptually with the second group of hormones that inhibit or promote adequate bone rejuvenation. The type and amount of steroids determines the message content for expenditure of available energy of a bone cell.

These cells need adequate molecular building parts constantly supplied by a highly functioning digestive tract. Wise nutritional choices are critical.

Joint Space

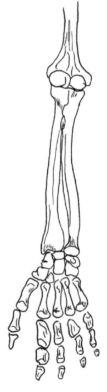

Hinged joints have an added layer of joint lining cells surrounding the joint cavity such as fingers, toes, knees, ankles, hips, elbow, and wrists. Contrasting these are the less moveable joints occurring in the intervertebral disc, sternum with rib articulations, hand and feet joints. Both types of joints have cartilage anchored over the bone ends and around the side by tough fibrous attachments that secure the two ends in close proximity.

Additional joint cells line the hinged joints and are like hollow sponges stuffed into a joint space. The secretion of these cells is a gel-like substance. The manufacture of this gel is one of the determinants of how well joints function. This gel is made from modified galactosamine that forms hylauronic acid. Gelatin is made from ground up partially digested cartilage. One of the components of cartilage is galactosamine.

When the joint cells are secreting this gel substance appropriately, the hinged joints are facilitated in their ability to glide with minimal friction during performance of their hinging action. Water performs magic when there is adequate supply. Only if there is an adequate supply of water during the ebb and flow of cleansing forces can water rinse off the gel that looks and feels dirty. This is one of the mechanisms for painful joints. When joints hurt drink abundant, clean water.

The cartilage overlying the bone ends adjacent to the joint space looks like shinny linoleum in the youthful state. As it ages, it becomes cracked and worn. Visualizing the additional joint lining cells occurring in the hinged joints as a grease forming carpet layer facilitates defending against some of these hostilities. This layer has its own blood and nerve supply that allows for a superior nutrition source. It also leads as a toxic waste site in the body for trash that must be removed. When this situation occurs, it is critically important that the garbage is removed. The owner usually perceives this as pain. Instead of consuming large quantities of clean water, many are trained from an early age to consume toxins like aspirin or acetaminophen (liver chapter). This contributes to more trash water. In addition concepts that are good for the cartilage are also good for the joint lining cells. The pain perceiving nerve fibers are not present in the cartilage, but in the surrounding fibrous anchoring ligaments that encases the joint and the joint lining cells themselves. It is the responsibility of these pain fibers to scream out if there is dysfunction in the joint. Processes that injure these nerves, like diabetes, diminish the ability to alert the owner of problems.

Bone Marrow

In some of the larger bones there is bone marrow. The potential for continued or the possibility of renewed vigor is contained here. This is the location of pure potential for the ability to rejuvenate the blood with new cells of all types. Processes that injure the potential energy contained in the bone marrow inhibit healing until they are corrected.

Some of the immune system cells have a life span of 6 hours. Without adequate maintenance of the bone marrow, there is depletion of vital cell lines that ensues and diseases follow.

Processes that are good for the bones are good for the bone marrow. The bone marrow needs informational content that directs use of available energy. Lack of quality information content leads to programed cell death of many potential cells.

Falling quality message content occurs when disease processes injure enough kidney cells that there becomes a diminished ability of the kidney to manufacture the hormone erythropoietin. Thousands of years ago Chinese physicians determined that sufficient kidney energy is necessary for the continued optimal function of the bone marrow. They also discovered that the kidney area (the adrenals that are attached to the kidney) and their dominance over the strength of the gonads all interact to generate sufficient message content directing energy expenditure within the bone marrow.

In western medicine there is a tendency to forget the holism of what the Chinese have known for thousands of years. In place of this are profitable approaches to treating failing bone marrow. This is found in the common practice of relying on recombinant DNA technology to manufacture the complex hormone erythropoietin. This doesn't mean that this expensive technology is never helpful, but that many diseased owners lack the ability to pay the astronomical fees for this treatment. Understanding the holism of what science has revealed often times allows for less costly alternatives.

It has been known for many years that adequate androgen content stimulates optimal performance of the bone marrow. The androgen class of steroid hormones is important to stimulate the different cell lines of the body to maximize potential performance.

Androgen type steroids stimulate the bone marrow to make new cells and increase the ability of the kidney to manufacture erythropoietin. Applying this knowledge in the clinical setting allows a way to avoid the costly approach to healing. There are some cases where this costly approach is warranted, but why not include the holism of more affordable options?

Holism discussions are incomplete until the energies that heal contrasted to the energies that maim, the seventh principle of longevity, are part of the healing plan strategy. The next section explains the seventh principle and how its healing properties can be realized. In addition, the health and needs of the brain, heart and muscles are reviewed.

SECTION VI

HEALTH IS A QUESTION OF BALANCE

Principle 7

The reoccurring body theme of balance is a prerequisite for true health. Balance reverberates all the way down to the opposing molecules that are interacting within a cell. Western medicine often ignores this because of the reductionism logic on which it is founded.

The seven principles of healthful longevity are largely about the balance between the opposing life forces; the creative forces versus the destructive forces. Where there is balance between the two, health can continue. In each of the five sections before this there has been an emphasis on one or two of the first six principles for healthful longevity. The central nervous system lends itself to the discussion of balance between all of these first six principles. This chapter concerns itself with how the central nervous system functions. The central nervous system, more than the other organ system, lends itself to explaining how the seven principles of longevity interrelate with one another.

The science is present to unite these holistic principles into a comprehensive assessment of what science has revealed. Reductionism of the logistical and detailed investigations into the biochemical reactions of life has merit. However, at some point it becomes devoid of the common interwoven theme of balance. When science becomes more unified it brings people to the realization that life is based on balance between opposing forces. Wherever there is imbalance, deterioration and disease eventually result.

In addition, this section prepares the reader for the hardest principle for the western mind to understand, the seventh principle. The seventh principle is about the energies that heal contrasted to the energies that maim. With this in mind, the central nervous system will be explored within the consideration of the seventh principle.

A few remarks about the seventh principle

Other medical scientific theories embrace the energetic understandings of balance. For example, traditional Chinese medical theory has the life energies quality at its foundation. The foundation of their energy science uses the concepts of Yin energy that directly opposes Yang energy in a harmonious way. The harmony between these two energetic entities is a prerequisite for health. The Chinese science of health embraces this reoccurring body theme; balance.

Conversely, the western system ignores the dynamic forces between Yin energy and Yang energy. These forces are mysterious energies that oppose one another. Thousands of years of accumulated evidence show that balance is necessary for health. Yin energy can be thought of as quiet, calm, contemplative, reflective, cool, deep, patient, and content. Yang energy is loud, rushed, hurried, hot, shallow, and explosive, on-the -move, action and inpatient.

Evidence has been accumulating for more than 60 years that the life force is an intelligent energy grid that permeates every cell. Every cell in the body is organized energetically by this living entity until death. The evidence seems to indicate that when this life force is evenly distributed and of the right vibration frequency all is well within the body.

In contrast, the western medical approach can best be described as the "slab of meat approach". The slab of meat is all that is left when the mysterious energies that organize the human form are ignored. The western scientific paradigm ignores the qualities of the life force. When life energy imbalances are the cause of disease then owners in these situations will continue to suffer. The western medical complex fails to consider energy aberrations that can cause a disease process. The Chinese are not the only medical theory that includes the life force energy.

Eastern Indian scientific theory has long understood the flow of optimal life giving energy through chakras in healthy individuals. Recently there have been some interesting applications of these imbalanced energy states, and how they correlate with disease. This evidence involves the other side of the story of what science has revealed but has been ignored. In this chapter, the ignored evidence will be reintroduced. The trouble with re-including it in the discussion of health versus disease is that many of the mainstream approaches and explanations of the inner-workings of the universe begin to look inconsistent and incomplete. Information about many of the alternative treatment modalities makes more mechanistic sense, and often appears less superstitious.

Down through the age's many wise men have contemplated the human condition. Dr. Paul Brand, author of the book, *Wonderfully and Fearfully Made* points out that knowledge is lost. The Egyptian physicians of thousands of years ago could perform surgeries that cannot even be contemplated today. High technology solutions can only go so far before one confronts the ignored energy of life. The life force needs to be considered and appreciated in order to carry healing over the 'bridge' that unites the mainstream with the alternative modalities.

The Intelligence behind the Intelligence

The body contains approximately one hundred trillion cells. The 46 chromosomes that contain the DNA within most cells are in some ways analogous to a computer encryption code. Without an intelligent operator the encryption code hides useful information. Something is missing at the encryption (DNA) level. Something else is needed to explain the precise and ordered unraveling and repair of DNA. The replication of DNA and RNA is superbly directed by some as yet unseen guiding principle. In addition, the RNA directed protein synthesis, which results in elaborate and unique protein architecture, needs direction. The direction of the construction of cell architecture involves many types of fat and specialized sugar groups. What directs how these all fit precisely together is not explained by the genetic code contained within the DNA. The DNA only contains the sequencing information for the construction of the amino acid sequence, which is contained within protein. It does not contain information, which regards the synthesis of the many different types of fat, and modified sugars added onto certain proteins. They need to be precisely arranged in three-dimensional space for life to continue. A plausible explanation for what directs these complex processes is currently beyond western scientific understanding.

There is interesting research, which regards the question of what the nature of the force is that intelligently directs the DNA. One of the early scientific pioneers was Dr. Harold Saxon Burr, a long time researcher at Yale University. In the early 1920's his research began documenting the electromagnetic field properties, found to occur in all living things. Dr. Burr later named this electromagnetic field, which is present in all living things, the life field. He pointed out that if one hadn't seen their friend in over six months, new molecules during the intervening time period, would have replaced every molecule in their friend's face. The fact that the body replaces all soft tissue molecules frequently is secondary to the body's ongoing cellular rejuvenation program. The cellular rejuvenation program occurs throughout life at varying degrees of efficiency. His research led him to conclude that it was the life field that served as an organizing template. He theorized that the electromagnetic field, which he measured, was the organizer of the structure contained in living things. He concluded that the electromagnetic 'template' preserves the pattern in the friend's face. The underlying energetic template reproduces a consistent appearance, even though the molecules themselves are different. He extended this concept to explain the mystery of embryological cells, knowing how to organize, divide and differentiate into fetal form.

Conversely, mainstream science is unable to explain these two fundamental life processes, because they ignore theories like Dr. Burr's. Specifically, there is no mainstream explanation for why one's face stays recognizable after the molecules are replaced. In addition, mainstream science is still baffled about the process of embryogenesis. Embryogenesis denotes the organized process of cell differentiation, spatial arrangement and orientation of the embryo's development. Dr. Robert Becker, in his book, **The Body Electric**, elaborated on this research. Dr. Becker comments, "Embryo genesis is as if a pile of bricks were to spontaneously rearrange itself into a building, becoming not only walls but windows, light sockets, steel beams and furniture in the process." Later on he summarized this mystery that led to his life research," As I contemplated their findings and all of biology's unsolved problems, I grew convinced that life was more complex than we suspected. I felt that those who reduced life to a mechanical interaction of molecules were living a cold, gray, dead world, which despite its drabness, was a fantasy. I didn't think electricity would turn out to be any élan vital in the old sense, but I had a hunch it would be closer to the secret than the smells of the biochemistry lab or the dissecting rooms preserved organs." Dr.'s Burr and Becker are in good company. Another scientist agrees with their line of thinking in regards to solving the mystery of an organizing energy field. Albert Szent Gyorgyi won the Nobel Prize for his work on tissue oxidation and the elucidation of the molecular structure of vitamin C. According to Dr. Becker, while addressing the Budapest Academy of Science on March 21, 1941, Dr. Gyorgyi pointed out that when these scientists broke living things down into constituent parts, life slipped through their fingers and they found themselves working with dead matter. Gyorgyi emphasized, "It looks as if some basic fact about life is still missing, without which any real understanding is impossible." For the missing basic fact Gyorgyi proposed putting electricity back into science's investigation of living things. More than sixty years later mainstream science is still trying to explain life within the limitation of molecular matter while ignoring the evidence for organizing energy.

The continued omission of the life force has altered medical treatment decisions. Some of the consequent treatment decisions have associated toxicities. Some of these toxicities are avoidable. In contrast, the alternative treatment modalities tend to address the importance of an owner's life force quality. This fact has resulted in alternative healing disciplines. This is a powerful common denominator between many of the alternative methods of healing. Some holistic physicians feel that the common denominator regards their common practice of improving, maintaining, and cleansing this life field. The alternative therapies believe that the life force functions more efficiently during health than in disease.

Some call the life force energy, (measured years ago by Dr. Burr), intelligent energy. Intelligent energy denotes the property of the life force to organize molecules into complex arrangements which life requires. This fundamental requirement of living things violates the science of physics third law of thermodynamics. The third law of thermodynamics states that molecular arrangements will tend to move in a random fashion towards more disorder. Again, mainstream medicine is unable to explain how living things violate this basic physical law of the nonliving universe.

Some newer mathematical theories predict that the life force swirls around at speeds faster than the speed of light. The faster-than-the speed-of-light requirement has merit because when energy moves this fast the math predicts it to behave with an organizational intelligence. Dr. Richard Gerber, in his book called, *Vibrational Medicine* explains quite well the math pioneered by Carl Muses. Carl Muses proposed in his work on hyper numbers, that when energy moves faster than the speed of light, organizational consequences occur. Dr. William Tiller of Stanford University expounded on these mathematical consequences and described this type of energy as difficult to measure within the dimension of the physical world, except that it would create a weak magnetic field. All living things studied, to date, create a magnetic field until death occurs.

The faster than speed of light property would help explain the above mentioned long-standing physic's enigma. Specifically, the third law of thermodynamics in physics states that energy naturally moves in a direction of more and more randomness (increased entropy). Life's complexly created molecules, which are precisely arranged so that life may continue, violate this basic tenant of physics. However, if one limits the third law of thermodynamics to a description of energy's behavior when energy travels at speeds equal to, or less than the speed of light, it remains consistent. Until very recently no mathematician or scientist had really thought about the consequences of energy moving at speeds greater than the speed of light.

Understanding the enigma regarding life energy violating physics thermodynamic law is best grasped by considering the chicken egg. If one dropped a million eggs on the floor, breaking each of the eggs, there would be a mess. There would be no chick formed. The physicist would say that the third law of thermodynamics was consistent in this case. However, it is only consistent because the act of breaking open the shell kills the life contained inside of it. Contrast this to successfully incubating any one of the eggs through its gestation time. The live chick would be formed. The baby chick is an example of increasing complexity, which is created from uncomplicated molecules inside the chicken egg. What was just a gooey mess inside the egg was energetically organized into the complex multi-organ and multi-cellular baby chick. What is the nature of this intelligent energy that violates the laws of physics? The theory of energy moving faster than the speed of light and behaving with an organizational intelligence is a viable explanation for how the life force may organize matter like the gooey chicken egg into a baby chick.[25]

Drs. Muses and Tiller were some of the first mathematicians to look into how energy behaves moving faster than the speed of light. They theorized that when energy travels faster than the speed of light it would behave with an organizational intelligence with only a weakly measurable magnetic field. They thought of the physical world, for which owners have sensory apparatus to experience, as the speeds equal to or less than light dimension. They further predicted that at speeds greater than light the measurement of the electrical properties of this type of energy would exceed today's technological capabilities. The one exception that their mathematical calculations predicted was the ability to detect a weakly measurable magnetic field. This theory is consistent with the measurability of a weak bodily becomes ignored in the mainstream world of medicine. Magnetic field, which changes in strength and polarization during different levels of activity and consciousness level. There is evidence, which would help explain life's mysterious energetic properties more completely yet, it is routinely ignored.

The life energy can best be thought of as moving within another dimension than the physical world. Current technologies cannot detect energy moving faster than the speed of light. In fact, this becomes the basis for claiming that it does not exist. The mathematical theory of matter moving faster than the speed of light, which predicts that it would create a weak but measurable magnetic field, tends to be ignored.

Interestingly, research looking into the organization of the body's magnetic field, has found an unvarying energy grid, corresponding to the ancient Chinese system of acupuncture meridian lines.

Science has come a long way in eloquently explaining cellular biochemical reactions. Scientific understanding is advancing about the understanding of the contents of the DNA program. However, the life energy evidence tends to be ignored.

Scientific theory, going back thousands of years in India and China, recognized the importance of living things containing optimal energy flow. The Indians call the life energy prana and the Chinese call it chi. In both scientific systems the attention to the overall quality and integrity contained within the life energy field is fundamental to health. In addition, the Chinese realized the quality of energy penetrating the body's trunk organs could be palpated in the peripheral pulse. This system quantitates the amount of chi contained within the various organs and is called pulse diagnosis. Pulse diagnosis was developed over the last several thousand years. Pulse diagnosis allows an elaborate understanding of the consequences of energetic excess or deficiency within each organ.

The electromagnetic lines, known as the acupuncture meridian lines, were painstakingly developed with their corresponding organ effects noted. Out of this several thousand years of observation, there developed an understanding of ways to increase or decrease the energetic meridian tone depending on what was needed. The energetic tone is composed of the opposing energies, Yin and Yang. When Yin and Yang are unbalanced an organ system dysfunction occurs.

The Chinese scientific theory regards chi as organizing life energy. This energy concept is worthy of some consideration. This theory predicts that Chi needs to be balanced by the forces of yin and yang within any organ system in the body or disease occurs. Investigations into chi energy could solve the mystery about the created perpetual complexity of living things.

The alternative idea of the existence of intelligent energy serving as the ultimate director of the cellular biochemical reactions of life has healing possibilities. Healing possibilities could be realized when the chi energy becomes improved. Improvement in the chi energy will improve the quality of the hormones secreted in a rhythmic and harmonious way. These alternative theories predict that the areas of body breakdown result from the chi energetic deficiency or excess. Chi is the Chinese description of intelligent energy, the life force, or prana.

The merging of energy theory and what is known about the biochemical reactions of life incorporates the intermediary step of the hormones and neurotransmitters. The hormones deliver the message, which was stimulated by the intelligent energy. The quality of the intelligent energy, within the body, becomes a determinant of how an organ is directed to spend energy. If the intelligent energy distribution and quality is favorable, this is communicated to the body's cells by the informational substances.

The informational substances include the hormones and neurotransmitters. The Chinese theory regarding chi predicts that practices that facilitate the life energy, will promote health by way of the informational substances. Any practice that injures the quality of the intelligent energy will promote aging and eventual disease. Western science can measure the diminished quality of informational substances. However, western science does not specifically appreciate or acknowledge the possibility of the life force energy being a determinant of these informational substances.

The Chinese and East Indians have developed theories that explain the life force energy. Western medical thought begins its treatment decisions at the level of the informational substances. Often times even this level of inquiry becomes less than adequate.

The theory of intelligent energy can best be thought of as the organizational template which directs the overall living body processes. The quality and completeness of this life energy determines which informational substances are secreted. Quality informational substances depend on a highly functioning intelligent energy field. This belief has long ago been appreciated and incorporated into Chinese and East Indian scientific medical thought. The belief that these energies are moving faster than the speed of light provides an explanation for why they are difficult to detect by conventional technological means. Similarly, before the understanding of television and radio waves, the presence of these wave energies in the natural environment largely went unnoticed until the technology was developed to measure their existence. The key to understanding this possibility regards an appreciation of the fact that television and radio waves existed down through the ages. Their properties of existence were not affected because humans were unaware of their presence. Today the upper limits of scientific study concerns energies which move slower than or equal to the speed of light. However, the evolution of mathematics considers the consequences of what energy would behave like when moving greater than the speed of light. Part of these consequences includes the possibility that would explain how life organizes matter into complex arrangements. If an owner can be open to this possibility, then a mechanism for why alternative therapies improve owner vitality becomes possible.

Chapter 24

The Physical Health of the Brain and Nerves

The brain has a unique protection system that is commonly known as the blood brain barrier. This barrier is created by the blood vessel lining cells (the 'tiles' discussed in the blood vessel chapter) within the brain, forming a tight interconnected barrier. The barrier is very selective on what it allows to pass in or out of the brain blood vessel. This barrier is complete except in a few areas deep within the central underside of the brain. These four small areas where the blood brain barrier doesn't exist are called the circum-ventricular organs. These small areas provide a window for the brain to more directly interact with the body environment and it allows an area of vulnerability for unwanted substances as well.

Physicians treating for possible brain infections have to constantly keep in mind that only a few antibiotics can penetrate beyond the blood brain barrier. This is a problem when attempting to medicate brain function. Illnesses like Parkinson's disease can be benefited if more dopamine makes its way into the injured neurons responsible for its manufacture. The trouble is dopamine cannot cross the blood brain barrier. Scientists circumvent this by providing a synthetic dopamine precursor, L-dopa that penetrates the blood brain barrier. Once the blood brain barrier is penetrated, L-dopa can be converted to dopamine.

The blood brain barrier creates a challenge for the brain cells. The challenge for brain cells is their continued procurement of all the needed molecular building blocks. The brain needs more molecular building parts because it is an area of high metabolic activity. High metabolic activity means that molecular parts wear out and need replacement more quickly. All this active replacement requires the use of lots of fuel and oxygen. The combustion of fuels and oxygen necessitates an increased need for efficient waste removal and rust prevention. In addition, only some of the most powerful body hormones can gain access to the entire brain. This fact has powerful repercussions when one wants to know how to keep their brain functional.

Keeping in mind the physical blood brain barrier will facilitate the understanding of nine determinants of physical brain health. These are:

1. Availability and completeness of neurotransmitters in the brain
2. Availability and direction for the use of molecular building parts
3. Adequate fuel delivery
4. Blood vessel health in the brain
5. Informational directions regarding cell architecture and rejuvenation
6. Anti-oxidant versus oxidant activity

7. Quality of the force field that the individual nerve cells are able to generate
8. Toxin accumulation
9. Status of the energy that heals contrasted to the energy that maims. There will be greater ability to make better choices in the day-to-day little decisions that promotes brain health when one considers the nine determinants to brain health.

It helps to organize the seven principles of health and how they relate to the nine determinates of brain health. The brain is somewhat unique and expanding from seven to nine will facilitate healing the mind.

1. Principles 1&2: Blood vessel health (4 and 6 above)
2. Principle 3: Hormone message content (5 above and 1 above)
3. Principle 4: Molecular replacement parts (2, 3, and 1 above)
4. Principle 5: Taking out the brain trash (8 above)
5. Principle 6: Cellular charge of brain cells (7 above)
6. Principle 7: Energy that heals contrasted to energy that maim brain cells (9 above)

THE NINE DETERMNANTS OF BRAIN HEALTH

1. Neurotransmitters

The many different neurotransmitters within the mind convey specific information to the neighboring nerves. A discussion of the numerous different neurotransmitters can get really complicated. Some of the most basic considerations will help to avoid gullibility about the medical business complex. It becomes important to get an overall feel for the different types of neurotransmitters. Neurotransmitter's availability is dependent on certain nutritional and biochemical factors. These nutritional and biochemical factors need to be present in order for a happier and more efficient brain function.

The first group of neurotransmitters is called the biogenic amines. These same neurotransmitter molecules (epinephrine, nor-epinephrine, dopamine, histamine and serotonin), when they occur within the blood stream, are known as hormones. A large proportion of this group of informational substances has blood vessel effects on tone when acting as hormones. Thus the terms neurotransmitter and hormone are thought of as a distinction of where in the body their action occurs and not as different molecules.

The bioactive amines are found in the nervous system and blood stream. These same molecules are called hormones when they are within the blood stream and neurotransmitters when they are within the nervous system. Someday some contrary guy is going to successfully propose that the simplified and unifying term, informational substance, take the place of this confusing arbitrary semantics drama between hormone and neurotransmitter. Until that far off day it is probably wise to get a grasp of this duplicity and understand the two ways of saying the same thing in as complicated a way as possible.

Examples of the precursors, which form the biogenic amine types of the neurotransmitters, are the amino acids: tyrosine, tryptophan, and histidine. Tyrosine can be manufactured into epinephrine (adrenaline), nor-epinephrine and dopamine. Tryptophan can be manufactured into serotonin and melatonin. Finally, histadine can be manufactured into histamine. There are a few others that will be discussed later in the chapter but in order to keep the discussion less burdensome this is all for now.

The biosynthesis of these neurotransmitters is, to varying degrees, all dependent on a number of nutritional cofactors (synthesis facilitators). Without sufficient cofactors these neurotransmitters manufacture becomes impossible. When was the last time that anyone heard of a mainstream physician inquiring about the nutritional adequacy of a given owners ability to manufacture these essential neurotransmitters? This is yet another example of how what is being taught within medical schools is deficient when compared to the holism of what science has revealed.

The conversion of tyrosine into the above neurotransmitters occurs in an orderly fashion. Each step of the progression requires certain molecular cofactors. The assembly line order of progression is dependent on adequate molecular replacement parts for each step of manufacture. Health consequences follow when any one of these parts becomes deficient. Tyrosine gets first converted to dopa, then into dopamine, then on into nor-epinephrine and finally into epinephrine. This may sound really boring and dull but underneath a superficial veneer of these qualities lays an exciting youth preserving mechanism. This is because when one understands the simple cofactors that are needed in order to make proper amounts of each one of these neurotransmitters one can get on the brain functioning advantage track that leads to vitality.

In the order of need, the above listed assembly line progressions of neurotransmitter manufacture are: tetrahydrobiopterin (made from folate), vitamin C, vitamin B6, and finally S-adenosylmethioine (SAMe). These are the basic cofactors that are needed in their active form or synthesis along the assembly line from tyrosine to epinephrine comes to a halt. It should be emphasized that for each neurotransmitter molecule made: one to two vitamin C's are used, one tetrahydrobiopterin is unloaded, and one SAMe is unloaded. Unless a highly functional molecular re-supply system operates, then these cofactors rapidly become depleted. In addition, SAMe can only be recharged when adequate folate, vitamin B6, vitamin B12, and the amino acid serine is available. It is more important to realize the need of a real food diet than to memorize all these picky facts.

The demands for newly manufactured bioactive amines are much greater within the blood stream. The blood stream needs more bioactive amines because these informational substances only exist for about 2 minutes. These informational substances have two minutes to convey their message, once released into the circulation, before being deactivated and then eliminated within the urine. This is in contrast to their ability, within nerves, to be released and recycled many times once they have been manufactured.

When owners become mentally, not what they used to be, the cause could be from one or more of the above nutritional deficiencies. SAMe and the molecules that recharge it each time it donates a methyl group is called collectively, the methyl donor system. The methyl donor system is used at the rate of one billion times per second. An owner is only as good as the least present nutrient within their methyl donor system.[26]

Serotonin

One of the most likely bioactive amines to be depleted comes from the amino acid tryptophan. The unique reason for this will be explained shortly. This amino acid is found in high concentrations in eggs, dairy products, and turkey. This obviously shows why vegans develop far ranging mental impairments. (This really isn't true, It was included just to add joy to all those that are not vegans).

Serotonin deficiency becomes more likely, compared to the other bioactive amines, because some of it becomes depleted in order to make melatonin each day. In contrast, the other neurotransmitters are more efficiently recycled each time they are released into the synapse. Serotonin within the brain is felt to be involved in arousal. Deficiency in the arousal state leads to one of the types of clinical depression. This is a business opportunity that has been well realized with the skyrocketing sales of drugs like Zoloft, Paxil, and Prozac. These drugs work by keeping the serotonin that is released between nerves around longer in the active little space between nerves called the synapse. These prescriptions poison the enzymatic machine, which pulls serotonin out of the synapse. Without these enzyme machines being poisoned every day the serotonin would only affect arousal for a normal time per excretion of it into this little space. However with the advent of these drugs, that are able to go beyond the blood brain barrier, this enzymatic machine becomes incapacitated for a while. The serotonin in this little space between the arousal nerves sends the arousal message for a longer time. It should be mentioned that two of the three most popular drugs in this class contain the most powerful oxidizing element on the planet (stronger than the oxygen radical). This cannot be good when it penetrates the blood brain barrier by being attached to the carrier molecule. How much of this breaks down within one's brain setting off a frenzy of rust production? The most powerful oxidizing element of all is fluorine and will be discussed latter in this chapter. It is mentioned here to help facilitate learning in regards to the other side of the story that science has revealed about the potential down side of what is for sale by the complex.

Here comes the protest and rationalizations about how these types of antidepressant drugs saved Aunt Sally, a vegan, who no one could help before. What isn't being said is that the rate-limiting step for serotonin manufacture is the amount of tryptophan delivered into the blood stream. Science has long ago revealed that serotonin levels within the brain are directly related to three factors. First, the amount consumed in the diet. Second, the ability of the digestive tract to absorb the tryptophan presented to it. Third, concerns the necessary presence of vitamin B6, which converts tryptophan into serotonin. This means that supplementing with tryptophan, vitamin B6, in the diet, and making sure that the digestive process is operative will do what these expensive prescriptions will do.[27]

The reason tryptophan is not readily available in America today is a result of suspect policies occurring within the FDA. How convenient, right when these new serotonin uptake poisons were to become the depression drugs of the nineties, a single source of a contaminated batch of tryptophan was discovered. Later it was found that the only reason that this batch caused severe muscle toxicity was that a single Japanese company tried to save money by changing the standard protocol by which it was traditionally made. Since the FDA answers to no one, they have used this excuse into the present time and thus limit effective strength tryptophan to prescription only. The prescription only designation makes this natural treatment much more expensive.

Serotonin depletion occurs because of two general processes. First, within the pineal gland there is the daily need to manufacture melatonin from available serotonin. Second, depletion occurs if there are not enough cofactors or dietary derived tryptophan present within the brain and the pineal gland. Cofactors are needed to convert tryptophan to serotonin. The essential cofactor, as far as melatonin synthesis, is SAMe. SAMe is part of the methyl donor system, mentioned above, which is depleted within the body at the rate of one billion molecules a second.

The previous discussion mentioned the need for vitamin B12, folate and serine to keep SAMe recharged. SAMe needs to be recharged each time it makes a new melatonin molecule. When healthy owners go to bed, serotonin release slows within the brain. Conversely, melatonin made during the day and stored within the pineal gland is released into the blood stream with the onset of sleep. In young children the amount released is much higher and this gradually decreases until melatonin release becomes quite diminished in old age. Adequate melatonin is cornerstone to a good nights sleep. The high levels occurring with sleeping children may explain the soundness of their sleep. The above daily drains off of serotonin within the brain in order to make new melatonin each day, explains the first reason why serotonin deficiency is more likely than other neurotransmitter deficiencies.

The second mechanism for brain serotonin depletion occurs when there is inadequate typtophan available to satisfy the body's serotonin and melatonin needs. Serotonin deficiency can occur from either poor dietary choices or a decreased ability of the digestive tract to properly dismantle proteins. The dietary deficiency of niacin (vitamin B3) will accelerate the body's need for tryptophan. Tryptophan usage accelerates because it is used to make niacin. Niacin deficiency causes the disease pellagra.

Melatonin release into the blood stream, from the pineal gland during sleep depletes brain stores of this substance. Melatonin is lost each night when it is rhythmically released into the blood stream, from the pineal gland, and performs its mysterious sleep enhancing activity. The melatonin released eventually degrades and then the kidneys remove it. The continual drain off of melatonin from the brain causes the perpetual need for new sources of tryptophan. Tryptophan is continuously depleted and therefore needs to be replaced by the diet.

In contrast, the other biogenic amine neurotransmitters operate under a theme of a highly effective recycling system. The other biogenic amines recycle more efficiently because they are without a drain off for other uses within the blood stream. The other neurotransmitters are released and recycled into the synapse. Here they deliver a message that each of their unique shapes imparts. Shortly after message delivery has been completed they are recycled back to where they came, the nerve ending. Because of this recycling system there isn't the same rate of depletion occurring with these other biogenic neurotransmitters.

The majority of serotonin in the body occurs outside the brain. The platelets and digestive tract contain the majority of serotonin within the body. Within the digestive tract it is used as a hormone that instructs this tube how it should behave. The serotonin message contained within the blood platelets involves the orchestration of clotting parameters. In addition, it encourages blood vessel spasm (vasoconstriction).

The three above additional serotonin purposes utilize greater than 90% of total body serotonin content. Therefore, when owners take drugs that keep serotonin around longer, then a percentage of the effect is within these areas! This fact explains the common experience of increased gastrointestinal distress while taking these drugs. It should be acknowledged that there are 7 different types of serotonin receptors. The drug companies research findings, which sell SSRI's, documents that the highest affinity for these drugs occurs within the limbic system in the brain. The limbic system contains only type 6 and 7 receptors.

Serotonin levels affect the amount of the hormone prolactin released from the pituitary. Prolactin may sound like another boring hormone at first. However, a higher prolactin level leads to inhibition of gonad function. Re-inclusion of this little detail helps explain the high rate of sexual dysfunction that commonly occurs when owners take these prescriptions. This does not mean that serotonin re-uptake inhibitors are never warranted. In fact, once someone is prescribed them, it is a pretty tricky business to safely navigate their discontinuation. However, the risk of decreased gonad function underscores the need to consider nutritional deficiencies early in the depression presentation. There are no side effects when one heals.

While an owner takes these types of medications they should monitor their prolactin levels. If sexual dysfunction occurs, a well-run 24-hour urine test should then be run and analyzed by a competent physician. If the gonad steroids are found to be low and continued serotonin re-uptake inhibitors are still warranted then natural sex hormone replacement therapy could be considered.

Histamine

The next neurotransmitter, in the bioactive amines class, to be discussed is histamine. Histamine is manufactured from the amino acid histadine. This is an important neurotransmitter and hormone. The role of this important informational substance is largely ignored. Histamine likely is ignored because there is a lot of money at stake, which revolves around the popular drugs known as the anti-histamines. This has far reaching implications on how physicians and owners are groomed in their thinking patterns.

Histamine secreting nerve cells (neurons) have their center (cell body's) within the tuberomamillary nucleus of the posterior hypothalamus. From here the neuron cell body sends projections (axons) into all parts of the brain and spinal cord. The axons carry the nerve impulse to the next nerve synapse where histamine is released. This small group of histamine secreting neurons, which connects to all parts of the nervous system, has a broad scope of influence. Some examples of histamine secreting nerve influences are: consciousness, blood pressure, pituitary hormone secretion, thirst and sexual behavior.

Mast cells are one type of immune system cell that tends to concentrate within the pituitary gland. Mast cells contain histamine. This is important because the pituitary gland is commonly known as the master hormone gland. Under the direction of the higher brain structures, the pituitary secretes powerful hormones that control the activity of the gonads, adrenals, thyroid, pancreas, placenta, and thymus. Adequate histamine within the pituitary modifies the release of many of these master hormones (ACTH, FSH, LH, prolactin, TSH and GH). In addition to histamine, dopamine and serotonin in the pituitary, all exert a modifying effect on how the pituitary responds to commands from the higher brain centers. The textbooks imply that it is the interplay between these three neurotransmitters, which influence the response of the master hormone gland to higher brain commands.

The bigger picture of histamines role within the brain includes its role in consciousness level, sexual behavior, regulation of body secretions, regulation of the release of the pituitary hormones, blood pressure regulation, drinking fluids behavior, and in pain thresholds. Histamine is especially important in activating the sleep center within what scientists call the diencepahlic sleep zone.

This doesn't mean that the popular anti-histamines are of low value in some medical conditions. Rather the implication is that the public deserves a better understanding for the consequences of chronically consuming a substance that affects powerful nervous system activities. Anti-histamines become unnecessary when one corrects the cause of the problem. For example, the use of DGL licorice root for gastritis was discussed in section three. Ways to evaluate the adrenal deficiency, which causes allergies, were discussed in the adrenal chapter.

Epinephrine

The neurotransmitter, epinephrine conveys a sense of alertness within one's mind. Epinephrine is the crowning glory of what can only be manufactured when all the previously listed biochemical cofactors are present (the methyl donor system plus vitamin C and tetrahydrobiopterin). Epinephrine's unique message properties have gone largely unrecognized and in its place there is a tendency to lump epinephrine's actions into those of nor-epinephrine and dopamine as well. Add to this the biochemical sloppiness that regards the common practice of trying to explain these three above listed bioactive amines in a complicated and arbitrary system of different types of receptors. Commonly these are referred to as: alpha 1, Beta 1, and Beta 2 receptors. This method of limiting the discussion regarding each of the above three's actions by this arbitrary nomenclature keep many a well-meaning physician confused.

Sometimes it helps to ignore the discussion of these arbitrary methods of 'pigeon holing' these informational substance receptors. In its place one can begin to glean an overall picture for why the body would prefer one of these neurotransmitters to the other. One complication of ignoring the interplay between the different neurotransmitters is the over prescribing of anti-histamines when the real problem is diminished epinephrine production.

Most allergies occur by a peripheral action of histamine acting as a hormone and not as a neurotransmitter. When owners take many of the anti-histamines they are potentially affecting the neurotransmitter availability and the peripheral acting histamine that produce allergies (among other things). This approach always has side effects because of the central role that histamine plays in the brain. In the immune chapter it was discussed how often times it is safer to take epinephrine like medicines for allergy control than the anti-histamines so commonly utilized. The mantra about blood pressure elevation resulting from herbs like ephedra becomes largely the hype of clever little sound bytes of disinformation when the other side of what science has revealed is included (immune and blood pressure chapters). Never the less, when taking powerful medicinal herbs like ephedra it is wise to be followed closely by a physician just in case there is even the slightest chance that one's blood pressure could become elevated. In addition to epinephrine like medication for the short-term control of allergies it is always a good idea to check these owners' adrenal gland function (adrenal chapter).

Perspective is added when one realizes that more people die from the complications of aspirin like medication in one week than have ever died of ephedrine or epinephrine treatments. Another possible role for epinephrine like medication involves the treatment of depressive illness. Epinephrine is safer than nor-epinephrine because it does not raise the blood pressure as avidly. However, before this possibility can be realized, there needs to be adequate studies performed.

Nor-epinephrine and epinephrine

In regards to the neurotransmitter role of epinephrine and nor-epinephrine, these substances can only be manufactured, when the previously mentioned cofactors are available. Briefly these are: tetrahydrobiopterin, vitamin C, vitamin B6 and SAMe. SAMe is consumed at the rate of one billion times a second within the body. It needs folate, vitamin B12 and serine to recharge it each time it donates a methyl to make epinephrine. Because nor-epinephrine and epinephrine are some of the major neurotransmitters, this is an important consideration. When one realizes the extent of the continual need for the above nutritional cofactors it helps one to be open to yet another cause of some cases of clinical depression. Depression is often the result of a nutritional deficiency. These deficiencies affect the ability for these parts of the brain to manufacture these important molecules (nutritionally-caused depression below).

Dopamine

Dopamine is the last, for now, of the bioactive amines needing to be discussed. Dopamine can be generalized as being involved with pleasure and fine motor coordination. When the part of the brain stem concerned with fine motor coordination fails in its production and release of dopamine, Parkinson's disease begins. Cocaine usage is generally felt to result in the increased presence of dopamine within the pleasure centers of the brain. This happens because cocaine poisons the ability to re-uptake dopamine between the pleasure nerves synapses. Therefore more dopamine is in these spaces. The higher the dopamine level within the synapse the more communication is conveyed for the pleasure message.

There is an additional important role of dopamine as a neurotransmitter within the brain that was previously briefly alluded to. This is in regards to dopamines effect on pituitary hormones when its level increases. Like serotonin and histamine, mentioned above, dopamine as well affects the pituitary responsiveness from higher brain centers. Dopamine levels increase within the pituitary gland when the nerve endings within the hypothalamus release it. The hypothalamus is the area of the brain immediately above the pituitary, which controls the pituitary secretions. In turn higher brain centers control the hypothalamus. As dopamine increases, within the pituitary, growth hormone release is encouraged and prolactin release is discouraged. Conversely, as serotonin increases within the pituitary prolactin release is encouraged and growth hormone release is discouraged.

A pivotal point in the understanding of how one keeps younger far longer than his numerous peers now occurs. To better understand why, one needs to recall two things. First, increased prolactin levels directly correlates with decreased gonad function. Decreased gonad function means a lowered steroid tone and pressure will occur. When steroid tone and pressure are lower the wear and tear changes inflicted by life fail to get repaired properly. Failed repair accelerates the aging process. The second point was more completely explained in the liver chapter. However, briefly stated growth hormone has many youth conserving properties. As owners age, growth hormone levels gradually decline to low levels and get really low just before death. Processes that increase growth hormone levels will tend to increase cellular rejuvenation activities described in the liver chapter.

Applying Biochemistry to Longevity

Millions of Americans' depression symptoms are treated with SSRI's. SSRI's raise the level of serotonin within the brain. Increased serotonin within the brain has the potential to raise prolactin and decrease growth hormone. It is instructive now to return to the consequences of an increased prolactin secretion and decreased growth hormone secretion within the pituitary. This situation results when serotonin levels become increased in the brain. The aberrations in growth hormone and prolactin levels can injure certain body tissues. One example of potentially vulnerable body tissue secondary to these types of hormone imbalances is heart valve tissue.

Cardiac heart valves are made from specialized cartilage tissue. As was discussed earlier in the joint chapter, a big part of the continued health of cartilage relies on the quality of the message content it receives. When high quality message content occurs these types of cells are instructed to invest appropriate energy in rejuvenation activities. (Cont.)

(Cont'd) The big players in this regard were said to be adequate androgen and growth hormone. When these two hormone groups reach cartilage tissue cells, rejuvenation activity becomes possible.

A few years ago certain pharmaceutical companies expressed great surprise and remorse when it became obvious that some owners who took the popular diet drug, fenfluramine (commonly known as the fen-phen diet of which fenfluramine was one of the components), developed heart valve damage. A common denominator for how these owners' heart valves were injured emerges if one applies the previous discussion in regards to increased serotonin levels within the pituitary gland. This is because drugs like fenfluramine raise pituitary levels of serotonin. It becomes more alarming when one realizes that some of the popular SSRI antidepressants are all structurally related, to varying degrees at the molecular level, to that of fenfluramine. These types of drugs tend to raise pituitary serotonin levels. It is important to recall that higher serotonin levels, within the pituitary, have been noted to raise prolactin levels and decrease growth hormone levels. It is important to apply the above previous discussion, which regards the role of increased prolactin and decreased growth hormone on tissues like the heart valves. First, the increased pituitary serotonin causes increased prolactin release that inhibits gonad function. The inhibition includes androgen release and production from the gonads. Second, when there is decreased growth hormone and androgen message content reaching cardiac valve tissue, there is a diminished message to instruct these cells to rejuvenate. The heart valve cells need instruction to invest appropriate energy into repair and rejuvenation activities. With low growth hormone and high prolactin in operation some owners' heart valves will succumb to disrepair. This scenario provides a likely mechanism of injury to the heart valves of patient's who take these types of medications.

The PDR does not group fenfluramine as a serotonin re-uptake inhibitor like the other antidepressants, which have a similar molecular structure. However, if one examines their molecular structures and active sites it becomes probable that the PDR division is arbitrary. The PDR and pharmaceutical text discuss the possibility of growth hormone secretion decrease for all of these substances including fenfluramine. In addition, the basic medical physiology text, link increased pituitary serotonin levels to an increase in prolactin secretion and to a decrease in growth hormone secretion. It is important to point out that because fenfluramine has been known to damage heart valves, this drug probably raises pituitary serotonin levels more than the others do.

Very few doctors or patients are made aware of these potential dangers. Some of the confusion occurs because of the likely arbitrary divisions in classification between fenfluramine and the other SSRI's. The risk is really unnecessary if the public still had affordable access to tryptophan. (Cont.)

(Cont'd)   Alternatively, owners who need these medications should be followed for elevated prolactin and decreased growth hormone levels. These same owners should also have their heart valve function checked until the actual risks are quantitated. When either of these test results become abnormal then supplementation could be considered to correct the deficiencies of either androgen or growth hormone.

A comment on a safer way to treat depression with medication

Some anti-depression medications work by raising brain dopamine levels. Increasing dopamine levels within the brain will decrease prolactin and raise growth hormone levels. The downside to this medication is a slight risk for seizure while taking this drug. There is the additional need to monitor thyroid status while on this medication.

The benefit of this approach from raising growth hormone levels and suppressing prolactin levels concerns the youth conserving properties of these two types of hormones. Specifically these hormones increase the tendency for appropriate message content delivery to the body's cells to invest in rejuvenation activities. The scientific name for this medication is burprion (Wellbutrin).   Stopping short of abusing cocaine, with all its predictable sad consequences, this is one of the most reliable methods for raising brain dopamine content. Dopamine is the neurotransmitter responsible for pleasure.

If one chooses the Wellbutrin route of treatment, they need to have their thyroid monitored. Thyroid monitoring becomes necessary because whenever dopamine levels rise within the pituitary thyroid function may be depressed. When this medication causes a depressed thyroid function, the conventional test for TSH will be unreliable as a measure of thyroid function. The axillary body temperature is a supportive step but an twenty-four hour urine, for thyroid function, will be helpful. The important point here is that Wellbutrin has potential advantages, in the treatment of depression, when its side effect profile is understood. Monitoring patients for possible thyroid dysfunction will avoid missing thyroid dysfunction caused by this medication. Thyroid dysfunction is more easily treated than when the gonads and growth hormone status become compromised. Until dietary tryptophan again becomes available, the Wellbutrin method of treating depression is less risky to one's health than the SSRI's. In addition, there is a group of owners who will dramatically respond with nutritional supplementation of the necessary vitamins that manufacture the needed neurotransmitters discussed above.

2. The brain's molecular building parts replacement program

Brain molecular building parts include unique components. Some of the need for unique brain molecular components arises because the brain is composed of more fat than nerve in its makeup. In turn, the fats, which make up one's brain, are constructed with unique components.[28] Unique components are needed within the brain because fat serves as insulation to prevent electrical cross firing between the different nerve cells. Adequate molecular supplies are also necessary to rebuild the brain structures that wear out. In addition, there is the continuous need to replace the nerve cell enzymatic machines that begin to breakdown. The high metabolic rate of the brain increases the rate at which molecular parts become defective. Because the brain burns about 25% of the oxygen within the body at normal basal conditions, it is more vulnerable to 'rusting' (oxidation damage) than many other body tissues. As stated above, the brain is composed of more fat than nerve by weight. This fact increases the rust vulnerability many times. The increase in vulnerability results from the rusting processes creating rancid fats within the brain.

It is accurate to describe the brain as a fatty bag of hormones and neurotransmitters. In health, the fatty bag releases in a rhythmical manner the appropriate amount of informational substances between the various nerves (the neurotransmitters). Concurrently, there is a rhythmical release, from the brain, of other informational substances into the blood stream (the hormones). The rhythm of the brain's release of information breaks down when there is a failure to provide ongoing replacement parts as they wear out. This subsection concerns what the brain needs to regenerate. Since fat is the number one component which makes up one's brain its procurement is emphasized next.

Fat is the Major Building Block that Makes Up the Brain

The brain is really just a bag of fat. Brain fat has well connected nerve cells within it. Within the fat are some specialized areas that secrete powerful informational substances into the blood stream. Therefore the quality of this fat is pivotal to intelligence.

Some owners make the procurement of molecular replacement parts for their fat bag a difficult process. No one is counseling these owners about how all the brain fat is kept in the right place. In addition, they usually have no clue about how to take out the fat trash that begins to stink. Anyone knows that when fat is bad it begins to smell rancid. Fat within the brain serves as support and cushion for the delicate connections. In addition, fat keeps the electrical activity confined by its effective insulating abilities. Because the fat in the brain has so much to accomplish, it makes sense that these fats are special. Because brain fats are special they have unique needs in order to keep them from rotting.

Myelinated nerves are examples of how the integrity of fat in the brain relys on the continued replacement of myelin fats that have rotted. Scientific writings frequently mention myelinated nerves and their importance for optimal brain and nerve functioning. In fact, the disease of multiple sclerosis, results from injury and breakdown of the myelin coating around these nerves. Myelin serves as an example of one of the specialized fats occurring within the nervous system. There are some important nutritional factors that need to occur in order for myelin fat to remain healthy. There are additional informational substances that need to be around in adequate amounts in order for optimal myelin synthesis to be maintained. Progesterone is central, for example, in the directing of adequate myelin sheath formation.

Another example of the unique needs of the brain for its ongoing molecular replacement program is the neurotransmitter, acetylcholine. The choline half is a specialized fat component needed in large quantities within the mind for neurotransmitter formation and specialized fat formation, including myelin sheath formation. The need for choline is underscored by its role in the synthesis of the neurotransmitter acetylcholine. This use of choline is in addition to the important, already mentioned, synthesis of the myelin sheath.

Now that the discussion is centering on the fat, which builds one's brain, it is important to include the neurotransmitter, acetylcholine. The choline half in addition provides a component of the specialized fat for the structural and insulating properties within the brain. Ample supplies of choline are also necessary for acetylcholine biosynthesis. Acetylcholine is the major neurotransmitter of the brain and nerves of the body. Ample supplies of choline are easily obtained with a high fat diet.

Conversely, owners on a low fat diet make their nervous systems acquirement of choline difficult and draining to other body systems. In order to make one choline molecule from scratch, three SAMe molecules are used up, plus all the recharging cofactors. This is in contrast to owners who regularly ingest quality sources of choline. Eggs and fish are really good sources. In addition, another important molecular building block for structural brain fats is called phophatidylcholine. Laypersons commonly call phosphatidylcholine, lethicin. The important point here is that all the brain and nerves in the body need a continuous and adequate supply of this essential building block or neurological efficiency becomes compromised.

The nervous system continually needs new sources of choline for its building block role. The nervous system uses choline for many construction processes. Because these processes are so numerous in the brain, not including them in one's diet could eventually deplete the methyl donor system (SAMe, vitamin B12, folate, serine, and methionine). The methyl donor system is depleted at the rate of one billion times a second. When was the last time a western trained physician counseled a middle aged patient, who was concerned about brain function, about this basic scientific fact? Again it is not a mean spirited conspiracy but rather a result of yet another evisceration from the mainstream medical education in regards to the importance of basic preventative and nutritional advice.

How one makes more intelligent choices on how to get their brains supplied with the highest quality fats is the topic of this subsection. In general terms, regular consumption of olive oil is a start. The essential fatty acids found in wild fish and green algae supplemented chicken eggs are important. In addition the lethicin found in eggs is important. Finally, the vitamins that make up the methyl donor system are fundamental, as well, in order to preserve or regain mental function.

The point is that brain structure maintenance has particular and unique molecular building part needs.[29] Owners who make it easier on their brains to acquire these basic essentials have an advantage for brain longevity. This information is contained within basic medical textbooks in a scattered and confusing way. The time has come for a re-inclusion of these basic scientific facts, in a way that physicians and patients can understand. The uniqueness of the fuel delivery requirements for brain function further explains how the brain is vulnerable when molecular parts replacement becomes compromised.

3. Fuel delivery to brain cells is crucial

Many owners are walking around on this planet that are mentally not as clear as they once were. Complaints of brain 'fog' early on in these patients typify the presentation. Later they go on to develop hypoglycemic events. In the extreme cases fainting and seizure disorders can result. Many of these patients have in common fuel delivery problems within their brain. Brain cells are more vulnerable to fuel delivery interruptions than other body cells. There are two central reasons for the brains increased vulnerability to fuel interruption. First the brain can only burn sugar for fuel. Therefore the brain becomes vulnerable to injury when the blood sugar falls. Second, the brain has a high rate of fuel usage (high metabolic rate). If fuel supplies are interrupted brain cells function are quickly impaired.

The brain is different than most other body tissues in that its ability to uptake sugar is independent of insulin and IGF. Thus unlike most other body cells the brain can take up sugar without either IGF or insulin's message content.

Many owners suffer from various vague forms of mental dysfunction. Sometimes these conditions occur only because their physician fails to consider issues of fuel delivery to the brain. Fuel delivery problems to the brain largely result from imbalanced hormones.

The problem for most owners that suffer from low blood sugar is a failure in their body's ability to mount an effective counter hormone response to insulin. The counter response hormones become necessary to counter insulins desire to direct the liver to suck every last sugar molecule out of their blood stream. Hormones operate on a system of balance. Balanced blood sugars only occur when the proper balance between insulin and the four counter response hormones exist. The counter balance hormones to insulin are glucagon, growth hormone, epinephrine and cortisol. By far the most important counter regulatory hormone to insulin is cortisol (liver and digestion chapters).

Healing these owners usually requires restoring hormonal balance. When was the last time a western trained physician was seen counseling about hormonal balance being central to healing these symptoms? Again this is not meant as a criticism of the many fine physicians desiring to help their patients but rather as an observation of yet another evisceration of what the holism of science has revealed. Instead, in the place of healing, western physicians are trained to prescribe frequent feedings of carbohydrates, which predictably results in a fatter patient.

A return to hormone balance allows healing brain fuel delivery problems. This approach is contrasted with constantly loading the 'antique weight scale' with insulin and then constantly re-supplying the body with more sugar before insulin sucks the blood sugar down again. Healing the brain fuel delivery problem requires a more effective counter weight. Owners whose bodys for one reason or another become enfeebled in their ability to secrete the ever increasing 'counter weight' of cortisol to the 'weight' of increasing insulin required by high carbohydrate diets, get low blood sugars.

Physicians who recognize the fundamental body theme of hormonal balance in the healthful state can counsel their patients to restrict carbohydrates. A restriction of carbohydrates lowers the need for insulin. Lowered insulin leads to a lessened need for the counter hormones, like cortisol. Exercise also has a profound stabilizing effect on one's blood sugars (muscle chapter).

Lifestyle changes make mechanistic sense if one is cognizant of balance. In other words if there is less counter weight (diminished adrenal function) one needs to decrease the need for making the weight (insulin) getting secreted into the blood stream. Attention to this basic understanding allows the 'antique weight scale of hormonal balance' to return to optimum. When this occurs then the symptoms of 'brain fog' anxiety, secondary to roller coasting blood sugars, seizure disorders from low blood sugar, and weight gain from the commonly prescribed hypoglycemic diet begin to resolve.

4. The blood vessels in the brain

The next physical determinant of brain health is the blood vessels. Much of what was discussed in the blood vessel chapter is applicable to the cranial blood vessels. However, that discussion requires additional material that emphasizes the particular vulnerabilities of the brain's vessels.

The first vulnerability of the brain vessels results from the volume of blood flowing within the brain. The brain contains 25% of total volume of blood in the basal state. The brain blood vessel lining cells have a higher rate of exposure to rust producers (oxidizing agents) than in other parts of the body. Owners who have elevated levels of oxidizing agents (rust producers) and/or low levels of anti-oxidants are vulnerable to cranial blood vessel injury.

The second vulnerability of the brain's blood vessels is due to these vessels coursing through a closed box (the skull). Blood that leaks from a brain vessel has nowhere to go without squishing delicate nerves and ripping them from their precise connections. Processes that weaken the blood vessels do more damage to the brain than similar insults elsewhere in the body.[30]

Last, nerve cells are the most vulnerable of all cell types to an interruption in oxygen and nutrient supply. One minute after an interruption in blood flow occurs, because of their high metabolic rate, neurons start to die. Even the high energy consuming heart cell can be oxygen and nutrient starved for up to 4 hours before it dies (myocardial infarction). This fact is partially explained by the high-energy requirements that neurons demand in powering up their force fields (cell charge) to propagate their action potentials and keep out injurious ions like calcium. The brain creates a higher electrical charge than other parts of the body. The high electrical charge of the brain is used to power the nerve transmissions between one another (the action potential). The neurons become vulnerable when the energy for current generation becomes compromised.

4. The hormones giveth and the hormones taketh away the brain

The right types of informational substances (hormones) direct the process for how one preserves their nerve cells physical integrity. Only when the proper mixtures of informational substances courses through the brain blood vessels will the nerve cells be directed to rejuvenate and repair themselves. Adequate repair and rejuvenation activities mean the nerve cells receive the proper directions to spend their cell energy wisely. Some of these hormone mixtures direct appropriate absorption of minerals, vitamins, molecular building parts and fuel. Still other brain hormones promote adequate cellular infrastructure investment and rejuvenation activities. Cellular infrastructure investment activities include: new cell machines (enzymes); new cell factories (organelles); toxin and waste removal, etc. Nerve cell rejuvenation activities regard repair activities. Examples of repair activities are: new outside the nerve cell support framework where it is damaged, rotten fats replacement, DNA repair and stabilization, etc.

The steroids like hormones are the only hormones within the body that can go within any body chamber. Once these most powerful hormones penetrate one's brain they then instruct the nerve cell DNA programs. Which DNA programs are activated or repressed centrally determines how that nerve cell spends its energy. All other hormone types (levels 2 through 4) are limited to where they can penetrate. Many other hormones cannot penetrate the blood brain barrier. However, all the steroids, thyroid, and vitamin A can penetrate into the central nervous system. Once inside the quality of their type and amount determines the appropriateness of the many different nerve cells DNA programs. The DNA program contains the genes. Which genes are turned off or on at any given time is a central determinate of how a cell spends its available energy. Lousy steroid amounts or types in the brain result in poor genetic program activation.

Processes that increase the steroid pressure and tone will give owners a longevity advantage. Processes that decrease the steroid pressure and tone within the brain will allow deterioration to occur more quickly.

Owners who have optimally functioning gonads and adrenals will have the ability to direct the wise use of nerve cell energy within one's brain. Optimally functioning gonads and adrenals can do this because they are capable of creating an optimal steroid pressure and tone. In addition, the brain can make some of its own steroids. This means that even when the gonads and adrenals begin to fail in some owners their brain has a back up system of it's own for the manufacture of steroids. The brain therefore has a degree of protection not afforded to other systems when the adrenals and gonads fail. However, all three areas of steroid production (adrenals, gonads, and brain) become potentially compromised when the body perceives stress. Stress redirects the nervous system energy into survival activities and away from repair and rejuvenation activities within one's brain.[31]

Modern life's complexities are stressful: time deadlines, financial worries, job security worries, relationship worries, keeping up with the Jones etc. Stress damages certain brain tissues involved in learning and memory. Stressful living increases the lifetime exposure of these brain tissues to cortisol (one of the main stress hormones). Cortisol is a major player as an informational substance involved in redirecting cell energy into survival pathways and away from cellular maintenance activities. The cells can't discern if the stress is real or imagined.

When stress is either real or imagined cortisol levels will increase. Cortisol is one of the important informational substances that make up message content delivered to cells during stress. Excessive exposure of these brain structures to cortisol has been implicated as a major mechanism of cell death in the brain. The cortisol message channels energy into survival pathways. When energy is directed into survival pathways there is a postponement in rejuvenation activities. If stressful events occur occasionally or are otherwise mitigated by adequate periods of behavioral and environmental restorative activities, then some delayed effects are noted in the degenerative process (section 2). If stress becomes chronic, the daily cortisol message continuously defers the rejuvenation, which keeps the brain in peak performance.[32]

Chronic high cortisol production rates direct, nerve cell energy away from rejuvenation activities and towards survival pathways. The lack of rejuvenation activities leads to an increase in brain wear and tear changes. This results from the chronic message of survival being delivered to one's nerve cells. During the stress response the learning and memory centers in the brain are not a teleological part of the emergency cell team. The emergency cell team is the cells in the body, which preferentially obtain ample energy during the survival response. Examples of these areas within the brain are the cerebellum and vision centers. Some examples of other cells, which are part of the emergency cell team, are muscle, heart, and lungs. The emergency response team cells get channeled metabolic energy to mount the bodies perceived survival challenge. However, they are asked by cortisol message content to put on hold critical cellular maintenance activities. The difference is that the emergency response cells receive ample fuel delivered during the perceived emergency. Thus cortisol causes deferred maintenance throughout the body and the shunting of fuel away from the memory and learning centers further contribute to brain aging.[33]

The effects of chronic stress on the brain are exacerbated when the stressors are of an unpredictable nature in timing and intensity. The additional promoters of chronic stress changes are a feeling of hopelessness, and the personality of the owner is emotionally reactive. Finally, the brain will age more quickly when there is less than optimal social support, as well. In the end all three of the above exacerbations of the stress response accelerate the brain-aging rate by increasing cortisol levels.

The destructive effects to one's brain from the chronic elevation of cortisol can be somewhat mitigated when there is a counter balance from the androgens. Balance between the catabolic effects (body wasting effects) of cortisol (and the other stress hormones) with regular secretions of the counterbalancing anabolic hormones (the rejuvenating and strength giving hormones) has restorative potential. The anabolic class of hormones (the androgen steroids) plays a central and powerful role in the brain restorative process. Its important to remember that cortisol is a steroid hormone but is catabolic (uses up body structures for fuel generation) in its effects. In addition, it is important to remember that all steroids have the powerful ability to instruct one's cells DNA program on which genes to turn off and which genes to turn on. Therefore, the quality, timing and amount of each steroid type interacting with a given brain cell is a central determinant of how wisely that cell is spending its energy.

All steroids are synthesized from cholesterol stores in the adrenal, gonads, and to limited extent the brain. However, each steroid has unique message content in how it directs body energy usage. Some of the steroids increase buildup activities within a given cell type and these are called anabolic. Some of them encourage burning different body structures for fuel to maximize survival during emergencies and these are called catabolic. Finally there are the steroids concerned with maintaining the minerals within the body at an optimum level for structure and maintaining the cellular force field (aldosterone and vitamin D). The brain, like other tissues, needs balance between all three types of steroid message content.

In the brain, the anabolic steroids are DHEA, progesterone, androstenedione, testosterone, and dihydrotestosterone. Different body tissues respond preferentially to the different anabolic steroids. Blood vessel health seems particularly responsive to DHEA and possibly progesterone. Brain myelin producing schwaan cells need a steady message from progesterone to optimize their nerve cell protective effects. GABA producing neurons in the spinal cord need adequate progesterone or anxiety and irritability occurs. DHEA is concentrated within the brain at five to six times the blood level when the brain is healthy. Each body tissue has a specific anabolic steroid, which it is particularly responsive to. The take home point is that the androgen class of steroids is necessary in their optimal amounts if return or maintenance to the healthful state is desired.

The anabolic steroids direct nerve cell energy into cellular infrastructure investment activities. Examples of this can be summarized in a broad way: toxin removal (taking out the cellular garbage), enzyme replacement (new cellular machines), rejuvenation of the cell membrane, and the manufacture of new organelles (cellular factories unique to each cell type). For longevity considerations the trick is to have enough anabolic tone influence (optimal amounts of DHEA, testosterone, progesterone, etc.) to counterbalance the possible deleterious effects of chronic stress elicited cortisol release. As mentioned earlier certain brain structures with their increased metabolic rate, are particularly vulnerable to increased cortisol message without adequate counterbalancing of the anabolic steroids.

Achieving adequate anabolic steroid levels within one's brain becomes possible only if several things are occurring regularly within the owner's body. First, there needs to be adequate functional capabilities in the gonads and/or adrenal glands. One or both of these paired glands needs to be sufficiently capable of producing the factory order of increased anabolic steroid production. If the bank vault is empty (ill or near dead adrenals and/or gonads) a response to stimulants towards increasing anabolic steroid production is not possible. Unfortunately, there are many owners who through toxic, surgical procedure, lifestyle, or poor genetic constitution of these glands have some degree of gonad or adrenal failure, which needs to be addressed before improved anabolic steroid output becomes possible. Second, there needs to be an adequate regular stimulus, to produce optimal anabolic steroids. Healthy sports competitions, regular aerobic exercise, warm nutritive relationships that are emotionally supportive, as well as positive emotions (happiness, joy, forgiveness, singing, and love) all directly stimulate more optimal anabolic steroid amounts. Of course amorous romantic sexual attractions can get the bank withdrawals going in the capable gonad.

Finally, it should be stressed that the steroid hormones are all derived from cholesterol or more rarely from plant derived sources containing high progesterone content (natural progesterone can serve as a precursor for most other steroid biosynthesis). Progesterone can easily, once inside the adrenal or gonad tissues, be converted to many of the other types of steroids including estrogen if the body's intelligence sees fit. This turns out to be a practical consideration because as bodies age there is a decreased ability to manufacture steroids from the cholesterol precursor route. The failing rate-limiting step seems to be in the freeing up of cholesterol within the cell so it can be delivered to the mitochondria (the site of the first chemical reactions in the synthesis of the steroid hormones). Deficiencies of panothenic acid and vitamin A seem to greatly diminish the ability of these tissues to manufacture steroids. In the immune and adrenal chapters reasons why these nutrients are so important was explained. Beyond the repair and maintenance of the neurons are the always-lurking destructive forces, which gain access to one's brain. One example of such destructive processes are those molecular substances, which tend to promote rust within one's brain. Thankfully the properly nourished owner has adequate molecules to counter the rust promoters.

The rust promoters versus the rust retardants

The next determinant of brain function regards the level of rust promoters versus rust retardants. Rust promoters are called oxidants. Rust retardants are called anti-oxidants. Alternatively there is the duplicity of saying the same thing by discussing a given elements electro-negativity. Electro-negativity denotes in chemical jargon the ability of a specific element to grab electrons (oxidize or rust) other elements or molecules. This is very important not to lose sight of these interchangeable terms if one is to avoid becoming the victim of what is not being said.

The top four rust producing atomic elements on the planet (out of more than one hundred) are fluorine, oxygen, chorine and sulfur. The ability of an element to produce rust regards their power of electro-negativity. The higher the electro-negativity of a certain element determines the ability of that element to rust or oxidize other molecules. This electro negativity scale gradates the rust promoting abilities relative to an interaction with all the other elements and molecular combinations possible within the world. The most powerful electron hog (rust promoter) on the planet is fluorine followed by oxygen then chlorine and finally sulfur.

When any of these oxidizing elements are present within the brain they had better be happy (stable) or the cellular consequence of rust formation results. Because human bodies are greater than 60% water, there is some protection. Protection occurs when elements like chlorine are bathed in sufficient water and then become largely free of a tendency to bind to body structures. Sufficient water creates a way for chlorine to associate loosely (dissolve) with oppositely charged elements within body fluids (sodium, potassium, and calcium).

However, this quality is largely absent for oxygen and fluorine in the ionic form. Much attention regarding less potent oxidizing agents is given within the media. It helps to be less gullible when one stays mindful of the big four electron hogs on the planet. These are the radicals of: fluorine, oxygen, chlorine, and sulfur. Most of the time the oxygen and fluorine ion are the main rust promoters to be concerned with in one's mind. A prime example of the reactivity of fluoride occurs with its propensity to react with tooth and bone tissue. Sure it makes these tissues harder but what is often left out is that fluorine makes these same tissues more brittle, as well. Brittleness is one measure of oxidation within body tissue. Here lies the concern of elements like fluorine and oxygen in the unpaired state within one's mind.

Oxidizing agents can damage one's mind by two different mechanisms. First, and more common with oxygen but less common with fluorine, is the unstable radical. The oxygen radical denotes the state of unpaired oxygen before it steals an electron(s) from a weaker atom. This occurs with oxygen because of the process described in chapter 1. Briefly, chapter one describes oxygen cleavage explosions within the mitochondria of numerous cells. Because tremendous amounts of oxygen get cleaved each day in an owner's life there will be a small amount of oxygen radicals generated. Oxygen radicals occur whenever the split of the two atoms, O2, get outside of the 'armor' of the mitochondria chemical reaction chamber. Owners who lack sufficient ability to deal with oxygen radical leakage get diseases resulting from oxygen radicals injuring cells. One proto-typical disease associated with this defect, in the unpaired oxygen mop up team, is Lou Garrig's disease (amyotrophic lateral sclerosis). Amyotrophic lateral sclerosis kills the motor nerves within the spinal cord because there is either an increased production rate or decreased ability to neutralize oxygen radical formation.

The second way that oxidizing agents (rust promoters) injure nerve cells occurs after the radical has hogged an electron. For example, the second mechanism occurs after the electron hog like oxygen and fluorine have already stolen an electron from somewhere else. Scientists denote this state by acknowledging a negative charge to these elements. Oxygen in this state is called oxide. Fluorine in this state is called fluoride. Even after their radical form has hogged an additional electron, they then still tend to bind to a positively charged body structures. When these hogs bind in this manner they alter the molecules properties and shape. The fluoride and oxygen ion can do this. One needs oxygen for life and therefore curtailment here is only possible by limiting intake of the salts of oxygen (blood vessel chapter) and in attempting to breath air that has less oxidizing properties (commonly called clean air). Fluorine is the same as fluoride except this designates that it already has hogged an electron of its own. Already mentioned was the popular example of fluoride binding the tooth enamel and bone readily. What is not being said is that it becomes harder but often these tissues become more brittle as well. Brittleness is another example of the rusting process (aging process). Fluoride and oxide within one's brain are a concern.

The example of fenfluramine needs to be recalled because it contains fluoride. The fluoride contained within fenfluramine has the potential to release fluoride within one's brain. The brain's number one protection from outside toxicities is a highly functioning blood brain barrier. Pharmaceutical agents that are capable of penetrating beyond this barrier can cause great harm if they contain injurious atoms. The fluoride content of fenfluramine provides such an example.

A journal of the American Medical Association article disclosed direct evidence that fenfluramine (one of the components of the popular fen-phen diet) damages neurons cultured in Petri dishes. About the same time of that discovery it was discovered that fenfluramine was injuring heart valves (earlier discussion). There are three fluorine atoms on each fenfluramine molecule. There are other widely used prescription drugs, which deliver fluoride to the brain. Prozac has the same amount of fluorine as fenfluramine. The other popular and related antidepressant, Paxil, has a single fluorine per molecule. In addition, if one inquires into the chemical structure of these mentioned SSRI's, commonly prescribed to treat depression, they all possess an aromatic ring. Fenfluramine has this same aromatic ring structure where the fluorides are attached in the same position as Prozac. These facts point to the possibility that the popular SSRI's are more related to the recalled, fenfluramine than the medical literature reveals. Awareness of this possibility makes it worthwhile to consider more completely how one heals nutritionally from depression.

The Politics of Scientific Information

The take home point here is not to vilify the profit driven scientific community that is operational in America today. However, the point is to alert the reader to yet another consequence of the fact that the science that gets popularized is only a small fraction of what science has revealed. Gullibility in this regard has health consequences and the above is only minimal examples of many. This will begin to change for the better as more people begin to realize that they have been the recipients of clever advertising campaigns. The PDR (physicians' desk reference) is actually less complete than it should be in regards to what science has revealed. It is worded so as to accentuate the upside of what is for sale and simultaneously minimizes the risks involved. Anyone who doubts this trend can read for himself or herself about any new drug that still has a patent advantage. (Cont.)

(Cont'd) The reason that it is important to read the patentable drugs that regard this trend is that one method for increasing new drug sales is to slam on the patent expired varieties.

In addition these advertising campaigns have been designed to steer thinking in a beneficial way. The benefits are larger profits for their most lucrative products. When one understands the down side then there will begin to be a demand, at the consumer level, for a more complete discussion regarding the options for a given ailment.

One further point about the PDR regards the realization that it has largely become an effective marketing strategy towards patients and physicians. These descriptions of the different drugs are sometimes without a picture of the chemical structures. The lack of a chemical structure becomes very disabling, when one wants to understand the basics on the safety within.

One needs to stay mindful about the way drugs are classified. Drug classification can lead physicians' thinking into erroneous avenues of understanding. The fenfluramine example being grouped outside the serotonin reuptake inhibitors (selective serotonin reuptake inhibitors) when they share many suspicious overlapping structural and activity related characteristics illustrate this point.

There is always the long held suspicion about under reported side effect profiles. This suspicion becomes more justified when one is cognizant of the often-harried physicians' workday. How much time do most doctors really have to read the fine print of these subtle PDR pieces of work? However, when the under reporting is outlandish, physicians eventually get suspicious and then warnings are printed. More common is the chronic under representation of the potential to harm a given group of owners who take different medications. If owners were again taught some of the basics about what the body processes are about, devoid of the complex abstractions, they would better be able to alert their physicians at the first signs of trouble.

Mercury as a rust promoter needs to be discussed while on the subject of scientific incompleteness and inconsistency. It is a long known fact that mercury is a nerve toxin. Less well appreciated, even within the medical community, is the duplicity of ways that pharmaceutical companies include mercury within vaccines by identifying mercury as a side name that few physicians and patients can recognize. This nasty little fact has finally come to light thanks to many doggedly stubborn owners who kept up the campaign against the mercury contained within these vaccines even while hidden under the ingredient name, thimerosal. This revelation has forced the manufactures of many childhood vaccines to agree to reduce the mercury content within these injections to 5% of the previous amount. They now say that much less mercury is needed in vaccines to stabilize the ingredients. This means that for years countless children have been injected with a known neurotoxin that was unnecessary. (Cont.)

(Cont'd) The common flu vaccine is another injection that contains mercury. In addition some types of testosterone injections contain mercury as well.

Arguably it would be advantageous for physicians to get their primary scientific information from unbiased sources of scientific inquiry. This probably will only become possible when enough patients stand behind their doctors and begin to demand a little house cleaning from the grips of the FDA and rampant corrupt funding of university research by silent pharmaceutical interests. Socialized medicine has many of the same problems inherent in the current system because of the lobbying protectionism of any 'complex' interest before passage would be possible. In other words the new socialized system would tax the citizens to ensure continued 'complex' profits.

Healing paths are probably most likely to originate outside of the current system. Movements like 'keep it simple' are such beginnings. Here doctors agree to charge less but accept no insurance or government programs of any kind for outpatient care. Patients pay in cash but at reduced charges because their doctor no longer has to generate huge sums of money to pay for all the paper work and time spent arguing with insurance programs. In systems like this the doctor patient relationship is again a private exchange and has a focus regarding the number one priority of getting the patient on a healing path.

Contrast this to the frenzied demands on a general practitioner's time today. Very little of his time gets to be focused on who the patient is, where he/she comes from, what hopes and fears they have and where they are going (someplace good versus someplace bad). In the end, when change comes to the way health care is practiced, it will come from the patient's demands. Politicians are scared to death of angry voters. This is why, despite the complex's best effort otherwise, there has been a gradual acceptance of alternative modalities. Patients have legitimized Chiropractic care, Acupuncture, Naturopathy, and massage therapy to their insurance companies. All the while, the various complex entities have been trying every dirty trick to attempt to marginalize the alternative therapies (appendices).

John Lee, M.D., summarizes the situation very well in the introduction of his book, *Some Things Your Doctor May Not Tell You About The Menopause*. He commented on how over the last several years there had been repeated attempts to marginalize the importance of his progesterone findings. However he communicated that the complex underestimated the power of the international women's network that regards what works. In the end, accurate scientific information will become available, only when consumers vote out those politicians that continue to receive 'honorariums' from the complex.

5. Taking out the brain trash

The unique power supply to the brain presents unique challenges to keep the brain free of toxins. The main vulnerability within the brain lies in the obligatory requirement of nerves to only burn sugar as their fuel source. Sugar is consumed within the nervous system at a high rate in oxygen's presence. Unlike most other organs, the brain can only burn sugar in its power plants. Failure of the power plant energy supply when blood sugar supplies fall, has toxic consequences to brain tissue. In addition, injury to delicate nerve cell content occurs, from the oxygen radical. Oxygen radicals create brain trash whenever there is an inadequate backup system. One back up system is the oxygen mop up enzyme machines. Oxygen enzyme mop up machines clean up the occasional unpaired oxygen radicals that get outside the 'armored' mitochondria. The nerve cell prevents the creation of oxidized cell components in two ways.

First, there needs to be an effective set of enzyme machines hanging around to process the oxygen radical (reactive oxygen species) situation when it occurs. The enzymes in the nerves, which neutralize reactive oxygen species, are called super oxide dismutase and catalase. Oxygen radical formation occurs because of the shear volume of oxygen being processed for life giving combustion reactions in nerve cell mitochondria. As stated previously, when this set of enzymatic machines are deficient, diseases like Lou Garrig's result. These types of diseases kill nerve cells when oxygen radicals are allowed to get outside of the protection of the mitochondria. When reactive oxygen species are outside of the mitochondria they damage the first structure that they contact. The damage from rust production processes eventually exceeds the best repair processes of the nerve cells.

A similar process occurs in the retinas of premature infants that require high oxygen content to remain alive. The high oxygen content that saves them, also in many cases, overwhelms the oxygen detoxifying systems and visual impairment results due to death of the nerves behind the retina. Scientists call this retrolentil fibroplasia.

The second form of brain defense with regard to oxidizing agents is more generalized. These anti-oxidants are able to neutralize many different 'rust' promoters within the brain. Glutathione, vitamin C, vitamin E, Garlic, and onions are all common examples of substances that perform this important task. They each work by stabilizing many different rust promoters when they react with them. Some of these anti-oxidants are rechargeable and others are only able to work one time. Nutritional deficiencies of these important protective molecules cause nerves to rust more rapidly. The brain becomes one of the most potentially toxic areas in the body because it has 25% of the body's blood at rest. This is especially true with regards to the blood vessel lining cells exposure to oxidation insults as the blood coursing through the brain.

There is an additional consideration in regards to 'rust' promoters. This consideration concerns what the nerve cell options are once a cell molecular component has been damaged. When nerve cell molecular components become injured a repair process needs to occur. Fat is the largest molecular component within the brain and hence is the most likely to get damaged. Therefore there needs to be an adequate cellular direction to invest in fat rebuilding activities. In addition to appropriate informational substances, which direct the repair of damaged intracellular contents, there needs to be a highly functioning land fill site (lipofucin deposits) or incinerator (peroxisomes). The incinerator burns the damaged fats. The lipofucin deposits within the nerve cells, as storage sites for damaged fat molecules. Lastly, concerns the requirement that there are adequate molecular replacement parts available to remanufacture the damaged structures. In the case of damaged fat replacement, the owner needs to have appropriate dietary fat supplies or have a highly functioning methyl donor system to make these specialized nerve fats from scratch.

Lastly, before leaving the toxin discussion, the owner is asked to remain mindful of ingested substances that have the ability to cross the blood brain barrier and move on into one's brain. Once they are inside they breakdown into elements like fluorine (fluoride usually in the body). Too many elements like fluorine place a particular strain on keeping adequate anti-oxidants around. Less anti-oxidants increase the rate of repair or replacement of brain molecular parts.

6. The cellular force field of the nerve cell

The concept of the cellular force field was discussed in section five. Because nerve cells require this property to function more reliably than in any other cell, a brief summary is in order. Recollect the analogy of the car battery. Car batteries operate on a similar principle, as do nerve cells. When the difference between certain mineral concentrations is maximized, these types of batteries charge up. The differences of electrolyte concentration are maximized about a membrane (or between the two posts in the case of the car battery). The greater the difference between the two minerals (across a membrane) then the battery will have more energy to perform electrical work. The nerve cell is similar in that the membrane lining the cell maintains a concentration gradient between different minerals, which allows it to perform the work of living things.

There are powerful hormones that are needed in adequate amounts, which direct the cell's DNA. Proper DNA direction allows the nerve cell to make the enzyme machines, direct repair to cell structures and direct the manufacture of force field generators (membrane mineral pumps) within the membrane. The force field generators (Na/K ATPase) are necessary for an effectively performing force field. The strength of a nerve cell's force field is directly related to the amount of force field generators, the minerals respective availabilities and the energy supply delegated to them.[34]

One example of the importance of the nerve cell force field occurs with its ability to prevent the inapropriate calcium ion penetration. The nerve cell membrane can only prevent the inappropriate penetration of calcium ion when it possesses sufficient strength of charge. Sufficient charge becomes possible only when adequate sugar makes its way into the nerve power plants. The power plants need sugar fuel and adequate oxygen to combust and eventually trap some of this energy. The energy trapped is then used to charge up the membrane by pumping certain ions against their concentration gradient. Any thing, which disrupts this process, allows the energy contained in the nerve membrane to run down. When the energy in the nerve membrane runs down harmful ions can gain entrance inside the nerve cell inappropriately.

Inappropriate calcium entry into nerve cells should not be confused with appropriately channeled entrance of calcium in order to perform cellular work. The difference with the later is when calcium enters appropriately it is tightly regulated and quickly pumped outside again. This movement of the calcium mineral about a membrane is similar to how a battery discharges and recharges. In contrast, inappropriate calcium entry into nerve cells is similar to when the battery post becomes oxidized. Battery oxidation results when the metals inappropriately leak outside the battery and react with the post. Visualize the gunk that accumulates on these aging battery posts. So it is with the inside of owner's nerve cells that for one reason or another are unable to keep calcium channeled within the appropriate pathways. When calcium penetrates outside of carefully gated channels then cellular gunk begins to occur. The cellular gunk occurs when calcium reacts with delicate inside the cell structures. The calcium reaction damages these nerve cell structures.

This is the main mechanism for nerve cell death when either oxygen or sugar delivery get compromised. In each of these cases the energy content of the nerve membrane falls (section five) and calcium rushes inside the nerve cell. Nerve cell death begins to occur in as little as one minute (usually four minutes and in cold water drowning it can be a lot longer). In other words, calcium is always lurking outside the cell wanting to get inside. The electrical charge keeps calcium out as long as the cellular force field is strong. When nerve cell energetics become compromised, as in decreased oxygen and/or decreased blood sugar, the force fields strength falls off dramatically. The energy contained within the nerve cell membrane is rapidly depleted when there is an interruption of its ability to recharge. A fall in membrane charge only takes a few minutes and when it occurs massive amounts of calcium are allowed to influx into the cell. Calcium can only flood into a nerve cell by the inappropriate channels when the force field is compromised. When the force field is compromised calcium will chemically react in harmful ways with intracellular contents.

Processes that increase a cells ability to generate a maximal force field give longevity and performance advantages to the nerve cell. Processes that compromise the ability of a given nerve cell to generate an optimal force field, lead to cell injury (old age). Nerve cells are particularly vulnerable if their force field diminishes for a short time.

The two main hormones within the body that determine how powerful a given nerve cell force field becomes is aldosterone and thyroid hormone. Thus a continued maximal nerve function only becomes possible when these hormones are present in sufficient amounts (section two). Over looking the central directive role, which these two hormones play, often allows owners' nervous systems to slip into the diminished energetic state mentioned above. The diminished energy state of one's nerve cells is best understood through the example of the common mineral imbalance of middle age. One important mineral imbalance particularly important to nerve health is potassium.

Potassium deficiency diminishes the cell force field and hurts nerves at eight different levels

Potassium is the main mineral within the nerve cells. Nerve cells, which possess adequate potassium, are afforded energy and protection. Unfortunately the importance of ample potassium within one's nervous system is often overlooked in the clinical setting. The failure to counsel owners on strategies, which will improve their nervous systems content of potassium, has many nerve health consequences. Fortunately once potassium deficiency is remedied the owner begins to heal.

The potassium-depleted nerve cells are irritable and weak. Many owners are misled by their annual lab test results, which clearly state that they have a normal blood potassium level. This blood stream measurement is known as the 2% tank of the body. This is because only 2% of total body potassium is in the blood serum. The other 98% is within the body cells. The confusion occurs when patients fail to appreciate that the 98% tank will greatly diminish before one ever sees a decrease in the 2% tank within the blood stream. The consequence of this misunderstanding is that there are a lot of owners with nerve cell potassium depletion but normal blood potassium test results.

The ability of a nerve cell to charge its force field is directly proportional to the availability of potassium inside the cell. Potassium deficiency often results from poorly informed diet choices. The consequences of poorly informed diet choices usually delays manifestation of the chronic disease expression until the onset of middle age.

The most common reason for potassium deficiency with the onset of middle age results from the American diet. Very little medical emphasis occurs in regards to the importance of the proper consumption of balanced mineral intake. Balanced mineral intake will promote the maximal nerve cell charges.

Conversely, the chronic imbalance of mineral intake, leads to the tendency for mineral imbalanced related diseases around middle age. The reasons for this have been discussed in other sections but a review as they pertain to nerve health is warranted.

Real food diets (natural food that has not been processed) tend to be high in magnesium and potassium. These foods are almost always low in sodium as well. They tend to be intermediate in their calcium content. When an owner consumes real food the minerals are rather easy to obtain in the optimally needed ratios. In general, 4000mg of potassium, 2000mg of sodium, 500mg of calcium, and 300mg of magnesium a day will suffice. Owners that live in hot climates will need more sodium. Owners that live in colder climates may need less sodium. In addition owners that sweat while either working or exercising may need more sodium. These mineral intakes only apply for those with normal kidney and adrenal function. Owners, who chronically have been fed the reversed mineral ratios of the processed food diet, have nerves that become fatigued and irritable around middle age.

Nerve problems occur around middle age in America because processed food has had much of its potassium and magnesium removed. Compounding the problem is the addition of large amounts of sodium to preserve the shelf life of processed food. When owners eat these altered mineral contents for years the nerves become less able to hang on to or procure the necessary potassium.

The nerve cell potassium deficiency process greatly accelerates in those owners who are under chronic stress. This occurs because the stress hormone, cortisol, increases potassium loss and conserves sodium. This is the second tier of a complex problem. It would be very difficult for this to occur if a given owner ate a real food diet because there would be sufficient potassium around to accommodate the increased loss.

The third tier of the nerve cell potassium deficiency problem occurs when the kidneys become damaged from chronic potassium deficiency. It has long been known for many years that low potassium intake is a risk factor for kidney damage (hypokalemic nephropathy). Paradoxically very little is said to patients in the clinical setting. The blood pressure begins to rise when the kidneys start to become damaged in this way.

High blood pressure is hard on the brain cells. If the doctor understands nutrition at this early stage he will begin to counsel his patients regarding the importance of a more balanced mineral intake contained within real foods. However, when the physician misses this healing opportunity, the patient will go on to develop more kidney damage. Once the kidney becomes damaged, blood pressure will be less responsive to a better diet. At this stage high blood pressure medication may be necessary on a permanent basis. One of the reasons high blood pressure medication becomes necessary is to protect the brain.

The fourth tier of the nerve injury caused by the potassium deficiency problem concerns the associated insulin resistance. Insulin resistance predictably occurs in the processed food diet situation around middle age. Insulin cannot facilitate sugar uptake in most cells without a one for one association between sugar and potassium. This means that for every sugar taken into a cell, their needs to be corresponding potassium taken up as well. When potassium availability is deficient then the secondary system within the liver gets activated. The problem here gets exaggerated as well because the pancreas senses the delay in the blood sugar falling when potassium deficiency is the problem. So in these situations the pancreas eventually secretes even more insulin for a given sugar load as more potassium becomes available from within the cells. This is one of the reasons an owner still gets fat even though they are eating less carbohydrates. A given owner will always secrete more insulin for a given amount of sugar when their total body potassium is diminished. The delay of blood sugar normalization damages nerves.

The liver receives a larger insulin message from the potassium deficient state, contributes to the fifth tier of potassium related illness that damages nerves. The liver only needs insulins message for it to begin sucking sugar out of the blood stream. In contrast, other body tissues require potassium as well to suck up sugar out of the blood stream. When insulin levels increases, as in the case of potassium deficiency, the enzyme HMG CoA reductase will be activated. This enzyme machine begins the process of turning sugar into fat and cholesterol. Here lies yet another simple explanation for how cholesterol tends to increase around middle age. High levels of liver manufactured fat and cholesterol (LDL) tend to damage the blood supply that feeds the nerves of the body. The blood vessels in these areas plug up when the macrophages lining the arteries stuff themselves chronically on LDL cholesterol.

The sixth tier of damage which low potassium states cause to nerve cells arises from the lessened tolerance for aldosterone within the body. Alsosterone is a fundamental player for two important nerve processes. One it tells the nerve DNA that it is important to invest in updated cell charge components within the cell membrane. Second, it is the steroid, which determines the rate at which cholesterol gets converted to pregnenolone. Aldosterone levels become the rate-limiting step for steroid biosynthesis within the gonads and adrenals. Nerve cell health depends on adequate steroid tone and pressure. Adequate steroid tone and pressure cannot occur without sufficient aldosterone levels which tell the steroid producing tissues of their body to begin the process. The steroid producing tissues of the body are: the gonads, the adrenals and the brain. Unless adequate aldosterone message content reaches these areas, the rate of steroid synthesis declines. A fall in steroid synthesis means that the steroid pressure and tone will fall as well (section one). The nerve cells consequently have diminished message content to rejuvenate.

The nerves of the body rely on adequate aldosterone levels to help keep the steroid production rate at youthful levels and the nerve cell charge sufficient. The processed food diet common in America today only compounds the difficulty of the body's steroid producing cells to receive adequate aldosterone message content. Aldosterone deficiency will occur for two reasons. First, is in the treatment of high blood pressure states with ACE inhibitors (section one). Most of the time these drugs are only necessary if one fails to catch the low potassium diet injury to kidneys early on. It also occurs when an owner continues to eat a processed food diet. Chronic subsistence on a low potassium diet will injure the kidneys. When the kidneys are injured, blood pressure will rise. Not until over fifty percent of the kidney is dead will the common kidney function blood test (creatinine) begin to rise into the abnormal range.

ACE inhibitors work in part by decreasing aldosterone and therefore conserving potassium. Potassium has long been known to lower blood pressure. The other mechanisms of ACE were reviewed in chapter three. The important point in this subsection concerns the many owners that are not aware of how their processed food diet is central to their nerve disease process at multiple levels. If these people change their diets early on, their nerves will benefit in multiple ways.

The second way that potassium affects aldosterone and therefore the nervous system steroid levels regards the fact that in some owner's atrial naturetic peptide (ANP) gets activated early on. This powerful hormone released from the heart of some owners overrides the stimulus to release aldosterone when a high sodium diet prevails. This hormone in these situations keeps these owners blood pressure low at a price to their health. The first price to health arises in that less aldosterone is made and therefore there will be a consequent reduction of the other steroids production rates. Second, there are consequences other than high blood pressure from diminished total nervous system potassium.

The seventh tier of potassium deficiency and the resultant nerve dysfunction arises from the diminished force field. When nerve cells are diminished in their force field generating abilities they become irritable. Different owners are more susceptible to this side effect. It comes down to the fact that different bodies handle potassium deficiency in their own prioritized way. Some do a better job at conserving potassium within the nervous system until late in the deficiency process. The important point to recognize is that some cases of anxiety or irritability have their origins in potassium deficiency states.

The eighth tier of potassium deficiency produced nerve disease present as weakness and fatigue. This situation occurs because total body potassium content serves as a determinant for the amount of cell protein possible within body cells. Nerve cells need protein for their function and health even more than other cells. Potassium within the cells has been known for many years to stabilize proteins by its association. Without adequate potassium, body protein is lost. Nerve cell health relies on the ability of potassium content to stabilize nerve cell proteins.

The eight ways which potassium injures one's nerves serves as an introductory example for how dietary deficiencies or excesses can alter nerve function. In addition, multiple other nutritional deficiencies cause clinical depression. Clinical depression therefore can be healed when the nutritional problem resolves.

Nutritional Deficiency Caused Depression

Imbalanced amounts of the different neurotransmitters often result in clinical depression. Mainstream medicine tends to lump all these cases into the umbrella of these owners having a biochemical imbalance. While the biochemical imbalance accurately describes the cause of their clinical problem the solution often becomes nutritional. However, instead of applying even a little effort for how a lousy diet might contribute to depressive illness, antidepressants are prescribed. Many patentable prescriptions therefore have been created to address deficiencies here in a peripheral ways. These medications achieve their usual circuitous improvement by keeping the deficient neurotransmitter around for a longer time in the synapse. However, proper nutrition will increase the amount of neurotransmitters available within the different nerve cells of the body. In addition, proper nutrition avoids side effects.

The science of neurotransmitter production and what nutrition is needed has been understood for years. Instead of advising owners on ways to increase their own neurotransmitter production, prescription medications are the treatment of choice. Certain nutritional factors need to exist before sufficient neurotransmitters can be manufactured which prevent depression. When certain neurotransmitter manufacture fails, predictable mental symptomotology follows. Paradoxically, rather than augment the deficiency through nutritional intervention, these owners are counseled that they have a biochemical imbalance.

The symptom control approach prescribes the various drugs that increase the length of time that the neurotransmitters occur in the synapse. These prescriptions do nothing to increase production of the deficient neurotransmitter. They only prolong how long the neurotransmitter gets to signal its message in the synapse. In marginally depleted states this approach has potential to help, but with a price. The price is dependent on the class of antidepressant agent given. Very few owners receive counseling with regards to what needs to happen nutritionally for normal neurotransmitter production to occur. Instead they are told that they have a biochemical imbalance and the implication usually is that it is genetic in its causality.

Some owners prefer a trial of nutritional supplementation before they embark on symptom control medicine. Nutritional supplementation covers the other side of the story of what science has long ago revealed about the cause of some depressive illnesses. The largely untold facts involve the central nutritional molecular building parts and chemical reaction facilitators (vitamins). These molecular building parts and chemical reaction facilitators are necessary within the brain for neurotransmitter biosynthesis to occur. If these factors are delivered in reliable and constant supplies to the central nervous system the need for prescription medicine often disappears.

Many conventionally trained physicians have little education into the importance of the pathways that bring about optimal neurotransmitter levels. How convenient to leave some basic nutritional science out of the educations of the certified experts.

Earlier in this chapter the most common neurotransmitters were reviewed and some of their manufacture requirements were discussed. A brief summary follows on what nutritionally needs to pass into the brain in order for different neurotransmitter biosynthesis to be allowed.

Serotonin (arousal states): Adequate tryptophan in the diet to provide the basic building block precursor.

Vitamins needed for manufacture: Tetrahydrobiopterin (made from folate) and pyridoxal phosphate (vitamin B6).

Dopamine (pleasure and fine motor coordination): Amino acids tyrosine and phenylalanine can serve as the basic precursor building blocks.

Vitamins needed for biosynthesis: Tetrahydrobiopterin (made from folate), pyridoxal phosphate (vitaminB6)

Norepinephrine (mental alertness): Dopamine is needed as the building block precursor.

Vitamin C is needed for its biosynthesis

Epinephrine (mental alertness): Norepinephrine is the building block.

SAMe is needed to allow its biosynthesis to occur. One SAMe is used for each epinephrine made, it is rapidly depleted without the methyl donor system adequately recharging it back into its active form.

Methyl Donors recharge system includes; vitamin B12, Vitamin B6, folate, serine, and methionine.

Tyrosine and phenylalanine lead to the sequential manufacture of first dopamine, followed by norepinephrine and lastly epinephrine. Epinephrine deficiency is most likely because deficiencies anywhere along the assembly line will prevent its manufacture. Where the nutritional deficiency occurs becomes the point neurotransmitter manufacture stops. In other words epinephrine deficiency is most vulnerable because it is reliant on the most vitamins for its manufacture.

Histamine (consciousness and arousal): histadine is the amino acid building block. Pyridoxal phosphate (vitamin B6) is needed for its biosynthesis.

GABA (calm states): Glutamic acid is the building block amino acid precursor needed.

An aside about GABA is that its production in the central nervous system is dependent on adequate progesterone levels. People that have diminished progesterone levels for too long tend to be anxious and irritable. This situation commonly occurs in peri-menopausal females up to two weeks before their periods (PMS).

The other irritability factor that always needs to be considered is the amount of sodium relative to potassium intake. Potassium has a calming affect within the CNS. It probably has to do with an adequate force field.

Pyridoxal phosphate (vitamin B6) is the vitamin needed for biosynthesis of GABA to occur. The advice of a nutritionally competent physician will facilitate the correct replacement dosages and regimens. In addition, some attention needs to be directed at the integrity of the digestive tract. Improperly functioning digestive tracts will frustrate attempts to heal nutrition deficiency caused depression. In some of these cases intravenous vitamin therapy may be warranted while the digestive problem resolves.

A caveat now occurs regarding supplementation to correct certain neurotransmitter deficiencies here. The salt of glutamic acid is known as glutamate. It is popularly known as monosodium glutamate and it is often hidden within ingredients such as vegetable flavorings, hydrolyzed protein and spices. Glutamate is the most powerful neurotransmitter for nerve excitation. Too much glutamate can excite a nerve cell to death. Nerve cell death results from over stimulation. Over stimulation of a nerve cell leads to a draining down of the nerve cell force field. When the nerve cell force field becomes depleted, the massive in rushing of unwanted charged particles like calcium, mentioned earlier, follows.

Just eliminating this salt from one's diet can often enhance memory. This is because nerve cells need to generate an adequate force field to be able to work efficiently. Molecules like glutamate continually discharge the force field's energy. The memory nerve's force field becomes depleted because the over stimulation of their membrane leads to the discharge of the concentration difference between important minerals. As the concentration difference between these important minerals about the nerve cell membrane decreases, the protection energy becomes depleted (the force field has run down).

Acetylcholine (abstract thinking ability): the first building block precursor comes from consuming adequate choline in the diet mostly from fish and eggs. The second building block precursor is acetate, which can be derived from all fuel sources (protein, fat and carbohydrates) only when adequate vitamin levels are present (nutrition caused heart disease). However, in the brain, it is usually only derived from carbohydrates (fuel discussion).

Low fat diet adherents make it hard on their methyl donor system. With appropriate types and amounts of fat intake, the methyl donor system is used at approximately one billion times a second. Unless low fat diet adherents have even more methyl donors available than normal their acetylcholine levels will tend to fall off. The acetylcholine levels will fall off because deficient fat intake leads to an increased need for the methyl donor system to synthesize choline from scratch. The more severe the fat deficiency is, the greater the burden on one's methyl donor system. Therefore the amount of methyl donor that one needs will sky rocket to much higher levels per second.

There is an additional potential problem that regards the procurement of acetate within the brain for the manufacture of acetylcholine and other fat building blocks within the brain. This problem arises from the fact that the brain only uses carbohydrates for acetate creation. This limitation means that all five nutritional cofactors need to be present in order for the brain to convert glucose to acetate. Specifically the rate-limiting step in question is the conversion of pyruvate to acetate. The enzyme complex that performs this is called, pyruvate dehydrogenase.

This enzyme needs five additional co-factors or acetate formation will not be possible. The five co-factors necessary are: vitamin B1, B2, B3, panothenic acid, and lipoic acid. Processed food is notoriously deficient in pantothenic acid and lipoic acid. So the fact that it has been re-fortified with a little of the B vitamins is not really helpful in this case. This is because as with other chemical sequenced reactions of the body the depleted nutrient is the broken link and everything stops at this point. What makes this situation even more alarming is that vitamin supplements are often deficient in these two needed nutrients unless they are specifically taken on their own.

The Energies that Heal Contrasted to the Energies that Maim

Science has not been pure in the pursuit of knowledge or understanding. Politics, social acceptance, vested interests, prejudice, money, etc have effected the conclusions and holdings of scientific inquiry. Consequently, some scientific theories have been based on incorrect analysis of the data. The data has been manipulated to serve many unscientific purposes. In the second half of this century the data was manipulated by the tobacco industry for monetary purposes. Five hundred years ago the data was manipulated to appear consistent with the canons of a powerful religious system. Scientific theories that were prevalent during the renaissance are laughable today because the data is reinterpreted in view of new knowledge. Einstein's cosmological constant has been interpreted and reinterpreted several times during the century of its first postulation because of new data, observation, or the persuasive power of the most recent and prevailing theory.

The most consistent element of scientific inquiry has been the intellectual tenacity of some members of the scientific community. These people did not accept a popular scientific theory that was inconsistent with the data. Their curiosity and intellectual integrity was stronger than their sense of professional survival; and in cases such as Galileo, their personal survival.

Ptolemy lived in the first century A.D. He noted certain inconsistencies in the scientific dogma that the sun revolved around the earth. He methodically explained his conclusions. When he proposed the novel idea that the earth revolved around the sun he and his theory were rejected and ridiculed by his scientific peers. For the next fourteen hundred years the world's top scientist clung to the belief that the sun revolved around the earth.

More than 1400 years after Ptolemy, Capernicus (1473-1543), noted similar inconsistencies. He methodically studied the data and observations. Capernicus reached the same conclusion as Ptolemy. The Church initially persecuted him. Capernicus' tenacity eventually won acceptance for his preposterous theory.

Galileo (1564-1642) made observations of unequally weighted falling bodies that were inconsistent with Aristotle's theories of gravity. Galileo's findings resulted in his dismissal from the faculty at the University of Pisa. Aristotle theory was still alive and powerful in the University of Pisa faculty. Today, basic physics include Galileo's observation that bodies of the different weights fall at the same velocity.

Dr. Ignatius Semmelweis, a Hungarian physician, who practiced in Vienna in the 1800's, demanded that his hospital colleagues and support staff wash their hands, especially when moving from autopsies and sick patient wards to the child birthing wards. The incidence of post-delivery fever and ensuing death from this illness plummeted to well below that of the wealthy women's childbirth hospital. The western germ theory was not even a speculation until Semmelweis perceived them; even before Lois Pasteur. Dr. Semmelweis had noted the inconsistencies of the scientific understandings of his day. He successfully developed this understanding into a primitive, but accurate germ theory.

Semmelweis was fired and ostracized from the medical community of his time. His ability to practice and his source of income was gone. Some say he cut off his finger and jammed the wounded stump into a corpse at autopsy. He then died from the infection attempting to prove his new theory. Others say he committed suicide from the despair and isolation.

Dr. Robert Becker, in the **Body Electric** says, "Science is a bit like the ancient Egyptian religion, which never threw old god away but only tacked them on to new deities until a bizarre hodgepodge developed. For some strange reason science is equally reluctant to discard worn out theories".[35] Later on Dr. Becker adds, "The healers job has always been to release something not understood, to remove obstructions (demons, germs, despair) between the sick patient and the force of life driving obscurely towards wholeness".

The material provided in this section offers a theory of health that is based on an energy theory. The energy theory proposed in this section is similar, in some respects, to the previously described historical antidotes. This theory is supported by scientific data and mathematical theory that is recognized by mainstream medicine. The conclusions described in this section have a devastating monetary impact on the medical industry. These conclusions also diminish the power and prestige of the medical industry. The energy theory of life will not receive immediate acceptance by the medical industry.

The Chinese medical scientists observed a pattern of energy flow within the human body. After thousands of years of observation these scientist decided that this energy pattern is invariable in the healthy human body. The early Chinese scientists determined disharmony or disruption in these energy flow qualities were associated with disease. After further meticulous observation the specific imbalances were correlated with certain chronic degenerative diseases. Heart diseases were one of these disease patterns. This Chinese system developed methods during the last several thousand years that are intended to restore the energetic balance found in the healthy state.

This Chinese medical system is popularly known as acupuncture. The western scientific community was ignorant of this medical system until the 1970's. An American journalist, in China, became afflicted with an acute appendicitis. The journalist was a high profile case because he was there to document President Nixon's historic tour. The journalist, following the removal of the appendix, was impressed by the pain control achieved by acupuncture techniques. He was allowed to witness Chinese citizens undergoing surgical operations with acupuncture needles as their only anesthesia. When the journalist published his experience and observations of acupuncture techniques, the western scientific community was caught off guard. Western scientific medical theory could not offer an explanation for the medical phenomenon described in the article.

According to the western medical theory, needles placed in the skin would not have an anesthetizing effect during surgical procedures. Western medical theory contradicted many documented cases where Chinese patients undergo various surgeries without any injected or inhaled anesthesia. Instead, they receive strategically placed needles. These surgical patients remain conscious and conversant while the operation occurs. When the operation is over they walk to the recovery room. These observations are well documented. The western scientific medical theory, however, does not have an explanation for this phenomenon.

The National Institute of Health was mobilized to remedy this embarrassing deficiency of western scientific understanding. One of the scientists engaged by the NIH was Robert Becker, M.D., of Syracuse, New York. Dr. Becker's credentials are impressive. He was instrumental in discovering the electrical device used in the healing of fractures when they would not respond to mechanical or surgical techniques. His work also led to the understanding that fracture sites need to generate an adequate electric field in order for the bone to heal.

When Dr. Becker began to work with acupuncture, he discovered the existence of electrical grids on or in the body. Dr. Becker proved the existence of the meridians themselves. He did this by measuring the electrical resistance difference between the meridians and the surrounding skin. He also developed a method to document the existence of these unvarying electrical grids. These grids were present within all the numerous subjects tested. He noted the presence of periodic "jump stations" along these electrical pathways. He documented that these "jump stations" corresponded to the acupuncture points of the ancient Chinese system.

One of Dr. Becker's theories was that the acupuncture meridians carried injury messages electrically to the brain. The brain responded by sending direct current to stimulate the healing process in the injured area. He postulated that the conscious mind perceives these messages as pain.

He knew that any electrical current grows weaker as the distance from the source of the electrical current increases. This is due to resistance along the transmission medium. He also knew that the smaller the amperage and voltage of the electrical charge then the faster the current would diminish as it moved away from its source. Electrical engineers solve this problem by building booster amplifiers along a power line to restore the strength of the electrical current. For currents measured in nano-amperes and microvolts, however, these boosters would have to be no more than several inches apart from one another.

He had more elaborate experiments planned when the NIH withdrew funding for further research into the matter.

A metal needle placed in an amplifier will short it out and stop the pain message. The Chinese believe that balanced circulation of energy through this constellation of points is a prerequisite to health. Proper placement of various patterns of needle placement brings these currents into harmony.

Western medicine has no corresponding anatomical structures to Becker's grid. Western science is based upon molecular structure and the forces contained within these structures. This reductionism approach is too narrow to include an explanation of Becker's grid. The western scientific theory needs an anatomical structure to explain the energy moving within the meridians. The effectiveness of acupuncture without a convincing western scientific explanation is an ongoing credibility problem for western medicine.

The western medical approach can be likened to the slab of meat approach. The slab of meat is all that is left when western medical theory ignores the existence and effect of life energy. Alternative medicine addresses ways to re-invigorate the flow of the life energies within a human body. This often is the common denominator between chiropractic manipulation, acupuncture therapy, message modalities, yoga and prayer. Each of these disciplines in their own way has the ability to effectuate a healing response by imparting a more harmonious energy flow within a given owner.

Many a good scientist's life work continues to collect dust because their work reintroduced the concept of an organizing energy contained within living systems. In contrast the western scientific approach preoccupies itself with DNA and the information that it contains. However, the information contained in the DNA is not useful within the body unless the life energy directs its activation and silence in a coherent way. Coherence of informational direction is how life violates the laws of physics. The life process violates the laws of physics because living things convert simple molecules to complex molecules in a coherent manner. The western scientific explanation has no explanation for this basic fact of life. Modern science asked its devotees to believe the similar analogy that there is this wonderful computer encryption program that can produce meaningful information without the direction of an operator. In other words garbage in is equal to garbage out. If DNA is the computer hard drive, then where is the operator?

The Chinese system of acupuncture theory directly addresses the importance of honoring the need for a healthy 'operator'. The operator contained within living things is the proper flowing of this 'intelligent energy'. The possession by living things of an intelligent energy, which organizes and directs life's complex processes, is one theory that explains the ability for life to violate the physical laws of nonliving systems. Intelligent energy is responsible for satisfying the ever present need to organize the flow of how the body is spending its energy.

The theory of intelligent energy being a determinant of health involves the concept of whether there is rhythm or chaos within the energetic template. The energies that heal contrasted to the energies, which maim owner's cells describe this process. Healing energies are thought to contain rhythm while harmful energies impart chaotic forces on owner's cell. Examples of healing energies are the positive emotions, such as: joy, forgiveness, love, kindness, and courage. Conversely, examples of the negative emotions are: hatred, fear, jealousy, and self-entitlement. The heart being a rhythmical organ can facilitate an understanding of the effect of these energies on one's health.

Chapter 25

The Heart

The mainstream explanation of the life process begins to look incomplete when one starts to examine the scientific evidence for what the life rhythms involve. The mainstream viewpoint, in regards to life, looks incomplete because its explanation of the universe does not include the evidence for the life rhythm energies. There is strong evidence that the life process contains rhythmical energies. This evidence points to the fact that rhythmical energies make life possible.

The mainstream scientific assumption started years ago. The western paradigm of how one stays alive was thought to be explainable by the molecules that make up the body structure. Hence, the energies that heal contrasted to the energies that maim were relegated to the religious belief systems. When the rhythmical energies are discussed, they are only discussed in a peripheral way. However, there are many good scientists who have demonstrated the folly of this approach (intelligence behind the intelligence).

Understanding the matters of the heart is about keeping one's personal power (rhythm). In order to understand healing paths of the heart, a discussion of rhythmical energy versus' chaotic energy needs to be undertaken.

The heart is a rhythmical engine. The performance of the body cells is affected when rhythm is diminished. Processes that facilitate rhythm energize the body. Processes that diminish rhythm do so by harming the integrity of the body cells. The body cells, including heart cells, become harmed by chaotic energies. The chaotic energies inflict harm by their effect on body rhythm. Each of these harmful energies is chaotic in nature. These chaotic waves have unique ways of injuring cells. Cells become diseased when the disorganizing energies are present in quantities that exceed the body's ability to neutralize them. Energies that maim cause injury to the rhythms of life. Rhythmic energy originates within the heart. Therefore, the heart serves as a major source of rhythm for all other cells.

The heart involves much more than a pump for swishing blood back and forth. When rhythm occurs within the heart it can provide the background energy, which the body cells need. Rhythm causes the oscillations necessary for the efficient transfer of molecules from one cell to another cell. In addition, the body cells outside of the blood stream use the pressure wave generated by the heart. The pressure wave generated beyond the blood vessels determines much about the health of body cells. All too often mainstream medicine ignores the obvious consequences when this energy wave is sub-optimal at the level of the cell.

The cartilage cell dilemma illustrates the necessity of the pressure waves ebb and flow. The dilemma of a cartilage cell describes the consequences to body health when rhythm fails. The cartilage cell does not have a direct blood supply (section five). These types of cells rely on the ebb and flow of fluids within the joint. The pressure wave created by the beating heart causes the ebb and flow of fluids to the cartilage cell in the body periphery. This ebb and flow causes the exchange of nutrients and waste. Most other body cells are closer to the blood vessels. They still depend on the pressure wave created by the beating heart.

The pressure wave created by the heart creates squishing forces. Squishing forces describe the mechanical squeeze, within body cells. These squishing forces are similar to the forces of gravity that augment the processes of nutrient delivery and waste removal to the cartilage cells. When gravity is applied and then released to joint tissue the ebb and flow of molecules occurs. A similar ebb and flow occurs in the body cells from the mechanical effects of the heart rhythm. When the heart is in rhythm, there are forces created that result in improved energy transfer beyond the obvious movement of blood.

Sometimes truth is so simple that it is overlooked. In medicine when truth becomes overlooked healing possibilities fail to be realized. The red blood cell's deformability process, (chapter two) when it arrives at the level of the capillary, is one example. Capillaries are a tight squeeze for red blood cells. In order for a red blood cell to go through the capillary it needs to be sufficiently deformable. All red blood cells must do this or they will plug up the capillary. When this happens it is called micro-vascular disease (chapter two). The consequence of decreased deformability of the red blood cells is high blood pressure. Only when the heart elevates its pressure will the stiffened red blood cells squeeze through the tight capillary spaces. Healing requires attention to the reasons that red blood cells become stiff (chapter 2). Healing does not involve lowering the blood pressure without understanding the reason for the elevated blood pressure.

The presence or absence of the heart rhythm and the consequent pressure wave is an important determinant of a healthy cell. Healthy cells receive adequate nutrients. Healthy cells also coordinate an efficient reloading of waste onto the red blood cells. Processes that encourage the effectiveness of the heart rhythm will enliven the body cells because they facilitate these two processes. When body cells receive the heart's rhythm they become more alive because they can receive nutrition and eliminate waste more effectively.

Ignoring the importance of the energy wave reduces the discussion of the heart to its pump function. The seventh principle of health is about the quality of this rhythm inside the body. Specifically, the seventh principle concerns itself with the presence or absence of balance between the energies that heal contrasted to the energies that maim cells.

The understanding and restoration of rhythmical energies is the common denominator of the alternative healing modalities. Alternative healing modalities include: chiropractic, acupuncture, homeopathy, meditative prayer and body massage. Each of these modalities, using its specific techniques, addresses the life rhythms. Paradoxically theses energies are almost always ignored by the mainstream view of the universe.

Rhythm

There are several common themes among the great violinist, athletes, poets, and songwriters. There is a concept, which they all employ to achieve greatness. Without mastery of this single principle advancement beyond mediocrity is impossible. All great performers or every great performance includes rhythm. Rhythm is an important element contained in every great performance.

Rhythm is not a linear skill that can be learned. It must be felt, used and exercised. Consistently the great performers possess a mastery of rhythm. Great violinists must feel the rhythm of the music before a remarkable performance exudes from their instrument. Likewise, great athletes tap into a higher rhythm that shows their grace. Rhythm causes the efficient use of available energy. The less wasted energy then the greater the achievement possible. When cells feel rhythm there is a minimal wasting of precious life energy. Ample life energy allows for a peak performance in the pursuit of happiness.

Healthy cells have rhythm. Healthy owners have rhythm in their lives. The heart is the metronome that creates a harmonic resonance throughout the body.

Doc Childre and Howard Martin of Heart Math Institute, point out that the heart is the body's main energetic oscillator, and in health there is an efficient, heart generated, pressure wave penetrating each organ.

The energies that heal are the energies that promote rhythm. It helps to conceptualize the power in rhythm by considering different emotional energies and their effect on body rhythm qualities. For example, the emotion of forgiveness imparts energetic rhythm. In contrast, the negative emotions contain chaotic energies which are destructive to body rhythm. Many owners waste precious life energy carrying around the energetic baggage of past grudges, guilt feelings, failures, and fears.

Emotions can be understood as thought forms. Thought forms have energy. The presence of rhythm or chaotic waves depends on the thought form. With the passage of time the chaotic energies tend to localize in their preferred body tissues. The energies that maim do so by imposing chaotic forces on the body's underlying rhythm. As the chaotic energies accumulate within the body they become clinically evidenced as stiff and sore body tissues. Many of the alternative medical therapies have their healing effect by facilitating the removal of accumulated chaotic energies within the body.

The negative chaotic energies begin in the mind. The importance of this fact explains why coaches often spend considerable effort in attempting to clear the athlete's minds before a performance. When the athlete's mind becomes cleared the rhythm of their performance improves. It is the rhythmical energies that help them to enhance their athletic performance.

As life happens most owners tend to accumulate significant negative, chaotic energies within their body tissues. All owners experience periods of emotional pain. The seventh principle of health promotes life rhythm energies in the face of adversity. The rhythmical energies are promoted by minimizing accumulation of the chaotic energies such as hate, anger, jealousy, impatience, and sadness. Secondly, maximizing rhythmical energies such as forgiveness, love, thankfulness, kindness and patience in important. An increase in rhythmical emotional energies can be thought of as spiritual growth. Increasing chaotic energies can be thought of as spiritual wilting.

Spiritual growth is painful but it will not harm the body. Spiritual growth can be described as the process of energetically releasing old toxic patterns of chaotic energies. The transition from accumulated chaotic energies to the ability to release them from the body is a painful cognitive process. However, spiritual stagnation creates physical pain. It is a congestion of chaotic energies within the body tissues.

Staying stuck in one's illusions requires increasing life energy to maintain until one day the owner is pushed off into another painful reality check. Reality checks are growth of the spirit. A growing spirit manifests as increased ability to forgive, love, give, accept, help and be kind.

Doctors see the common thread between pain release and the process of spiritual growth among their patients and themselves. Some have concluded that owners are here to learn. Some owners learn their lessons faster than others. Some waste less life energy. Reducing chaotic energy also reduces the waste of life energy.

The minimization of these chaotic energies turns out to be a very selfish understanding when pursuing health and longevity. Owners who can stay fresh in the rhythm of the moment have the health advantage of the seventh principle of longevity. Owners who can do this are able to release the energies that maim, and have more energy for the present. More energy for the present day results from the increased body rhythm that the positive emotions confer. When an owner has internal rhythm, they are intensely alive. They are alive down to the level of their vibrating cells.

Master owners down through the ages have consistently maintained their own rhythm while adverse life experiences occurred. Awareness of their own rhythm during painful times allowed them to stay centered. Centeredness is a state of maintaining one's personal rhythm despite the temptation for the chaotic energies to arise. Staying centered is a way for the masters of life to refrain from reacting emotionally in ways that have negative energetic consequences to their body tissues.

Healing into longevity, despite adverse life events, involves the understanding of how one deflects the chaotic emotions. In contrast, the common unhealthy experience is reacting to each and every crisis. The indulgence in constant negative emotional reactivity leads to the accumulation of the chaotic energetic debris. The chaotic energetic debris weighs down the cells. Eventually it accumulates to the point of affecting inner rhythm. The masters understood that no matter what happens one has a choice to react or not to react. It comes down to keeping personal power (rhythm).

The Energetics of Enlightenment

In general, as human beings progress towards enlightenment there seems to be an increased conservation of energy within their body cells. The energy conservation within these body cells arises from their optimizing the rhythmical vibrations. Optimal rhythmical vibrations occur when the energies that heal are the predominant emotion. The 'masters' knew the secrets of maintaining their personal power in the face of negative events.

The masters were aware of the temptation to experience negative emotions. The masters viewed these temptations as learning opportunities. In adverse circumstance, the master knew how to choose personal power. Personal power is the rhythm of living energy that occurs when one is healthy. Healing involves allowing the processes that facilitate increased rhythm to penetrate to the level of the body cells. So much disease results from the disharmonious chaotic energies. The chaotic energies can be thought of as stagnant and swirling in nature. Chaotic energies are absorbed into the body tissues when the owner indulges in negative emotions. When negative emotions are absorbed beyond one's tolerance threshold, disease results.

Many owners become involved in a vicious cycle of emotional highs and lows. Owners caught in this drama of emotional reactivity have good days. However, the willingness to indulge in negative emotions guarantees there will certainly be bad days. It becomes an increasing challenge to have a good day as more emotional negative baggage accumulates within the tissues. 'Gray' emotional tone typically sets in around middle age. Survival mode occurs at this time. These owners feel trapped in a gray and cold world.

Listening to a heart felt path is of great value in some cultures. These societies place great importance on its members discovering their uniqueness. They believe this is a teaching planet and that humans are created to learn. They believe that there is only one human worry and that is that a given owner is honoring his reason for asking to be born. They believe in asking to be born into the human domain. They believe that each person is given unique talents and abilities. In these cultures it is up to the individual to re-discover why they are here. The only worry is about whether they are honoring their gift. All other worries in these societies are an illusion. The orientation within these cultures is to channel conscious energy into discovering why an owner chose to be born and what it is he can contribute

The western mindset is much different. The life of being a doctor in clinical practice reveals that most adults are stressed out. Most of the time owners are in a series of days typified by the need to hurry. The hurry is in pursuit of what they believe will make them happy.

There are exceptions to this common observation. These exceptional people keep physicians going to work. These exceptional people make a difference in all who are sensitive enough perceive their beauty. These are the owners who have not lost their rhythm (personal power) and, therefore, are alive to what life has to offer. Often they are described as exuding a particular freshness.

As a culture, the relationship between happiness and rhythm has been forgotten. Without rhythm operating in one's life there can be no happiness. Perhaps other cultures have something to teach western people about more fulfilling lives. These cultures possess knowledge of the importance of rhythm and its relationship to health and happiness. These cultures possess knowledge of processes that facilitate rhythm. These cultures look within and understand the kind of emotional baggage that destroys health and happiness.

The energies that maim are contained within certain body tissues. These chaotic energies tend to accumulate with the passage of time. If one understands this a healing path becomes possible. This path does not have to wait until an owner becomes enlightened. Rather there are alternative medicine modalities that facilitate a flushing out of the tissues of the energies that maim (the painful and chaotic energies). These methods include chiropractic craniosacral therapy, acupuncture, and various types of massage therapies, homeopathy and prayerful meditation. Each of these modalities has the common denominator that, in there own unique way, cleanses the life field. Each in their own way, cleanse the body of the emotional baggage of the energies that maim.

These techniques can be applied as an owner is working consciously to learn how to forgive. These modalities also buy time while one learns how to avoid the reactive indulgence of the negative emotions. These treatment modalities offer a way of keeping things in an energetic balance. It becomes a personal choice as to how one feels most comfortable flushing their chaotic energetic debris.

There will come a time in each owners life where the ability to forgive is enhanced. This ability allows the experience of freshness and openness to life. Many theologians believe this is where one begins to awaken to life and its true meaning.

Without forgiveness, joy in life is not possible. The Chinese have known for several millennia that joy is the preferred emotion of the heart. When the heart is in rhythm there is ample joy operating in ones life.

The peculiar thing about life that physicians witness first hand is that the owners who choose joy each day often have some of the most difficult lives and circumstance. This is one of the truly awe-inspiring advantages of a life devoted to helping owners to heal. There is often an opportunity to witness a joyful owner who confronts the painful moments in life with a faith that things will get better. Accompanying this faith is the belief that what seems like misfortune often turns into an opportunity.

An old parable illustrating this point goes something like this: There was an old poor man living high in a mountain valley with his only son. One day he and his son came upon a group of horses corralled in a narrow canyon. The young son was so excited and exclaimed 'father what wonderful luck to have come on these horses trapped in this canyon'. The father was older and wiser and he took this opportunity to say 'good luck or bad luck who knows'. The son was quite puzzled by his father's words. The next day the son was attempting to work with the horses when suddenly he was kicked and suffered a terrible fracture to one of his legs. To this he cried out to his father 'oh what terrible luck'. His father patiently responded while splinting up the son's leg, 'good luck or bad luck, who knows'. The son just looked at his father in disbelief at this statement. Then in the next little while a terrible war broke out in the kingdom and while the young man was lying in his bed recovering an emissary for the king came to recruit all young men to fight in the war. When he left because he saw that this young man would be crippled for quite some time the son said to the father 'good luck or bad luck who knows'.

What does an openness and freshness to life look like in every day terms, so that an owner can apply the principles to a more healing life rhythm? Cultivating a consciousness of the energy that they, and those around them, exude provides a meaningful clue. Conceptually it is a question. Is there 'lantern' energy or 'vacuum' energy in operation? Most people are a blend of both. Very few are on either extreme of the energy spectrum.

The lantern energies result from those who have accessed the gift of their hearts, allowing joy to touch those that they contact. Almost all owners have encountered people that have an abundance of love, courage, passion and faith. It is truly a joy to be in their presence. They become the trusted friends that people seek out and rely on during the challenges of the life experience. These people have accessed the gifts of the heart and are able to touch others lives in a powerful way. Less obvious is the energetic rhythm that those that possess this wisdom exude.

The energetic lanterns of the world have accessed the gifts of the heart. Doctors see these owners. Many have had challenging lives. Many are materially poor. Many have ongoing problems that they face with courage. The difference between them and the energetic vacuums seems to be that they choose to forgive and therefore greet each day with freshness. They realize that hanging on to the negative emotional energies did them harm. Freed by this understanding, they have the ability to touch the lives of those all around them.

There are those who seem to suck energy from all they contact. This is the other extreme on the energetic spectrum. A powerful component of the healing process is gained when an owner becomes sensitive to the energetic dynamics in operation and consciously begins to promote ways to facilitate their own rhythm.

It takes all types of energetic shades, between the vacuum and lantern types, to make up a world.

It takes an openness to see this dynamic played out in so many ways between so many different owners each and every day. Less obvious is the rhythm-versus-chaos that is transferred with each interaction, down into owner's cells. Healing can begin to occur when a given owner begins to make conscious decisions that facilitate the healing energies.

The energies that heal contrasted to the energies that maim are a difficult concept for the western mind to grasp. Jesus' Sermon on the Mount summarizes, in many ways, the path to the healing energies that confer a rhythm to the cells. The love chapter in Corithians 11 also helps one to grasp how to access the gifts of the heart.

It comes down to living the truth of the gifts from the heart. What does it look like when one is living in heart wisdom? Mother Theresa provides an inspiring example. She was able to live out her life in the wisdom of the gifts from the heart and give to those in need. Mahatma Gandhi lived a life of non-violence and tolerance through which he was able to accomplish much good for his fellow countrymen. Patch Adams, M.D., whose message of laughter and non-violence, has led to a hospital providing for free patient care. Patch has continued to live on minimal dollars a month and the rest he donates to the gift of his free clinic. He decided many years ago that he was never going to have a bad day again. Here is a man living in the gifts from the heart.

Physical Health of the Heart Muscle

The seven principles of longevity have unique application within one's heart. The principles, which need additional clarification as they pertain specifically to the heart, are briefly expanded below.

Principles 1 and 2: Prevention of Rust and Hardening

What is good for the blood vessels is also good for the heart (section one). However, the heart blood vessels are unique in two ways. First, the heart receives its blood nourishment in diastole. Diastole is the resting phase while the heart chambers are filling with blood that will be ejected with the heart's next beat, systole. When the blood pressure is lowered too far the heart blood supply may become vulnerable. In contrast, other body tissues depend on systole for their nourishment. Systole describes the forceful ejection of blood from the heart out into the body. Systolic pressure is measured by the upper blood pressure value. Diastolic pressure is measured by the lower blood pressure value. The heart vulnerability occurs when there are blockages within the blood vessels that supply the heart. The blockage tends to increase risk because they tend to produce a pressure drop past the area of constriction. The lower the pressure, then the lower the perfusion pressure is. As a rule, this warrants a more modest decrease of diastolic pressure when one already has heart disease. This will tend to keep the perfusion pressure adequate past the diseased segment of the coronary artery. This fact results because what ever the pressure is before the blockage, it is always lower past the blockage.

The second unique feature about the blood vessels that supply the heart muscle regards the amount of immune scavenger cells that line the inside of these coronary vessels. These scavenger cells are called macrophages. These cells have a propensity to collect LDL cholesterol. This provides the heart with an adequate fat fuel supply when the owner exercises. However, well-fed and sedentary types of owners very rarely cause these cells to discharge their fat contents. Rather, in these sedentary types the fat slowly collects after each feeding event. The higher the insulin levels then the higher the message content within the liver to make and dump LDL cholesterol into the blood stream. The more LDL cholesterol in the blood stream then the more stuffed these macrophage cells become.

Around middle age these cells can become so laden with LDL cholesterol that they are called foam cells. Foam cells do not go anywhere. The larger they grow the more the coronary arteries are blocked. Congregations of foam cells are the earliest recognized lesions in the development of heart disease.

The ways to discourage foam cell growth in one's coronary arteries were reviewed in the blood vessel chapter, the digestion of fat subsection (section three) and in the liver chapter (section four). Attention to the ways one lowers blood vessel risk factors discussed in the first section will help to solve the foam cell growth problem. This can be followed by an accurately run cholesterol profile if one's profile was abnormal to begin with. This also applies to owners who have a more normal profile if they are taking a cholesterol-lowering drug. Cholesterol lowering drugs lower LDL cholesterol production. However, these drugs cause the owner's body to experience the side effects mentioned in the first, third and fourth sections.

Principle 3: The Hormones Giveth and Taketh Away the Heart

There are several hormones important in the regulation of the blood supply within one's heart. The ability to increase the supply of nutrient rich blood on demand is largely the role of the biogenic amine type hormones. Histamine is one such hormone, which is important to both blood supply and pump function of the heart muscle. Histamine seems to be the secret hormone within the heart.

One of the secrets about histamine regards its ability to increase the strength of the heart's beating. In fact, one of the benefits to the failing hearts that ACE inhibitors provide is their ability to increase the activation of the histamine receptors in the heart. When histamine receptors activate the force of contraction increases. The increased power of contraction increases the delivery of nutrients to the body.

Epinephrine is the second example of an important blood flow regulator to heart muscle from the biogenic amine hormone class. Increased epinephrine levels will cause the dilatation of coronary arteries to five times their resting diameter. During times of increasing demand the dilatation greatly enhances cardiac work output. Processes that ensure adequate epinephrine availability protect the heart from inadequate dilatation. Epinephrine deficiency decreases the ability of the heart to increase its work output. Epinephrine deficiency results from nutritional deficiency. Nutritional deficiency becomes common when one chronically subsists on a processed food diet. When epinephrine deficiency occurs the heart is unable to dilate its coronary arteries to increase blood flow.

Some of these dietary deficiencies result in the increased production of norepinephrine, which is much weaker and also less able to dilate the coronary arteries. The other consequence of increased nor-epinephrine production, with concurrent epinephrine deficiency, is that the systemic blood pressure rises considerably. Blood pressures rises considerably because without adequate epinephrine, the blood pressure elevateing effects of the sympathetic nervous system are exaggerated. The blood pressure increase places a tremendous extra strain on the heart. Epinephrine deficiency is usually related to a depleted methyl donor system (section three). A useful laboratory marker that the methyl donor system is depleted is an elevated blood homocysteine level. A homocysteine level is easier to interpret than twenty-four hour urine test for epinephrine breakdown products. In addition, since epinephrine has such a short half-life in the blood stream the testing for meaningful blood level averages become cumbersome.

Sufficient amounts of thyroid hormone are fundamental to normal heart function. Optimal thyroid message content directs the heart cells to do two important things. First, thyroid directs the heart cell DNA programs to make more epinephrine receptors. More epinephrine receptors allows the heart to increase work performance, increase the blood supply within the coronary arteries many fold, and burn more fuel in the presence of oxygen. Second, the heart is able to burn more fuel in the presence of oxygen because the thyroid message also directs heart DNA to invest in upgrades of the mitochondria (the power plants). The ability of the heart cell to receive the message content of the epinephrine is dependent on adequate thyroid hormone message content directing the formation of epinephrine receptors. The ability of the heart cell to burn fuel and oxygen within the power plants is dependent on adequate thyroid message. Adequate thyroid message directs the mitochondria (the power plant) to upgrade its ability to create energy packets for the work of heart cells. The mitochondria often number over two thousand per heart cell. This high number causes massive amounts of energy to be generated for useful work. Thyroid causes the energy generation abilities of the mitochondria to increase many fold (thyroid chapter).

Cortisol helps thyroid direct the heart cell DNA to manufacture the epinephrine receptors. Cortisol depletion results in Addison's disease and these patients present with a small and weakened heart. Thyroid and cortisol message content are needed to instruct the heart cell DNA to manufacture the completed epinephrine receptor. Cortisol and thyroid are level one hormones and are therefore able to direct DNA activity. Insufficient levels of either hormone will produce a decreased ability to respond to epinephrine. A decreased epinephrine response results in a diminished ability to increase nutrient supply within the heart muscle. A decreased nutrient supply results in a diminished ability to increase the work output of the heart.

Testosterone is the primary director of heart muscle cell build-up. The heart cell DNA receives the build up message from testosterone.

A corollary to this fact is that one of the most successful medications used to invigorate the failing heart, as a pump, are the digitalis medications. Digitalis medications' molecular structures are made up of testosterone like steroids attached to a few sugars. These patentable derivatives of the fox glove plant are second to no other heart medication in their ability to re-invigorate a failing heart.

Physicians are usually schooled about the peripheral effects digitalis of slowing conduction time. In addition this medication is presented with the abstraction of the Frank-Starling curve. This curve describes the improvement of pump function when digitalis-like medications are prescribed. The more powerful salient point that elucidates their mechanism of action is found in their molecular structure.

The molecular structure of the digitalis derivatives (cardiac glycosides) contains testosterone-like steroids. These molecular arrangements are similar to ginseng. However, the relation to digitalis and ginseng is obscured by the scientific nomenclature. The nomenclature changes when it describes ginseng's active components as saponins. However, both of these substances are technically glycosides.

The digitalis-like medications have the side effect of breast enlargement. One of the big obstacles to successful testosterone replacement in middle-aged males is breast enlargement. There are two common reasons this occurs in middle-aged males. First, is the often present increased body fat content. Increased body fat is a common feature in those owners that have a weakened heart. One of the problems with increased body fat is that it has a propensity to convert testosterone to estrogen. Estrogen is made from testosterone with the enzyme called aromatase. Aromatase is found in fat cells. The breasts of obese males are stimulated to grow by the increased estrogen that is created. Recently there has been increased interest in aromatase inhibitors. However, testosterone-like medications, like digitalis, is a common cornerstone prescription to invigorate a failing heart.

The second reason that the middle-aged heart disease afflicted male will tend towards enlarged breast is the fact that they are often methyl donor deficient. Methyl donor deficiency increases the conversion rate of testosterone to estrogen. This side effect occurs because this conversion creates methyl for other body processes. An elevated hemocystine level is a useful marker for methyl deficient owners.

Testosterone treatment is in the mainstream for treating a failing heart in other parts of the world. Several years ago there was a study done in England that convincingly showed the benefit of testosterone replacement therapy for heart disease patients. The caveat here is to avoid testosterone conversion into estrogen. One possible solution is to administer the more powerful dihydro-testosterone. Dihydro-testosterone (DHT) cannot be converted to estrogen.

There is an additional important caveat of administering DHT or testosterone to male owners. This concern is the mercury additive sometimes found in the injectible forms of testosterone. The code name for this additive is thimerosal. Mercury is toxic to body tissues and has no business being added to these preparations. Therefore any owner with heart disease considering testosterone therapy needs to obtain mercury free hormone. In addition, there is also the need to follow serial PSA's any time steroids are prescribed past middle age because of the possibility of stimulating abnormal prostate growth.

Principle 4: You are What You Supply and Absorb

There are other diet related deficiencies that impair the work performance of the heart.

Carnitine deficiency has long been known to produce a type of heart failure. Often physicians fail to even perform a rudimentary inquiry into a heart failure patient's carnitine status. Carnitine is a necessary carrier of most fatty acids into the heart mitochondria. Only when a fatty acid is successfully transported inside the furnace can it be further processed for combustion in the presence of oxygen. Heart cells are particularly vulnerable to carnitine deficiency because they prefer fatty acids for their fuel source. This is probably why the macrophage cells line the coronary arteries. These cells are probably storing fat for the next time an owner physically performs.

Carnitine deficiency leads to a diminished ability of the heart mitochondria to burn their preferred fuel, fatty acids. The diminished ability to combust fatty acids diminishes the work performance of the heart cells. When work performance diminishes severely then heart failure occurs. Healing occurs when the carnitine again becomes available.

Co enzyme Q10 (ubiquinone) is needed in the heart cells. However, the heart requires increased amounts of this nutrient (chapter one) because it combusts so much energy within its mitochondria. Only when owners eat a real food diet can they absorb this in sufficient quantities. Sushi is an excellent source.

The backup system is the liver's ability to manufacturer Co enzyme Q10. Statin like drugs compromises the backup system. These drugs work by poisoning the liver enzyme, HMG Co A reductase. This enzyme makes both cholesterol and Co enzyme Q10. This fact means that unless an owner absorbs sufficient dietary derived Co enzyme Q10 there becomes an increased risk for deficiency of this important nutrient while on the statin drugs.

There is the smoldering suspicion that owners on the statin drugs, who become deficient in Co enzyme Q10, are at increased risk for both heart failure and cancer development. The facilitation of cancer development is thought to be because the major advantage of the body's immune system against cancer cell formation is energy generation. Immune cells can generate energy much more effectively when adequate Coenzyme Q10 is present. This occurs because early on cancer cells often lack a blood supply and hence are living off anaerobic methods.

The heart failure is thought to occur because heart cells require the highest amount of this nutrient of anywhere in the body. Therefore a deficiency will show up here first. If Co enzyme Q10 becomes deficient while on the statin drugs, the powering up of both the immune system and heart function become compromised.

The statin drugs become unnecessary whenever the diet and lifestyle stimulate the secretion of appropriate hormones. In the case of HMG Co A reductase, cholesterol biosynthesis is stimulated by increasing insulin. Increased insulin is required when excess carbohydrates are consumed, potassium deficiency, or chronic stress with a sedentary lifestyle to name a few. This enzyme's activity towards cholesterol manufacture is retarded when increased glucagon is present. Glucagon levels are encouraged by a low carbohydrate diet. Increased insulin levels inhibit glucagons release. Potassium deficiency increases the need for insulin. Finally stress decreases the ratio between glucagon and insulin. It is the lowered hormone ratio at the level of the liver that makes cholesterol synthesis more likely. These three common culprits are often the cause of abnormal cholesterol profiles. Each one has been discussed in the previous sections of this book. However, potassium deficiency is important to review because it pertains specifically to heart performance and longevity.

Principle 6 and the Heart

Potassium deficiency will damage the heart in eight different ways

Potassium deficiency can show clinically as a diminished EKG voltage. Potassium deficiency is common by the onset of middle age. Many owners are unaware of this fact because their laboratory slip from their annual blood work clearly states that their serum potassium is normal. The serum potassium is only a measurement of the 2% tank that regards body potassium. The other 98% of body potassium is contained within the body cells. The 98% tank is not measured by this common test. In addition the 2% tank (the blood stream) will not fall at all until total body potassium becomes severely diminished. A decrease in total body potassium content will harm one's heart in eight different ways.

The reason potassium deficiency is so common involves the fact that most owners in America consume processed food. Processed food in general has a greatly diminished potassium and magnesium content. Also processed food tends to have huge amounts of sodium added. The sodium is added by the food industry to preserve shelf life. The body was designed to intake about three times as much potassium as sodium per day. Here lies the problem in America today. The American diet is a processed food diet, in general. Unless food is unprocessed, the ratio of these important minerals will be altered (section one for relative food mineral concentrations table).

An altered mineral intake ratio eventually affects the heart cellular charge. Both the heart and nerve cells, which innervate the heart, are extremely vulnerable to altered mineral balance. This is because the heart and nerve cells operate on a principle of exaggerated rapid exchange between these minerals in their work cycle. The heart cells and nerve cells within the heart conduct more electrical activity about their cell membrane. When there is an increased amount of mineral flow these cells perform more work. The body, with the help of aldosterone and thyroid hormones, will direct the concentration of potassium and magnesium within these cells. Simultaneously, these hormones facilitate the concentration of sodium and calcium outside these cells. The functional ability of the heart cell relies on the preferred concentration of these four minerals about the heart cell membrane.

Physicians are educated in a manner that compounds the problem of a low potassium diet. The physician's education does not directly emphasize the importance and methods to achieve adequate potassium intake. There is a vague emphasis on trying a low sodium diet when a middle-aged patient begins to experience elevated blood pressure. Fruits and vegetables are high in potassium. However, when an owner continues to eat processed food the increased sodium diminishes the beneficial ratio. When stress occurs the diminished ratio sets the stage for increasing blood pressure. Unless both physicians and owners become aware of this fact, there will be a diminished likelihood of avoiding symptom control medicine.

Before the discussion on how potassium deficiency injures the heart in eight different ways, one additional point deserves emphasis. It is important to emphasize that the body's cells charge themselves by creating an optimal concentration ratio between four main electrolytes (minerals). The electrolyte ratio occurs between sodium, potassium, magnesium and calcium. In general if one eats about 1000mg a day of sodium, 4000mg of potassium, 500mg of calcium and 300mg of magnesium the optimal ratio is maintained. This is only valid when an owner has normal adrenals and kidney function. Sodium requirements will also increase with increased sweating or gastrointestinal losses. It should also be emphasized that there are individual variation in the need for these different minerals. Therefore the counsel of a competent physician is sometimes necessary if questions arise. One useful method to monitor this ratio is to monitor the blood pressure and also how one feels. These two, facts taken together, will go along way for developing an effective plan for improving the quality of one's mineral ratio.

The eight ways that potassium deficiency will damage the heart are:

1. Diminished heart cell charge generating abilities (section five)
2. Potassium deficiency accelerates syndrome X because it raises insulin levels (chapter three)
3. Chronic potassium deficiency damages the kidneys and this begins blood pressure elevation. Blood pressure elevation wears out the heart muscle (chapter three).
4. Potassium deficiency causes insulin resistance. Insulin resistance means that for a given sugar load more insulin will need to be secreted before blood sugar will come down. The delay in returning blood sugar to normal will tend to 'rust' heart blood vessels.
5. A body potassium deficiency will lead to an increased activity of the liver enzyme, HMG Co A reductase. This enzyme's activity increases with rising insulin levels. Low potassium with a given sugar load will tend to promote greater insulin release. The increased insulin level will tend to activate HMG Co A reductase and begin the synthesis of cholesterol particles known as LDL cholesterol. The cholesterol manufacture process becomes greatly exaggerated because of the increased insulin level when one is insulin resistant. Potassium deficiency is a major cause of insulin resistance. Elevated LDL cholesterol is a known risk factor for the development of coronary artery blockages. Remember the foam cells that eventually will form here.

6. Low potassium states diminish one's tolerance for aldosterone secretion. Diminished potassium will affect aldosterone in three possible ways. First aldosterone levels will fall off because aldosterone increases potassium loss. When a given owner is eating the correct mineral ratios then potassium loss involves a good thing. In these situations potassium loss allows the kidneys to flush out waste. However, when potassium becomes deficient then the increased sodium causes fluid retention whenever aldosterone increases.

   The second problem related to aldosterone and potassium deficiency is blood pressure. Chronic potassium deficiency will require the aldosterone level to come down in order to normalize the blood pressure. The blood pressure comes down either through medication or the body's wisdom. Aldosterone will need to come down or blood pressure will rise whenever there is increased sodium and decreased potassium within the body. The trouble with diminished aldosterone states caused by potassium deficiency or medication is that aldosterone is the rate determiner for all other body steroids biosynthesis. Owners with higher aldosterone secretion will make more steroids than owners with low outputs of aldosterone.

   The third consequence of diminished aldosterone with potassium deficiency is that aldosterone increases the heart cell's ability to fully charge its membrane (along with the help of thyroid hormone). Only when the body minerals are balanced can the increased aldosterone, needed by the heart's cell charging mechanisms, be tolerated without high blood pressure problems. The one exception occurs in those owners who possess high levels of the override hormone, ANP (hormone chapter).

7. Adequate potassium is needed within all body cells to stabilize protein content. When the heart cell content of potassium becomes depleted heart cells protein content becomes unstable. Therefore protein loss occurs from these cells. Both heart cells and other muscle cells contain high amounts of protein. This fact explains why a potassium deficiency leads to loss of muscle mass.

8. Potassium deficiency will make the nerves innervating the heart irritable. Irritable nerves are more excitable and therefore cause an irregular heart rate. Irregular heart rate is the cause of sudden death. Sudden death is less likely when there is an optimal mineral concentration about the heart nerve membrane. Owners that constantly push their luck by eating foods that will alter this ratio are at increased risk of sudden death for this reason.

Principle 7 and the Heart

The hormones carry out the message delivery. However, the intelligent energy in living bodies determines when and which body hormones are needed. Processes that facilitate the harmony of this life energy (intelligent energy) promote the best hormones. Processes that interrupt the life energy flow will also disrupt the hormone types and amounts. There are health consequences when this organizing life energy becomes static, disorganized, excessive or deficient.

The stasis, disorganization, or excessiveness of the life energy is the energies that maim heart cells. Processes that confer rhythmic flow and optimal amounts of the life energy are the energies that heal heart cells. These considerations are also important within the context of the next chapter. Muscles, ligaments, and joints are some of the major tissues that become congested with static energies.

Chapter 26

Muscles and Ligaments

Some physicians and alternative practitioners have noted the relationship between different life issues and different levels of back and neck pain. For example, emotional distress tends to disrupt level T9. More painful life issues can tend to disrupt T6. Career issues tend to be felt in C3. Relationship issues tend to be felt in L5. Of course, back and neck pains are also caused from trauma, strain and degenerative processes. In contrast, the above correlations tend to result from trivial movements in bed, bending over, or twisting while grasping an object. These patients then present with varying degrees of incapacitating neck or back pain.

East Indian energy theory regarding the charkas seems to correlate with these cases of incapacitating back and neck pain. Former NASA researcher, Barbara Brennan wrote an excellent introduction to these theories in her book, *Hands of Light*.

These ideas are the foundation of chiropractic theory. Chiropractic adjustment techniques facilitate the unbinding of the static energy (the energies that maim). The theory of static emotional energy collecting within the joint spaces explains a possible mechanism for these types of clinical presentation.

There is no western scientific explanation for why chiropractic medical modalities effectively relieve these symptoms. Western medicine fails to recognize that energy stasis is the cause of the energies, which maim tissues. The relief of pain by spinal adjustments is only one example of the powerful healing effect contained in chiropractic techniques.

The alternative treatment modalities such as chiropractic, Charka energy theory, acupuncture, and homeopathy understand the need to optimize the mysterious life energies flow before healing can begin. The life energy flow is important within the muscles, ligaments and joints. The stasis within these tissues produces pain and stiffness.

Many alternative treatment modalities address the relief of the stasis within one's body tissues. Stasis occurs when the flow of one's life energy becomes disrupted. Another description of static energy collection within body tissues is tension. Stressed owners tend to be particularly vulnerable to accumulations of static energy. When these aberrant energies are collected they lead, initially, to painful body areas and only later to diminished joint, ligament, and muscle function. The alternative modalities are effective at releasing these static energies.

Chiropractic adjustment theory applied appropriately in the clinical setting effectively addresses the aberrant energy collections. Aberrant energy collections tend to occur within body tissues as negative emotions collect. The supplementation of these treatments with a competent massage therapist is often synergistic.

As stated previously, the quality of the hormones reflects the health of an owner. However, the quality of life energy flow patterns determine which hormones become possible. For example, before stressed owners secrete cortisol, there is an aberration in the life energy, which causes the command for the cortisol secretion. Therefore alternative treatment modalities, which facilitate the normalization of energy flow patterns, will improve the hormone milieu in stressful situations.

On the opposite extreme, when considering muscle, ligament and joint health, are the healing powers contained within the positive emotions. Owners who have rewarding emotional experiences will tend to secrete optimal hormone mixtures. The alternative treatment modalities, like chiropractic, can be extremely helpful to those owners who experience chronic negative emotions in their lives. These owners have an increased likelihood of secreting sub-optimal hormone mixtures that reflect the distressed energetic state. The more quickly that the aberrant energy is released then the less damage caused by hormonal imbalance.

Different emotions have unique impacts within the body tissues. Emotions directly affect the types and amounts of hormones secreted into the blood stream. Athletic competitors have an elevated testosterone level just before a competitive event. The only players who continue to have elevated testosterone levels just after the competition are the winning team.

Another example occurs in those owners who feel overwhelmed and trapped within a negative life situation. These owners will tend to have a much higher blood cortisol level. The chronic elevation of the cortisol level will direct body energy into survival pathways and out of the rejuvenation activities necessary for continued vitality. While a given owner is learning to improve the emotional energy quality in his/her daily life, these alternative treatment modalities can often release some of the accumulating static energies. They accomplish this, each in their own way (i.e. chiropractic, acupuncture, homeopathy, neural therapy, massage therapy, yoga exercises, etc.), but the common denominator that they each have is in their ability to optimize the movement of the life energies into a direction of harmony.

Most owners agree that having a human experience is hard work at times. Many people find that there will always be new challenges and disappointments along the path of their life's work. Cultivating an awareness of the options of how to cope allows re-channeling of fresh new life energy. The use of new life energies, to reinvigorate one in times of hardship, allows healing paths to open up. The western medical model of health delivery is like the slab of meat approach. When the intelligent energy considerations are eviscerated from the treatment strategies human beings become slabs of meat. The slab of meat is all that is left when the life force has been removed.

Many owners are leaving mainstream medicine. Many of these owners sense something missing from their conventional treatment. Some holistic physicians would argue that the common denominator between many alternative treatment modalities regards their manipulation of the intelligent life energies towards optimum. The qualities of the life energies are an under-utilized approach in mainstream medicine today. Healing potentials, which consider the life energies, make more sense in the management of the numerous chronic degenerative diseases.

One adjustment technique, which has shown marked promise in the treatment of chronic degenerative disease, is called craniosacral therapy. Craniosacral therapy is a spinal adjustment technique that has great power to heal. It can be viewed as a mechanism for releasing static energy situations within the spine.

A Missoula Montana physician had an interesting encounter with the healing potentials within this discipline last year. Last year while training in a craniosacral therapy class he related the following story. Upon arriving, another M.D. addressed the class and informed them that he was only there because his wife insisted that he attend to help her. Apparently he reluctantly agreed. The Missoula physician was paired up to learn this alternative technique with this gentleman as his partner. While working on this man's spine in the mid-chest area the Doctor noticed an unusual energy release. According to charka theory, this is the center of heart energy. At first he didn't say anything because he suspected it was only his imagination. Suddenly this skeptical doctor asked if he had felt the energy release that he was experiencing. The Missoula physician told him that he did notice an odd sensation. The next morning this doctor came in and exclaimed that he had terrible asthma that required regular intervals of medicine or he would need a rapid intervention in the emergency room to stabilize his breathing. He then said that during the previous evening he had forgotten to take his breathing treatment and medicines. He woke up in the middle of the night remembering his medication. He was pleasantly surprised to notice that he had no breathing difficulty what so ever.

Craniosacral theory would explain that this man suffered from a static energy imbalance within his spine, which was affecting his lungs. The lungs were energetically imbalanced to the point that he was not able to breath without a constant symptom control medical regime. The power contained in moving life energy around is a very important point that this case illustrates.

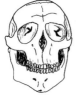
The western medical view has no explanation of this mans healing response. Scientific inconsistencies point the way to better methods of treating a disease. Craniosacral medical theory maintains that human beings contain intelligent energy (life energy). Health can only occur when the life energy flows rhythmically and optimally. When the life energy becomes static or imbalanced then the body becomes diseased.

The Physical Needs of Muscles, Ligaments, and Athletes

Muscle definition and strength provide tangible evidence of the power contained in hormone quality and proper nutrition. Directly observing these two important determiners of muscle and ligament function reveals that something very important is often missing from the physical exam in America today.

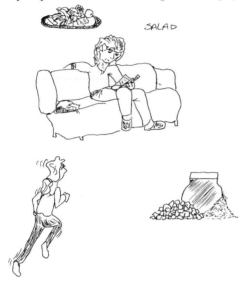

SALAD

The science exists which explains the importance of optimal hormone (types and amounts) and nutritional building blocks for muscle tissue. All other performance enhancers are only marginally effective without these primary determinants. The failure to include this in one's evaluation, in the clinical setting, often contributes to the unnecessary acceleration into old age.

The first determiner is the fact that muscle cells only perform as they are directed. The most powerful directors are the level one hormones. They instruct a muscle cell's DNA program. The types and amounts of these most powerful hormones determine which genes are turned off and which genes are turned on. The steroids, vitamin A, and thyroid hormones are the only hormones that contain this ability. The quality and amounts of the different steroids determine whether the message to the muscle cell DNA is coherent. Coherence or incoherence to the energy direction is analogous to a cellular 'melody' or cellular 'noise'. The incoherent message of noise leads to old age. One way of avoiding old age depends on which DNA programs are activated or suppressed. The quality of the message content determines whether a chaotic genetic program is present or absent. The DNA activity is a powerful determinant of how big and strong a muscle cell becomes.

Muscle cells are excellent examples of the importance of balance between anabolic and catabolic message content. Only when there is proper balance between these two opposing processes can the DNA program direct buildup activities appropriately in the muscle cell. Extremely high anabolic message content occurs in the body builder. These large muscles are only possible with high androgen message content. High androgen message content directs the muscle cell DNA to increase cellular infrastructure investment activities. Muscle development provides an example of the central role of anabolic steroids. Anabolic steroids direct the DNA program to increase cell build up activities.

The muscle cell response to steroids is no different than the other cells through out the body. Other cells in the body respond to appropriate amounts and timing of their preferred anabolic steroid. The difference between muscle cells and other body cells is that each body cell type has a preferred anabolic steroid. For example DHEA is the preferred steroid within the brain. DHT is the preferred steroid for nice skin. The muscles prefer testosterone for their maximal development message.

Muscle cell message content needs to be counterbalanced by the catabolic steroid, cortisol. Cortisol message content is important for maximizing energy while an owner is exercising. The cortisol message is also important to prevent excessive soreness following exercise.

Muscles need an adequate stimulus (exercise) before the gonads and adrenals are summoned to produce increased message content of the anabolic steroids. There is a relationship between muscle use and steroid message content. Maximal muscle development is dependent on both processes. Failure on either end of this equation leads to little muscles.

Exercise results in soreness and annoying injuries (strains) when adrenal and gonad function are impaired. Any owner who suddenly begins to become excessively sore following modest workouts needs a steroid hormone evaluation. Replacement with real steroids may be indicated when a severe hormone deficiency is discovered. Other cases respond nicely to improved diets and nutrients.

Once there has been a complete inquiry into the muscle hormone status of the level one hormones, the 'lesser' hormones can be considered. An example of a level 2 hormone is insulin-like growth factor (IGF). IGF is over one hundred times more plentiful in the blood stream of healthy owners than is insulin. IGF helps muscle cells obtain the nutrition within the blood steam. IGF facilitates the anabolic steroids desire to build bigger and stronger muscles. When IGF is low the anabolic steroid message has less ability to build cells like muscle cells. Muscle cells cannot build without the proper molecular building blocks. IGF and insulin facilitate the absorption of nutrition by muscle cells. Insulin needs increase when IGF falls because insulin becomes the backup system for muscle cell fuel intake.

The relative roles of IGF and insulin in muscle cell nutritional needs have been largely ignored within the mainstream medical approach. Even though in the healthy owner IGF occurs at one hundred times the normal insulin levels, the increase of insulin receives the advertising dollar. The trouble with this approach is that insulin produces many side effects, which IGF does not have. Examples of the differences of the insulin message content within the body are: insulin causes increased cholesterol and triglyceride synthesis within the liver, insulin is more rapidly destroyed without adequate IGF, increased insulin increases appetite, insulin rises after eating while IGF rises during fasting.

Insulin and IGF facilitate the uptake of muscle fuel. However, insulin facilitates a relatively small amount of fuel uptake within muscle cells because it is present in much smaller amounts (less than one percent of IGF levels). Additionally, insulin is only elevated following a carbohydrate meal. IGF levels in healthy owners tend to stay up between meals. Healthy muscles are dependent on adequate IGF levels.

IGF levels are dependent on two factors. First, the liver needs adequate direction from thyroid, DHEA and cortisol. When all three of these hormones are present, these level one hormones instruct the liver to manufacture IGF hormone. However, it is the second factor, which allows the release of IGF from the liver. The second factor is growth hormone (GH). Increased estrogen levels inhibit the release of IGF by GH. Owners who have healthy levels of IGF also have healthy levels of thyroid, DHEA, cortisol, estrogen and GH.

High blood sugar stimulates insulin increases but low blood sugar stimulates IGF release. The opposite is also true. High blood sugar decreases IGF but it is low blood sugar, which decreases insulin release. When IGF is released there has been a preceding release of GH. This is in response to a falling blood sugar, which causes stored sugar to be dumped by the liver into the blood stream. The released IGF then causes the released sugar to be used. IGF levels maintain body cell fuel levels between meals. Insulin maintains liver storage of sugar and fat levels following meals. In this way healthy muscles have access to fuel at all times.

Understanding the relative roles of IGF and insulin are an important biochemical marker of youthfulness within the muscles. It is also important to avoid the popular practice of receiving growth hormone injections without a proper evaluation of the IGF levels. Without a proper evaluation of the IGF levels, GH will tend to promote high blood sugars and therefore increase insulin output. Increased insulin output is associated with all the negative effects on body physique discussed in section two.

The level three hormones affect muscle performance by opening up or closing down the blood supply within the exercising muscle. Deficiency of the level three hormones leads to diminished muscle performance. Adequate supplies of the level three hormones are dependent on adequate protein meals and many vitamins. Examples of level three hormones are: epinephrine, nor-epinephrine, histamine, serotonin, and dopamine. All of these hormones have short active life spans of several minutes. Therefore, the tone of the blood vessels is constantly determined every few minutes by which level three hormones are dominant.

The useful analogy here is in the water system network that underlies many large cities. Fluctuations in demand because of time of day and location necessitate that water engineers open up or tighten down available water supply with numerous different and strategically located check valves throughout the city water supply system. Similar processes are in operation within the body. Understanding ways to direct maximal blood supply into the performing metabolically hungry areas of the body confers a performance advantage on its owner. Under optimal conditions, the body is able to reroute a tremendous increase in blood flow to the active area. Shunting blood away from the less active areas enhances the effect.

The adrenal gland contains two layers. The outer layer is the cortex. The adrenal medulla is the inner layer and manufactures some of the level three hormones.

In order to understand muscle performance the inner core of the adrenal gland's hormonal products needs to be understood. This part of the gland is called the adrenal medulla. It is here that powerful hormones are made that prevent unconsciousness from occurring when one stands up. It is the arterial muscle layer which contract when one stands. The arterial muscles will contract when there are enough level three hormones instructing them to do so. The ability for the arteries to contract or relax is determined in part by the adrenal medulla.

The adrenal medulla is largely responsible for performing the task of the body's 'water engineers'. The city planners design the water system underneath the city but it is the water engineers that constantly decide which valves are turned up and which are turned down. Incompetent water engineers on the staff create inefficient water delivery to certain areas of the city. This is a simplification of what the adrenal medulla does in regards to directing blood flow within the vessels.

The level three hormones task of directing blood flow can only be accomplished correctly if adequate amounts of certain molecular parts are available. Epinephrine is the most desirable of the level three hormones in exercising muscle. Exercising muscle needs sufficient epinephrine levels to direct the blood vessels to open. When the blood vessels supplying muscle open there is an increased supply of fuel and oxygen delivered. The other level three hormones presence competes with this process.

The second determinant of powerful muscles, alluded to above, is the nutritional status of the body. Epinephrine manufacture requires specific nutrients. The adrenal gland needs an adequate supply of either phenylalanine or tyrosine and also numerous cofactors (vitamins). If one or more cofactors is deficient then the adrenals cannot manufacture the most beneficial types of hormone within this class, epinephrine. The necessary cofactors needed for the synthesis of epinephrine are: tetrahydrobiopterin (made from folate), vitamin C, vitamin B6, and SAMe. Since SAMe is used within the body at the rate of one billion times a second, it needs to be recharged with the following nutrients: vitamin B12, folate, serine and methionine.

Epinephrine is a member of the bioactive amines, listed above. They are either called hormones or neurotransmitters. Their site of action determines which class they are in. If it is in between two nerve endings they are called neural transmitters. If they are being discharged into the blood stream (the adrenal medulla is a major site for this but there are other sites through out the body) they are known as hormones.

When bioactive amines are in the blood stream they act as the water engineers, discussed above. All water engineers are not created equal. Peak performance athletes predictably are getting only the best 'water engineers' directing their blood flow. Most owners fail to understand ways to enhance the level three-hormone mixture to obtain more competent water engineers. More competent water engineers lead to better blood flow in the exercising muscles. Nutritional deficiencies prevent the manufacture of adequate epinephrine, which leads to a prematurely diminished athletic performance.

For maximum performance abilities within the muscles epinephrine can be thought of as the master water engineer. It has the informational content to open up the blood vessel diameter leading to the exercising muscles, liver and the heart. Increasing blood flow within the areas of increased metabolic demand obviously allows for better delivery of oxygen, nutrients and the increased ability for waste removal (carbon dioxide, lactic acid, spent cofactors, etc.). The liver needs an increased blood supply during exercise because it is the site of removal and reprocessing of the huge amounts of lactic acid generated within exercising muscles.

Epinephrine is only made when all the cofactors are available because it is at the end of the assembly line for the bioactive amines manufacturing process. When nutritional deficiencies cause the synthesis of epinephrine to decrease there is less instruction for the blood vessels to open up during exercise. Normally during exercise the blood supply to the heart, skeletal muscles and liver is increased because epinephrine is present. However, when epinephrine becomes deficient nor-epinephrine levels will rise. The trouble with increased levels of nor-epinephrine is that its message tightens down the blood supply to the heart, skeletal muscle and liver. The consequence here is that less fuel is delivered to these metabolically active tissues during exercise.

When optimum conditions prevail (youthfulness) the adrenal medulla will make 90% epinephrine. Under healthy conditions, the adrenal only makes 10% nor-epinephrine and dopamine. This has important implications for those owners who desire to feel as good as good as possible when exercising.

One of the most common nutritional deficiencies within the adrenal medulla occurs in what is known as the methyl donor group of substances. When a methyl donor deficiency occurs within the adrenal medulla, there is the inability to convert nor-epinephrine into epinephrine. When these adrenals are stimulated, during exercise, to dump epinephrine into the blood stream they have a diminished ability to do so. Epinephrine release is inadequate because of the methyl donor deficiency. Only epinephrine contains the message to direct blood flow increases to exercising muscles, heart, and the liver.

.   Many owners take the expensive SAMe in a pill to recharge their methyl donor status. This is not always necessary. Supplementing with adequate serine, vitamin B12, vitaminB6 and folate often will recharge the deficient methyl donor state. It is important to remember that these bioactive amines within the adrenal are made from tyrosine or phenylalanie. A functional digestive tract needs to be involved (digestion section). There are other cofactors needed to manufacture epinephrine from tyrosine. These are tetrahydrobiopteran, vitamin C and adequate cellular magnesium.

The exercising muscles discussion concludes the organ systems and longevity principles contained within the manual. The last section provides a perspective of what needs to be checked before healing paths can be created. Most owners wait until at least mid-life before they have the revelation about their demise being somewhere in the future. This realization leads some to begin to want renewed health. Others could care less and that's OK. The last section is for the owners who want to know some of the basic tests that can better evaluate how bad off they are. The body report card so generated provides a baseline from which healing can begin.

SECTION 7

100,000 MILE EXAM AND TUNE UP

100,000-Mile Exam

Middle age to the body is analogous to a car with one hundred thousand miles on its odometer. How the car has been maintained, accident history, quality of replacement parts, quality of fuel, and how it has been used begins to show at the one hundred thousand mile point. It is the same with an owner's body at the middle age.

Many owners have experienced life-changing realizations at this point in the life cycle. Some receive their wake up when they take a long hard look at themselves naked in the mirror. They ask themselves the hard question that day that had been buried beneath layers of denial for years. How long will this body last? This question is usually followed by a second question regarding whether or not they will suffer as they near the end.

The doctor sees evidence that some things about the earthling experience are fairly typical. The hard question that occurs around middle age is one such example. Not all owners ask this question while they are naked in front of a mirror, but sooner or later they ask it. Sooner or later they also ask it honestly.

At this point of connection, with their need for a functional body, they usually seek guidance on how to repair some of the damage that one hundred thousand miles of living has inflicted. Who they trust and obtain advice from will be a big determinant of the success or failure of the achievement for healthy longevity.

This book has been about the other side of the story of what science has revealed. It concerns the maintenance of health. This section is about applying these seven principles when an owner reaches the point in their life where they are ready to ask the hard question. The one hundred thousand mile exam involves an assessment of where an owner stands in regard to the seven principles of longevity. If they can obtain a report card on all seven determinants, they are in a better position to take an active role in their own healing.

PRINCIPLE 1: An assessment of rust promoting mechanisms
History:
1. Deficiency of anti-inflammatory fatty acids
2. Diabetes
3. Obesity
4. Excessive consumption of oxidized fats
5. Nutritional deficiencies that promote rust
6. Excessive exposure to oxidizing agents
7. Abnormal hormone message content exposure history
8. Tobacco abuse
9. Male gender

Physical signs of rust:
1. Premature gray hair
2. Reading glasses before age forty-five when compared to normal vision when younger
3. Premature wrinkles
4. Shortness of breath
5. Protein in the urine
6. Retinal vessel changes
7. Certain nail changes
8. Leg hair distribution decrease

PRINCIPLE 2: An assessment of the loss of flexibility mechanisms

High blood pressure is a sign of this problem, but there are many fixable causes.

History for high blood pressure causality:
1. Magnesium deficiency
2. Increased insulin level
3. Increased sodium intake and/or decreased potassium intake
4. Stiffened red blood cells
5. Methyl donor deficiency
6. Nitric oxide deficiency
7. Syndrome X (duet to increased insulin and cortisol)
8. Abnormal hormonal fats

EXTENSION OF PRINCIPLE 1 is the opportunistic mechanisms that accelerate rust formation, but require its initial presence from some other rust promoter.

1. The additional abnormal hormones that direct the liver to manufacture the sticky fats (LDL and VLDL cholesterol)
   a) Additional nutritional deficiencies that inhibit the burning of fat for energy
   b) Nutritional deficiencies that inhibit carbohydrate fuel combustion in the presence of oxygen.

Lab that concern principle 1:
1. Fasting insulin levels
2. Fasting IGF-1 levels
3. Prolactin levels
4. HDL, LDL, and triglycerides level

    5.   Blood sugar level
    6.   Homocysteine level
    7.   Dark field microscopy of blood cells

PRINCIPLE 3: The Hormones Giveth and the Hormones Taketh Away

An assessment for the presence of obesity and the amount of involvement of the seven different hormones

    1.   High insulin states
    2.   High cortisol states
    3.   Diminished androgen states
    4.   Increased estrogen states
    5.   Diminished thyroid states
    6.   Diminished epinephrine states with increased nor-epinephrine
    7.   Diminished IGF-1 levels

The health of the adrenal system

    1.   An assessment of the stress level
    2.   An assessment of the six links of their adrenal chain of health
    3.   A twenty-four hour urine test for adrenal steroids quality and amounts
    4.   A valuable clue about adrenal dysfunction concerns the appearance of either an increased eosinophil count or a right shift in the white blood cells. A right shift is evidenced by an increased lymphocyte and decreased leukocyte count. These changes are consistently present with autoimmune disease but conventional medicine fails to unite these clues of association.

Ovary health in women

    1.   An assessment that defines the level of balance between estrogens and progesterone
    2.   An assessment includes how functional the androgen status is for muscles, joints and skeleton for cellular rejuvenation.
    3.   An assessment of the six links of the ovary chain of health

Informational substances: assess how wisely an owner spends available body energy. The informational substances (hormones) determine the direction of body energy expenditure.

Steroid tone and its six determinants:

1. Adrenal and gonad health
2. Nutritional adequacy
3. Genetics
4. Environmental toxins
5. Emotional qualities operating within
6. Secretogogues

The four misunderstood steroids inclusion in the evaluation by using a twenty-four hour urine test

1. Aldosterone
2. Thyroid
3. Vitamin A
4. Vitamin D

Thyroid health

1. The seven links in the thyroid chain of health need to be considered in all patients
2. Vitamin A adequacy - it is necessary for thyroid message content to manifest
3. Adrenal adequacy is a permissive determinant for normal thyroid function

Testicle health in men

1. Twenty-four hour urine test for testicle produced steroids
2. Assessment of estrogen mimics and estrogen status
3. IGF-1 levels interplay with the steroids
4. The joints, skeleton, skin, muscle mass, and personality provide valuable clues about testicle health

Hierarchy of hormones assessment

1. Level 1 - the generals of the hormones
2. Level 2 - the polypeptides
3. Level 3 – the biogenic amines
4. Level 4 – the 'vocal' hormones

PRINCIPLE 4: You Are What You Absorb (two components to this)
1. Digestive tract integrity
   a) Adequacy of the different juices in the different digestion chambers
   b) Proper hormones that communicate with other chambersInjury history or presence to digestive chambers
2. Nutritional adequacy of the molecular replacement parts
   a) Amino acid quality for all twenty different amino acids
   b) Essential fatty acid intake
   c) Fiber
   d) Bacteria helpers
   e) Adequate fats in the diet
   f) Intact vitamins and amount
   g) Relative mineral intake ratios and amounts
   h) Appropriate carbohydrates consumption for activity and fitness level
3. Quality of body protein
   a) Quality of body carbohydrate content
   b) Adequacy of the four different types of fat roles
   c) Cell structure and H20 retention
   d) Fuel
   e) Hormone precursors
   f) Brain fat adequacy
   g) Pancreas hormones and the opposing counter-regulatory hormones
4. Assessment of the torture chamber effect in the diet

PRINCIPLE 5: Taking out the cellular trash adequacy
The thyroid message content allows all six-trash removal organ systems to function properly.

1. Kidney
2. Lungs
3. Skin
4. Liver
5. Colon (section three)
6. Immune system (section five)

Steroid Pressure - signs of decrease show up on the periphery first.

1. Skin health
2. Joint health
3. Bone health

PRINCIPLE 6: the adequacy of cellular charge assessment

1. Cellular charge is dependent on the optimal ratios of potassium, sodium, magnesium, and calcium. After middle age this can only occur with a consistent real food diet instead of a processed food diet.
2. Cellular charge in the brain and heart will decrease around middle age if the above minerals are not consumed in the proper ratios.
3. Chronic stress depletes cellular charge because the mineral ratios become altered
4. Aldosterone levels need to be sufficient for the maintenance of cellular charge especially of the nerve and heart conduction systems
   a) A separate benefit of adequate aldosterone is the stimulation of continued steroids biosynthesis
5. Thyroid needs to be adequate for nerve and heart conduction health to occur.
6. Certain trace minerals like vanadium and chromium injure the red blood cells electrical charge by inhibiting the sodium and potassium ATPase pump. This increases serum potassium and is the reason that insulin sensitivity improves (insulin's fuel uptake role is dependent on available potassium).
7. The immune system is the prototypical organ system that illustrates the principle of cellular charge.
8. Fluoride and iodide inhibit energy packet formation in the red blood cell.
9. The digestive tract integrity affects cellular charge because it secretes over seven quarts of various concoctions of minerals daily. In all it absorbs over nine quarts of mineral and nutrients daily.
10. Pancreatic Beta cells release GABA, which hyperpolarizes (increases cellular charge) the alpha cells.
11. Calcium pummels sperm heads when cervical mucus contains progesterone.
12. Nerve cells relax and are fed when they encounter progesterone because GABA is released and these cells hyperpolarize with chloride.
13. Niacin intake leads to increased red blood cell cellular charge because of the increased formation of NADH (this can lead to decreased potassium availability secondary to potassium sequestration that can lead to insulin resistance).
14. Red blood cell deformability and cellular charge.
15. Vitamin deficiency and its effects on cellular charge.
16. Hypoxia in the EMF environment.

17. Toxemia of pregnancy is secondary to a progesterone deficiency that leads to decreased GABA and a diminished chloride channel activity
    a) Pancreas
    b) CNS
    c) Red blood cells
18. There is a electrical sucking grid that pulls in adequate water to inflate cells that otherwise would become squished flat by gravitational forces. When this system fails the owner begins to have the look of old age.
    a) Joints
    b) Skin
    c) Lining of the inside surface of the blood vessels
    d) Lining of the respiratory tract
    e) Lining of the digestive tube
    f) The space between neighboring cells called the intersitial space

PRINCIPLE 7: The Energies That Heal Contrasted to the Energies That Maim

The rhythm of the heart beat
1. The intelligence behind the intelligence
2. Life is vibrational
3. Homeopathy and how it expands understanding of life's underpinnings
4. Acupuncture another clue about defects in the western model of the universe
5. Emotional energies that confer rhythm on cells.
6. Emotional energies that confer chaos on cells.
7. The summation of the integrity of the energy template determines which hormones are secreted and therefore determines functional ability at the highest level.
8. Counseling on which of the alternative disciplines (chiropractic, acupuncture, homeopathy, yoga, prayer, message, or breath work) is right for releasing the chaotic energies that maim the body cells. Each owner has unique needs and the discipline that works for one may be uncomfortable to another.

Finding a holistically trained medical doctor is rare. As of this writing Naturopaths, Chiropractors, and Acupuncturist may be the surest way to begin the seven principled healing plan.   There are several thousand alternatively minded medical doctors scattered throughout the country.   Many belong to either the American Holistic Medical Association or the American College for the Advancement of Medicine.

Good luck and God bless.

APENDICES

Apendix A

HOMEOPATHY

Homeopathy is the simplest form of medicinal prescription and the most straightforward example of the scientific method applied to medicine. The origins of homeopathic medicine go back to 1796 when Samuel Hahnemann wrote his first article discussing the law of similar, in Latin "similia similibus" or "likes are treated by likes". He meant that if a pharmacologically active substance was capable of producing symptoms in a healthy individual, then it would cure those same symptoms in someone who is ill. (Essay on a New Principle for Ascertaining the Curative Power of Drugs Lesser Writings p.249). Before this time medicines were tested on animals or in the chemical laboratory. The assumption was that a medicine acts in the human body in the same manner as it acts in the laboratory. Hahnemann codified his method in the classic text, **_Organon of the Medical Art_**. This book is still the main text used to train homeopaths in the classical method. The underlying philosophy of homeopathy is that the vital force or the basic internal energy of the person is reflected to the outside world in the form of symptoms, whether mental or physical. This is the information, which the homeopath must obtain to find the right remedy each person.

Classical Homeopathy has 3 Basic Tenets

1. The Minimum Dose

This is the smallest dose necessary to create a healing effect. Hahnemann was incensed by the "un inquiring (sic) repetition of the inanities of the great grandfathers of medicine repeated by their great grandsons in regards to the use of dosages of medicines, let us ask nature" (from Lesser Writings, p. 385). He wanted to use healthy human subjects to ascertain the exact effects of small doses (i.e. 1/1,000,000 of a grain).

Claude Bernard (1813-1878) is credited with the idea of experimental medicine. It is clear that Hahnemann originated this idea, as early as 1801. His technique of giving a group of healthy people a medicine in a low dose and recording their symptoms is known as a proving. This method is still the way new remedies are discovered in homeopathy today. This allows nature to demonstrate how a medicine will act in the human body. Every medicinal substance has a particular vibrational affinity or resonance within the human body. Every medicinal substance will create specific symptoms when ingested. Hahnemann reasoned that if this affinity is true then a small dose of the same medicine stimulates the innate healing responses of the body. This hypothesis was tested, using the scientific method, and proved.

A Homeopathic dose may be written as 12c or 200x or some similar alphanumeric code. The process of serial dilution and succussion between each dilution step makes these medicines. Succussion is to strike the vial containing the medicine against a hard, but resilient surface, like a book. To create a remedy of the plant Arnica Montana one would first macerate the plant and mix it with ethyl alcohol and water. This helps to extract the medicinal properties while leaving behind the cellulose and other inert plant materials. The liquid is then strained off. This mixture is called the mother tincture and is the basis for all homeopathic remedies. To make remedies of the C or centesimal potency, mix one drop of mother tincture with 100 drops of alcohol. To make the X or decimal potency mixes 10 drops of alcohol with one drop of mother tincture.

The mixture is then succussed 100 times. Next a drop of the new mixture is added to either 10 or 100 drops of alcohol and the process is repeated. The number of the remedy indicates the number of serial dilutions and succussions. The letter is the Roman numeral of the type of dilution process used to create the remedy.

2. The Single Remedy

Hahnemann's single remedy did not imply a single chemical element. Each homeopathic remedy is composed of a single source of chemical molecules. (i.e. only using Arnica Montana leaves). Each of Hahnemann's homeopathic remedies had been proved by the homeopathic method, (e. g, to observe their effects on a population of healthy humans). The homeopathic method does not prescribe any medication, unless it has demonstrated its effectiveness for a symptom. The homeopathic method prescribes a medication, which has produced a specific response in a population of healthy people that is identical to the symptoms presented by the patient. The homeopath chooses the remedy that most closely matches the patient's symptoms and gives it in a very minute dose. These medications cause an artificial or sympathetic vibration that stimulates the defense mechanisms. The body's defense mechanism dissipates the symptom complex.

3. The Totality of Symptoms

Homeopathic medications can be used for their general effect. This use of homeopathic medication is not the homeopathic method. The classic homeopathic remedy must be prescribed using all symptoms that can be elicited from the patient. The more precise the symptom picture the more effective the prescribed homeopathic remedy becomes. Individuality is the key to the classical homeopathic prescription.

Remedies work by stimulating the internal energy of the body. The preparation of the remedies contains very little or no physical substance.

According to a principle of chemistry known as Avogadro's number there can theoretically be no physical substance left in the preparation after the twelfth dilution step. Most of the remedies used in homeopathy are well above twelve dilution steps. Some homeopathic remedies include thousands of dilutions steps.

These preparations carry very subtle vibrations that have a very profound effect on the human body. Physical ailments (such as pneumonia and tuberculosis) and emotional imbalances have been successfully treated with homeopathic remedies for over 200 years.

Homeopathy is clear and simple in its scientific explanation. It is one of the most challenging clinical practices because it demands the practitioner to proceed with an absolutely unprejudiced mind and extreme attention to detail. Only in this way can the homeopathic physician see the person as they are and prescribe the correct remedy.

Apendix B

ACUPUNCTURE

The correct remedy, acupuncture is one of the oldest forms of medicine in the world with a written history of more than 3,500 years. The therapy is accomplished by the insertion of fine needles into very specifically located points on the human body. These points may also be stimulated by burning moxa herb (Artemisia vulgaris) directly on the point, by using a cigar shaped stick held near the point or by attaching the herb directly to the needle.

The Chinese name of acupuncture is Jin Jiu, which means Needle/Heat. This expresses the way in which acupuncture was actually practiced. The name acupuncture comes from the misapprehension of the French Jesuit priests in the 1600s. When the Jesuits observed the practice in China they used the Latin "acu" meaning 'needle' and "punctura" meaning 'puncture' to describe what they saw. The Jesuits did not attempting to translate the Chinese name.

In the theory of Chinese Medicine, of which acupuncture is only one of many branches, the manipulation of the energy (Qi) of the body is the main purpose. Energy flows through the body on channels or conduits called meridians. Any disturbance in the flow is believed to be the cause of all illness or infirmary. This includes physical ailments and mental/emotional problems. The Chinese make no distinction between the mind, body, and spirit. The meridians, even though they each have a separate name and a distinct function are individual components of one continuous flow of energy throughout the body. They appear as separate entities but are an uninterrupted pattern of energy movement that encompasses the entire human energy systems.

One of the main theoretical foundations of acupuncture is called the Five Phase Law. This is also sometimes referred to as the Five Element Law. It holds that each of the twelve meridians of the body is ruled by an element: Fire, Earth, Metal, Water, and Wood. Four meridians are contained within the fire element and two each for the remaining four elements. Each of these phases or elements is a representative way to assess energy movement in the body. They are used to characterize very specific relationships between the different elements and the different meridians. These relationships are very exacting and have been reproducibly observable for millennia.

The two pillars of Oriental Medicine can analyze each of these elements and their accompanying meridians. The two pillars are diagnosis by looking at the tongue and feeling the pulse. The tongue is analyzed for its shape, color and coating, observing the tongue will reveal the character of the energy in each meridian.

The pulse is taken from the radial artery at the wrist in three positions and at two depths. Each of these positions and depths is a direct reflection of the movement and character of the energy of each individual meridian. The skilled acupuncturists can read the energy of the entire body by these two methods. He may then determine where energy may be stuck or obstructed and determine an acupuncture prescription to alleviate the disturbance.

An interruption or block to the energy flowing through the meridians can come from a physical trauma, a stressful event, dietary indiscretions or other causes. When the meridian flow is changed then the physical, chemical and mental/ emotional changes related to that meridian occur. These blockages or disturbed flows may be altered in a positive way by many methods including diet, herbs, massage, but most efficiently and directly with acupuncture.

Oriental medical practitioners realized centuries ago that every body process is controlled by energy from thought and movement on a macroscopic level, and by biochemical and cellular processes on a microscopic level. Acupuncture, with its specific energetic approach to the processes of the body, allows the practitioner to directly access the human energy system in away that is not possible by any other means. The acupuncturists can directly influence the function of the various internal organs, body processes, and emotional reactions by the judicious insertion of needles. These patterns of needle placement are a continuation of a tradition contained in thousands of years old oriental medical old Oriental medical texts.

Apendix C

The Chiropractic and Osteopathic Perspectives

Neuromechanical Integrity and Health

The art of joint manipulation dates back to antiquity and has been passed on for generations in many traditions. Hippocrates made extensive references to it in his treatises and it has always been an essential component of Chinese medicine. The first formalized institutions specializing in manipulation were not established until the second half of the nineteenth century. Osteopathy and chiropractic were founded in the United States in 1874 and 1895, respectively. Both professions use similar techniques and procedures, some of which were incorporated from the European tradition of bone setting. The theory and rational of the two professions is different. Early osteopaths operated on the premise that osteopathic manipulation restored health by improving circulation while early chiropractors believed that the chiropractic adjustment restored health by reducing interference to the nervous system. Modern research has suggested that both theories are partially true.

There are many similarities in the history and evolution of chiropractic and osteopathy. There are also many differences. Both professions tend to treat the body holistically. Osteopaths also include drugs and surgery in their practice, Traditional medicine strongly condemned both professions as being unscientific and dangerous, because osteopathy and chiropractic emphasized the role of proper joint mechanics with good health. Osteopathy abandoned many of its traditional practices in the 1960's in order to become more acceptable to mainstream health care. Currently osteopaths are the equivalent to medical doctors and very few practice manipulation.

This is paradoxical because the profession was innovative and published a great deal of novel research in the 1940's and 1950's. Many of the soft tissue techniques used today have their roots in osteopathy. Chiropractic, however, refused to abandon its basic paradigm and is still harassed by traditional medicine.

The AMA had evidence that chiropractic was more effective than traditional medicine in treating certain conditions, it made it unethical for member physicians to associate with chiropractors. It was considered unethical for members to accept referrals from chiropractors, teach chiropractors, or provide diagnostic services for chiropractors. The AMA publicly denounced chiropractic as an unscientific cult and court testimony revealed that the AMA used lies and fabrications to proceed with its agenda of eliminating chiropractic.

These confrontations reached a climax in the 1970's when a class action, anti-trust suit was filed against the AMA and several other defendants by members of the chiropractic profession. In 1990 the United States Court of

Appeals ruled that the AMA had engaged in an illegal conspiracy to destroy the chiropractic profession. As a result of the court decision, chiropractors now have staff privileges in hospitals across the country, work with physicians in numerous high profile, multi-disciplinary clinics, and, after a very successful trial period, are now commissioned in the United States armed services.

Even though spinal manipulation is one of the most validated forms of treatment for back pain and headaches, there are still those critics who denounce it as unscientific and dangerous. Ironically, Many of there critics, who claim to be champions of the scientific method, frequently make statements about chiropractic and spinal manipulation that are in direct conflict with the scientific facts. These critics have, however, motivated segments of the chiropractic profession to use critical thinking skills and engage in quality research.

During the past 25 years a great deal of research has gone into spinal manipulation and mechanical joint dysfunction. Mechanical joint dysfunction, called the osteopathic or somatic lesion by osteopaths and subluxation complex by chiropractors, can be caused by many factors. These include trauma, the compression forces of gravity, stress, repetitive motions, poor ergonomics, bad posture, and childbirth.

It is now becoming evident from the research that mechanical joint dysfunction occurs when movable (diarthrodial) joints become locked and restricted. This causes the pain generating tissue of the joint complex to become irritated leading to spasm, congestion, inflammation and pain. Subsequently, there is a buildup of inflammatory toxins (including leukotrienes, cytokines, prostaglandins, and lactic acid) that can damage the connective tissue and the sensory and proprioceptive nerves. The loss of normal motion also reduces mechanoreceptor stimulation, which results in propriaceptive loss. The aberrant and compensatory motion patterns that result, add further sensory irritation to the nervous system. Irritation of the nervous system causes a vicious cycle of pain, spasm, and inflammation.

Skillfully applied joint manipulation restores motion to the joint complex, which subsequently, decongests the area and flushes the toxins. When the normal mechanical properties of the joints are restored the irritation subsides and the tissues gradually heal. It is now generally accepted by the medical community that spinal manipulation is effective in treating many musculoskeletal conditions and relieving the symptoms associated with these conditions.

Chiropractors and osteopaths have noticed that their patients frequently report improvements in other areas of their life following their treatments. A Recent study in Sweden found that, overall, 23% of the patients adjusted reported improvement in the non-musculoskeletal symptoms. Of those patients whom had four areas of their spine adjusted, this number increased to 25%. Among the most common non-musculoskeletal symptoms included improved breathing, improved digestive function, sharper vision, improved circulation and improved menstrual function.

While there have been numerous studies published relating to the efficacy of spinal manipulation on musculoskeletal conditions, there have been relatively few published on non-musculoskeletal conditions. There have been a few studies suggesting that spinal manipulation may be of benefit in treating asthma, various pulmonary conditions, dysmenorrheal, otitis media, migraines, and certain types of visual disturbances. Some people believe it is outrageous to suggest that spinal manipulation can help anything other than musculoskeletal conditions.

There is abundant research to suggest a plausible mechanism that explains this phenomenon. It has been demonstrated repeatedly that sustained irritation to certain peripheral sensory nerves can lead to facilitation (stimulation) of the autonomic nervous system. The autonomic nervous system, which governs circulation and affects nearly every organ and gland in the body, has nerve reflex centers throughout the spinal cord. Certain types of pain receptors can stimulate these nerve centers. The constant firing of these receptors theoretically can cause and imbalance in the autonomic function.

Mechanical joint dysfunction is a source of sensory irritation to the spinal cord. This mechanical joint dysfunction may lead to facilitation of either the sympathetic or parasympathetic components of the autonomic nervous system, depending on the level or irritation. This might account for the wide variety of conditions that appear to have improved following chiropractic and osteopathic treatments. Osteopathic researchers coined the term "sustained sypatheticotonia" to describe this phenomenon while chiropractors prefer to call it a somatovisceral reflex. Our understanding of the intricate network of reflexes is in the central nervous system is in its infancy. Much more research is needed before we have a definitive understanding of the mechanisms involved.

Many soft tissue and ancillary techniques have evolved from the osteopathic and chiropractic professions. Perhaps the best known is CranioSacral therapy. At the turn of the century osteopathic physician William G Sutherland observed that the cranium consists of multiple inter-locking sections of bones that are capable of very small amount of movement. He postulated that when these bones become locked and restricted there is an interruption of the rhythmic flow of the cerebral spinal fluid from the brain to the sacrum. In 1977 osteopathic researcher Dr John E Upledger elaborated on the procedures developed by Dr Sutherland and others. He developed the technique known as CranioSacral.

This technique is a gentle, hands-on therapy that focuses on relieving restrictions in the sutures of the skull and connective tissues of the body, especially those surrounding the cranium and sacrum. It is theorized that these restrictions are related to chronic pain and emotional dysfunctions. CranioSacral has evolved into a very popular technique practiced by physicians and other trained health care professionals throughout the world.

There have been suggestions that spinal manipulation works on a level involving the subtle energies of the body. Chinese medicine has maintained that chi (the subtle energy that flows through the acupuncture meridians) does not flow well through diseased tissues. Other researchers have speculated that these energies flow poorly through disorganized tissues including scar tissue, fibrotic tissue, and inflamed tissue. Many of the most important postulated channels of subtle energy flow through or are adjacent to the spine. One theory is that using spinal manipulation to restore normal mechanics and vascular function to the spinal joints and surrounding tissues, the movement of energies through these tissues may be improved.

In summary, joint manipulation has a long, colorful history. Chiropractors currently provide 94% of the manipulation in the United States and carry the burden of substantiating its efficacy. With the increased acceptance and popularity of manipulation, the osteopathic profession has shown renewed interest in the subject. In Europe, many physiotherapists are trained in manipulation while in the Unite States physical therapists are now attempting to enter the field. These professions and modalities are evolving due to the creative professionals who are open to alternative forms of healing.

Apendix D

NATUROPATHIC MEDICINE

The foundations of Naturopathic medicine are found in medical models from around the world. Naturopathic medicine blends modern scientific knowledge with Natural Medicine.

The foundation of Naturopathic medicine is constructed from medical models of many cultures. Naturopathic medicine blends modern scientific knowledge with the centuries of medical experience from western and other cultures. All styles of medical practice have had good and bad aspects to them and Naturopathic medicine draws from the most effective aspects of all those styles. The growth of Naturopathic medicine has occurred like other structured organizations.

The growth of naturopathic medicine results from three factors. First, it has the ability to develop effective and ethical practices. Second, it involves the practice of methods that includes experimentation, observation, and deduction. Third, it conducts research towards testing the validity of current practices and developing new data, which serves as the basis for improved practices. The Naturopathic profession is based on the belief that growth, change, and creativity result in improved methods and modalities. The profession of Naturopathic medicine provides its practitioners an environment that encourages creative investigation and problem solving.

Historically, physicians and healers had an understanding of human health and the complex processes called healing. This understanding sometimes exceeds modern medical understanding. Simple, safe, non-toxic methods of treatment for many non-life threatening health conditions have been replaced by what is for sale by the complex. Modern physicians believe that if it is not taught in medical school, it is not valid. Naturopathic medical schools teach progressive modern medical techniques, and the older, still-valid healing techniques. These techniques are taught in medical history classes, therapeutic treatment classes, and in clinical settings.

The Naturopathic physician has comprehensive training in many different treatment modalities including:

The biochemical healing energies are used contained in herbs, vitamins, amino acids, lipids, glandulares, natural hormones, and general nutrition. These can be given orally and intravenously (IV-injected into a vein), depending upon the physical requirements of the healing process. Certain levels of degeneration or dysfunction require more aggressive intervention.

Enhancing digestive functions for healthy absorption, proper immune function, and healthy waste removal. Unhealthy intestinal function can be a source of toxin and inflammation stress.

Trash removal through enhanced liver, kidney, skin, intestinal, and cellular detoxification and drainage. Some toxicity can be treated simply. Others, such as heavy metals, need to be addressed more aggressively with special metal binding agents.

Enhancing Body System Communication on cellular, nervous system, hormonal, and emotional levels. This includes nutrition for cellular charge and biochemical function. Natural hormones are used to balance or enhance cellular, tissue, and emotional function. Acupuncture and Neural therapy improve autonomic (automatic) nervous system functions and normalize cell charge. Modalities such as homeopathy, Bach Flower remedies, and emotional and spiritual counseling are used to promote the health, healing, and life energies of the human body system and in eliminating toxic trash.

ND's learn the fine aspects of functional communication in the internal world of the patient and the external world of human relations. Quality cellular and organ system relations are dependent upon quality communication.

The training and medical practice of Naturopathic physicians is based on six principles which include:

1. **First do no harm (Primum no nocere) -** A universal tenant in medicine that is the primary principle of naturopathic medicine. All other principles of Naturopathic medicine support this principle.

2. **Treat the Whole Person -** Higher levels of health function and personal growth require harmony on all levels of being, including the mental, emotional, physical, biochemical, and spiritual levels. These are important components of the living cellular symphony that is the human life. The potential for health evolves as each body cell and multi-cellular section evolves. Many emotional markers measure the quality of cellular "music". These include: joy, happiness, love of life, lack of disease, high levels of energy, physical strength and endurance, quality sex drive and function, healthy skin and joints, good digestion, and emotional stability.

3. **Doctor as teacher (Docere) -** The Latin root of "doctor" is "teacher". An important part of healing is learning and understanding the disease process. ND's teach their patients about the disease process so that the patient can actively participate in the healing process. The doctor is also a learner. The naturopathic physician listens, observes, and conducts physical and laboratory examinations. The doctor will assess the patient presentation. The doctor analyses body chemistry, mental, emotional, and physical symptoms, habitual patterns, family patterns,

and psychological health of the patient. The final and most important part of the interaction is teaching the patient exactly what is happening, why it is happening, and how to promote higher levels of health function. The Naturopathic physician provides support to the patient during the challenges of healing, change, and life. It is the job of the physician teacher to help the patient resolve the victim mentality and become an informed and self-empowered person.

4. **Treat the cause (Tolle Causam) -** Instead of viewing symptoms as the enemy to be attacked, symptoms are viewed as interpretable expressions arising from an underlying cause. The body will not generally start expressing symptoms without a reason. This is where the doctor needs to be a detective in the process that is broader than diagnosis. Skin conditions, congestion, allergies, inflammation, fatigue, obesity, diabetes, heart disease, PMS, anxiety, irritability, to name a few, are usually secondary consequences to other treatable systemic conditions. Treating the causes of these conditions prevents decay of the quality of life and health. Treating only the symptoms allows the cause to continue festering.

5. **The Healing Power of Nature (Vis Medicatrix Naturae) -** ND's have been trained to honor the innate intelligent nature of life and health in all living things. Providing the right building blocks combined with removing the active causes will assist the cellular systems to regain and build higher levels of health and life.

   There is a world of biochemical and physiologic substances that come from Nature. ND's promote healing by using these substances. The ND physician is trained to understand the biochemical compatibility of medicines and to honor the intelligent nature of healing while using these medicines. Sometimes the healing process is a simple process. Other times it requires a more invasive, less natural, intervention. An objective physician can assess the patient's condition and provide the appropriate intervention.

6. **Prevention is the best cure.** The identification of risk factors, identification of biochemical imbalances, promoting healthy life-style choices, are used to relieve immediate symptom complaints and illnesses. These practices prevent the progression of the dysfunction on into a disease. The majority of all disease processes are preventable. The ND can assist the patient to develop the self-management of the patient's health. The ND can also provide alternatives to the unhealthy practices of the patient. The self-management techniques used by the patient can prevent the need for more complex body repair work.

   Prevention also includes maintaining a healthy physical and emotional environment. Chemical and emotional trash will poison our societies and physical environment. In order to minimize the accumulation of cellular (biochemical) and emotional (energetic) garbage we need to prevent the poisons from entering our environments and food chains. The Naturopathic profession is a vigorous advocate of ecologic and social health reform.

The practice patterns of Naturopaths are varied. The creative environment encouraged by the Naturopathic profession results in experimentation and investigation. This professional atmosphere allows NP's to rely on an eclectic and broad spectrum of modalities. This atmosphere also permits other N.D.'s to specialize, and limit their practice to a very narrow range, much like the specialists in traditional medicine. Due to the variety of treatment tools and philosophical beliefs within the profession, there are many types of naturopathic doctors to choose from. The patient must feel free to investigate the N.D.'s in his/her vicinity and chose the most appropriate physician for his/her individual needs. The naturopathic physicians who have been in practice for more than a few years will be able to proficiently assist the treatment of most general healthcare issues.

The licensing requirements of Naturopathic Medicine are currently in a state of flux. Not all naturopaths are created the same. The licensing issues have had a negative impact on the consistency of training required to practice naturopathic medicine, throughout the United States. There are loopholes that allow some mail-order type schools to offer unregulated doctorate degrees in naturopathy. These mail-order degrees are offered without any actual classroom education, clinical supervision, or laboratory experience. In the states that do not require professional licensing of naturopathic doctors (N.D.'s), these mail-order degree participants are able to call themselves doctors of naturopathic medicine without regulation. It is just important to distinguish between the quality and depth of expertise of ND's you may encounter, especially in the unlicensed states.

The profession of Naturopathic medicine proposes that safety and competency factors must continue to be associated and maintained with the term doctor. Licensing needs to be supported and incorporated on a national level. The licensing is needed to support freedom of choice and to help the public differentiate those with a true post-graduate doctorate education from the simpler self-taught natural healthcare provider.

The potential for growth, healing, and evolution are infinite. Each human being is a cell playing in the symphony of the human consciousness. Naturopathic medicine is committed to achieve high levels of health for patients, the social and physical environment. Naturopathic medicine's creative and holistic approach to treatment is a positive and effective contribution to global healing process.

Endnotes

[1] Schwarzbein, Diana, M.D. The Schwarzbein Principle. Deerfield Beach Florida: Health Communications Inc. 1999

[2] Sears, Barry, Ph.D., et al. *Enter the Zone.* New York: HarperCollins Publishers, Inc., 1995

[3] Lee, John R., M.D., et al. *What Your Doctor May Not Tell You About Premenopause.* New York: Warner Books, Inc., 1999

[4] Atkins, Robert C., M.D. *Dr. Atkins' New Diet Revolution.* 2nd ed. New York: Evans and Company, Inc. 1999

[5] Cooney, Craig, et al. *Methyl Magic, Maximum Health Through Methylation.* Andrews McMeel Publishing, Kansas City.

[6] Whitaker, Julian M.D. *Dr. Whitaker's Guide to Natural Healing.* Rocklin, CA: Prima Publishing, 1995

[7] Jefferies, William Mck. M.D. Safe Uses of Cortisol. Second Edition. Springfield: Charles C. Thomas Publisher, LTD, 1996

[8] Lee, John R., M.D., *idem*

[9] Pert, Candace B., Ph.D. *The Molecules of Emotion.* New York: Simon and Schuster, Inc., 1997

[10] Reiss, Uzzi, M.D., et al. *Natural Hormone Balance for Woman,* New York: Pocket Books, 2001.

[11] Shippen, Eugene, M.D., et al. *The Testosterone Syndrome.* New York: M. Evans and Company, Inc., 1998

[12] Sears, Barry, Ph.D., *idem*

[13] Sears, Barry, Ph.D., *ibid*

[14] Atkins, Robert C., M.D. *Dr. Atkins' New Diet Revolution.* 2nd ed. New York: Evans and Company, Inc. 1999

[15] Sapolsky, Robert M., *Stress, the Aging Brain, and the Mechanism of Neuron Death.* Cambridge, MA: The MIT Press, 1992.

[16] Whitaker, Julian M.D., *idem*

[17] Wright, Jonathan V., M.D. and Gaby, Alan, M.D. *Nutritional Therapy in Medical Practice.* Doubletree Seattle Airport Hotel, October 16-19.

[18] Wright, Jonathan V., M.D., et al., ibem.

[19] Bland, Jeffery S., Ph.D., ed. *Clinical Nutrition: A Functional Approach.* Gig Harbor, WA: Institute for Functional Medicine, 1999.

[20] Sears, Barry Ph.D., et al, *idem.*

[21] Sears, Barry Ph.D., et al, *ibed.*

[22] Lowe, John C., et al. *The Metabolic Treatment of Fibromyalgia.* Boulder, CO: McDowell Publishing Company, 2000.

[23] Cooney, Craig, et al., *idem.*

473

[24] Whitaker, Julian, M.D. *DHEA Helps Regulate the Immune System.* Health and Healing, September, Vol. 8, No. 9, 1998.
[25] Gerber, Richard M.D. *Vibrational Medicine.* Sante Fe: Bear and Company, 1996.
[26] Cooney, Craig, et al, *idem.*
[27] Wright, Jonathan V., M.D., et al., *idem.*
[28] Pert, Candace B., Ph.D., *idem.*
[29] Cooney, Craig, et al., *idem.*
[30] Sapolsky, Robert M., *idem.*
[31] Sapolsky, Robert M., *ibid.*
[32] Kasala, Dharma, M.D. *Brain Longevity*
[33] Sapolsky, Robert M., *idem.*
[34] Sapolsky, Robert M., *ibid.*
[35] Becker, Robert O., M.D., et al. *The Body Electric.* New York: William Morrow and Company, Inc., 1985.

References

Abou-Seif, MA., Youssef, AA. *Oxidative Stress and Male IGF-I, Gonadotropin and Related Hormones in Diabetic Patients.* Clin Chem Lab Med, July, Vol. 39, No. 7, 2001.

Abrams, William B., M.D., et al. *The Merck Manual of Geriatrics.* New Jersey: Merck Sharp & Dohme Research Laboratories, 1990.

Adams, Patch, M.D., et al. *Gesundheit!* Vermont: Healing Arts Press, 1993.

Adams, MR. *Oral L-Arginine Improves Endothelium-Dependent Dilatation and Reduces Monocyte Adhesion to Endothelial Cells in Young Men With Coronary Artery Disease.* Dept. of Cardiology, Royal Prince Alfred Hospital, Sydney, Australia.

Arvat, Emanuela, et. al. *Stimulatory Effect of Adrenocorticotropin on Cortisol, Aldosterone and Dehydroepiandrosterone Secretion in Normal Humans: Dose Response Study.* The Journal of Clinical Endocrinology and Metabolism. Vol. 85, No. 9, pages 3141-3146, 2000.

Atkins, Robert C., M.D. *Dr Atkins' New Diet Revolution.* 2nd ed. New York: Evans and Company, Inc, 1999.

Atkins, Robert C., M.D. *Dr Atkins' Vita-Nutrient Solution.* New York: Simon and Shuster, 1998.

Ames Company. *Modern Urine Chemistry.* Elkhart, IN: Miles Laboratories, Inc, 1982.

Aoki, Kazutaka, et al. *Dehydroepiandrosterone Suppresses the Elevated Hepatic Glucose-6-Phosphatase and Fructose-1, 6-Biophosphatase Activities in C57BL/Ksj-db/db Mice.* Diabetes, Vol. 48, August 1999.

Arndt, Kenneth A., M.D. *Manual of Dermatologic Therapeutics.* Boston: Little, Brown and Company, 1983.

Ballentine, Rudolph, M.D. *Radical Healing.* New York: Harmony Books, 1999.

Balch, James F. M.D., et al. *Prescription of Natural Healing.* New York: Garden City Park, 1990.

Barazzoni, R., et. al. *Increased Fibrinogen Production in Type 2 Diabetic Patients Without Detectable Vascular Complications: Correlation with Plasma Glucagon Concentrations.* Journal of Clinical Endocrinology and Metabolism. Vol. 85, No. 9, pages 3121-3125, 2000.

Bareford, D. *Effects of Hyperglycemia and Sorbitol Accumulation on Erythrocyte Deformability in Diabetes Mellitus.* Journal of Clinical Pathology. Vol. 39, Issue 7, 1986.

Bargen, J.A., M.D., et al. *Every Woman's Standard Medical Guide.* Indianapolis: American Publishers' Alliance Corp., 1949.

Bate-Smith, E.C., ed. *Chemical Plant Taxonomy.* London: Spotttiswoode, Ballantyne and Company Limited, 1963.

Bauer, Cathryn. *Acupressure for Everybody.* New York: Henry Holt and Company, 1991.

Becker, Robert O., M.D., et al. *The Body Electric.* New York: William Morrow and Company, Inc, 1985.

Becker, Robert O., M.D., et al. *The Direct Current Control System, A Link Between Environment and Organism.* New York State Journal of Medicine, April 15, 1962.

Beers, Mark H., M.D., ed. *The Merck Manual of Diagnosis and Therapy.* Whitehouse Station, NJ: Merck Research Laboratories, 1999.

Behrendt, H., M.D. *Chemistry of Erythrocytes.* Illinois: Charles C Thomas Publisher, 1957.

Bellack, Leopold, M.D., ed. *Psychology of Physical Illness.* New York: Grune & Stratton, 1952.

Bellamy, MF, et al. *Hyperhomocystinemia After an Oral Methionine Load Acutely Impairs Endothelial Function in Healthy Adults.* Circulation 98:1848-1852, 1998.

Ber, Abram, M.D., F.R.C.P. *Neutralization of Phenolic (Aromatic) Food Compounds in a Holistic General Practice.*

Berezina, TL, et. al. *Influence of Storage on Red Blood Cell Rheological Properties.* Surg. Res. January, Volume 102, No. 1, pgs. 6-12, 2002.

Bergman, Richard N., et al. *Free Fatty Acids and Pathogenesis of Type 2 Diabetes Mellitus.* Trends In Endocrinology and Metabolisim, 11, 2000.

Berkow, Robert, M.D., ed. *The Merck Manual of Medical Information.* Whitehouse Station, NJ: Merck Research Laboratories, 1997.

Bensky, Dan, et al. *Chinese Herbal Medicine, Materia Medica.* Seattle: Eastland Press, Inc, 1986.

Bensky, Dan, et al. *Chinese Herbal Medicine, Formulas and Strategies.* Seattle: Eastland Press, Inc, 1990.

Berkow, Robert, M.D., ed. *The Merck Manual 15th ed.* Rahway, NJ: Merck, Sharp, & Dohme Research Laboratories, 1987.

Bernstein, Richard K., M.D., F.A.C.E. *Diabetes Solution.* New York: Little, Brown and Company, 1997.

Bland, Jeffery S., Ph.D., ed. *Clinical Nutrition: A Functional Approach.* Gig Harbor, WA: Institute for Functional Medicine, 1999.

Bland, Jeffrey, Ph.D., *Nutritional Endocrinology.* Washington: Metagenics Educational Programs, 2002.

Bown, Deni. *Growing Herbs.* New York: Dorling Kindersley Publishing, Inc., 1995.

Bown, Deni. *Encyclopedia of Herbs and Their Uses.* New York: Dorling Kindersley Publishing, Inc, 1995.

Bradly, James, M.D, et al. *Dr. Braly's Food Allergy & Nutrition Revolution.* Connecticut: Keats Publishing, Inc., 1992.

Bratman, Steven, M.D., et al. *Natural Health Bible 2nd ed.* California: Prima Health, 2000.

Brennan, Barbara Ann. *Light Emerging.* New York: Bantam Books, 1993.

Brennan, Barbara Ann. *Hands of Light.* New York: Bantam Books, 1987.

Bricklin, Mark, ed. *The Practical Encyclopedia of Natural Healing.* Emmaus, PA: Rodale Press, 1976.

Bricklin, Mark, et al. *The Practical Encyclopedia of Natural Healing New, Revised Edition.* Emmaus, PA: Rodale Press, 1983.

Brink, Marijke, et al. *Angiotensin II Induces Skeletal Muscle Wasting Through Enhanced Protein Degradation and Down-Regulates Autocrine Insulin-Like Growth Factor I.* Endocrinology, Vol. 142, No. 4, 2001.

Bruce, Debra F., et al. *The Unofficial Guide to Alternative Medicine.* New York: Macmillian, Inc, 1989.

Burr, Harold S. *Blueprint for Immortality.* Essex, England: The C.W. Daniel Company Limited, 1972.

Brand, Paul, M.D., et al. *Fearfully and Wonderfully Made.* Grand Rapids, MI: Zondervan Publishing House, 1980.

Caine, Winston K., et al. *The Male Body: An Owner's Manual.* Emmaus, PA: Rodale Press, Inc, 1996.

Capra, Fritjof. *The Tao of Physics.* New York: Bantam Books, Inc, 1984.

Carey, Ruth, Ph.D., et al. *Common Sense Nutrition.* California: Pacific Press Publishing Association, 1971.

Cattaneo, L., et al. *Characterization of the Hypothalamo-Pituitary-IGF-I Axis in Rats Made Obese by Overfeeding.* Journal of Endocrinology, February, Vol. 148, No. 2, 1996.

Chopra, Deepak M.D. *Ageless Body, Timeless Mind.* New York: Harmony Books, 1993.

Chambers, John. *Demonstration of Rapid Onset Vascular Endothelial Dysfunction after Hyperhomocystinemia.* Circulation 99:1156-1160, 1999.

Childe, Doc L., *The HeartMath Solution.* New York: HarperCollins Publishers, 1999.

Choi, Cheol S., et al. *Independent Regulation of in Vivo Insulin Action on Glucose Versus K+ Uptake by Dietary Fat and K+ Content.* Diabetes, Vol. 51, April 2002.

Christ, Emanual R. et al. *Dyslipidemia in adult Growth Hormone Deficiency and the Effect of GH Replacement Therapy.* Trends in Endocrinology and Metabolism. Vol. 9, pgs. 200-206, 1998.

Clasey, JL., et al. *Abdominal Visceral Fat and Fasting Insulin are Important Predictors of 24-Hour GH Release Independent of Age, Gender, and Other Physiological Factors.* J Clin Endocrinol Metab, August, Vol. 86, No. 8, 2001.

Clemente, Carmine, Ph.D. *Anatomy A Regional Atlas of the Human Body.* Maryland: Urban & Schwarzenberg, 1981.

Cousins, Norman. *Anatomy of An Illness as Perceived By the Patient.* New York: Bantam Books, 1979.

Company, Merck &. *The Hypercholesterolemia Handbook.* Pennsylvania: Merck Sharp & Dohme, 1989.

Cooney, Craig, et al. *Methyl Magic, Maximum Health Through Methylation.* Andrews McMeel Publishing, Kansas City.

Cush, Keneth and DeFronzo, Ralph. *Recombinant Human Insulin-Like Growth Factor 1 Treatment for 1 week Improves Metabolic Control in Type 2 Diabetes by Ameliorating Hepatic and Muscle Insulin Resistance.* The Journal of Clinical Endocrinology and Metabolism. Vol. 85, No. 9, pgs 3077-3084, 2000.

Cusi, Kenneth, et al. *Recombinant Human Insulin-Like Growth Factor I Treatment for 1 Week Improves Metabolic Control in Type 2 Diabetes by Ameliorating Hepatic and Muscle Insulin Resistance.* The Journal of Clinical Endocrinology and Metabolism. Vol. 85, No. 9, 2000.

Danese, Mark D. Effect *of Thyroxine Therapy on Serum Lipoproteins in Patients with Mild Thyroid Failure: A Quantitative Review of the Literature.* Vol. 85, No. 9, pgs 2993-3001, 2000.

Davenport, Horace W., DSc. *A Digest of Digestion 2nd ed.* Chicago: Year Book Medical Publishers Inc, 1978.

DeBoer, H., et al. *Changes in Subcutaneous and Visceral Fat mass During Growth Hormone Replacement Therapy in Adult Men.* Int. Journal of Related Metabolic Disorders, June, Vol. 20, No. 6, 1996.

De Leo, Vicenzo. *Effect of Metformin on Insulin-Like Growth Factor (IGF) I and IGF-Binding Protein I in Polycystic Ovary Syndrome.* The Journal of Clinical Endocrinology & Metabolism, December, Vol. 85, No. 4, 2000.

Dessein, PH, et al. *Hyposecretion of Adrenal Androgens and the Relation of Serum Adrenal Steroids, Serotonin and Insulin-Like Growth Factor-1 to Clinical Features in Women with Fibromyalgia.* Pain, November, Vol. 83, No. 2, 1999.

Diamond, John W., M.D. *An Alternative Medicine Definitive Guide to Cancer.* California: Future Medicine Publishing, Inc., 1997.

Dobelis, Inge N. *Reader's Digest Magic and Medicine of Plants.* Pleasantville, NY: The Reader's Digest Association, Inc, 1986.

Dowsett, M. *Drug and Hormone Interactions of Aromatase Inhibitors.* Endocrine Related Cancer Vol. 181-185, No. 6, 1999.

Eden, Donna, et al. *Energy Medicine.* New York: Penguin Putnam Inc, 1998.

Ejima J et al. *Relationship of HDL Cholesterol and Red Blood Cell Filterability: Cross-sectional Study of Healthy Subjects.* Clinical Hemorheological Microcirculation. Vol. 22, No. 1, pgs 1-7, 2000.

Epstein, Donald, et al. *The 12 Stages of Healing.* California: Amber-Allen Publishing, 1994.

Erickson, Robert A., M.D. *Testosterone-Its Real Impact.* Journal of Longevity. Vol. 7, No. 9, 2001.

Fawcett, JP. *Does Cholesterol Depletion Have Adverse Effects on Blood Rheology?* Angiology, Vol. 45, Issue 3, 1994.

Ferril, William, M.D. *Molecular Mechanisms of Biological Aging.* Medicine Tree, 1998.

Ferril, William, M.D. *The Adrenal Mystery.* Medicine Tree, 1998.

Fitzpatrick, Thomas B., et al. *Color Atlas and Synopsis of Clinical Dermatology. 3rd ed.* New York: Mcgraw-Hill Companies, 1997.

Fottner, C., et el. *Regulation of Steroidogenesis by Insulin-Like Growth Factors (IGFs) in Adult Human Adrenocortical Cells: IGF-I and, more Potently, IGF-II Preferentially Enhance Androgen Biosynthesis Through Interaction With the IGF-I Receptor and IGF-Binding Proteins.* Journal of Endocrinol, September, Vol. 158, No. 3, 1998.

Frankel, Edward. *DNA: The Ladder of Life. 2nd ed.* New York: McGraw-Hill Book Company, 1979.

Frost, Robert A., Lang, Charles H. *Differential Effects of Insulin-Like Growth Factor I (IGF-I) and IGF-Binding Protein-1 on Protein Metabolism in Human Skeletal Muscle Cells.* Endocrinology, Vol. 140, No. 9, 1999.

Gaby, Alan R., M.D., et al. *Nutritional Therapy in Medical Practice.* Kent, WA: Wright/Gaby Seminars, 1996.

Gdansky, E., et al. *Increased Number of IGF-I Receptors on Erythrocytes of Women with Polycystic Ovarian Syndrome.* Clinical Endocrinal, August, Vol. 47, No. 2, 1997.

Gangong, William F., M.D. *Review of Medical Physiology 10th ed.* Los Altos: Lange Medical Publications, 1981.

Gangong, William F., M.D. *Review of Medical Physiology.* Los Altos: Lange Medical Publications, 1971

Gangong, William F., M.D. *Review of Medical Physiology. 19th ed.* Stamford, CT: Appleton&Lange, 1999.

Gangong, William F., M.D. *Review of Medical Physiology. 20thed.* McGraw-Hill Companies, Inc., 2001.

Gardner, Joy. *Healing Yourself.* Freedom, CA: The Crossing Press, 1989

Gerber, Richard M.D. *Vibrational Medicine.* Sante Fe: Bear and Company, 1996.

Gerras, Charles, ed. *The Complete Book of Vitamins.* Emmaus, PA: Rodale Press Inc, 1977.

Gerras, Charles, et al. *The Encyclopedia of Common Diseases.* Emmaus, PA: Rodale Press, Inc., 1976.

Giller, Robert M., M.D., et al. *Natural Prescriptions.* New York: Ballentine Books, 1994.

Glowacki, Rosen CJ, et al. *Sex steroids, The Inuslin-Like Growth Factor Regulatory System, and Aging Implications for the Management of Older Postmenopausal Women.* J Nutr Health Aging, Vol.2, No. 1, 1998.

Gokce, Noyan M.D. *Long Term Ascorbic Acid administration reverses Endothelial Vasomotor Dysfunction in Patients with Coronary artery Disease.* Circulation, Vol. 99, pgs 3234-3240, 1999.

Goldberg Group, Burton, ed. *Alternative Medicine The Definitive Guide.* Washington: Future Medicine Publishing, Inc., 1994.

Golden, GA, et al. *Steroid Hormones Partition to Distinct Sites In A Model Membrane Bilayer: Direct Demonstration By Small-angle X-ray Diffraction.* Goodman, David, 'Soy toxins', press release, 1998.

Goodman, Paul. *Compulsory Mis-Education and the Community of Scholars.* New York: Vintage Books, 1962.

Gori, Francesca, et al. *Effects of Androgens on the Insulin-Like Growth Factor System in an Androgen-Responsive Human Osteoblastic Cell Line.* Endocrinology, Vol. 140, No. 12, 1999.

Graham, Ian M. *Plasma Homocysteine as a Risk Factor from Vascular Disease.* JAMA, June, Vol. 27, No. 22, 1997.

Grant, William, Ph.D. *The Role of Milk And Sugar In Heart Disease.* The American Journal of Natural Medicine, November 1998.

Greenspan, Francis S., M.D., eds. *Basic and Clinical Endocrinology.* Stamford, CT: Appleton&Lange, 1997.

Griffin, Tom, M.D., et al. *The Physicians Blueprint Feeling Good For Life.* Arizona: New Medical Dynamics Inc., 1983.

Grinspoon, Steven, et al. *Effects of Androgen Administration on the Growth Hormone-Insulin-Like Growth Factor I Axis in Men with Aquired Immunodeficiency Syndrome Wasting.* Journal of Clinical Endocrinology and Metabolism, Vol. 83, No. 12, 1998.

Gurnell, Eleanor M. *Dehydroepiandrosterone Replacement Therapy.* European Journal of Endocrinology, Vol. 145, pgs 103-106, 2001.

Guyton, Arthur C., M.D. *Textbook of Medical Physiology* 7*th* ed. Pennsylvania: W.B. Saunders Company, 1986.

Halmos, Gabor, et. al. *Human Ovarian Cancer Express Somatostatin Receptor.* The Journal of Clinical Endocrinology and Metabolism, Vol. 85, No. 10, pgs 3509-3512, 2000.

Hamel, Frederick G., et al. *Regulation of Multicatalytic Enzyme Activity by Insulin and the Insulin-Degrading Enzyme.* Endocrinology, Vol. 139, No. 10, 1998.

Hanley, Anthony J.G., et al. *Increased Proinsulin Levels and Decreased Acute Insulin Response Independently Predict the Incidence of Type 2 Diabetes in the Insulin Resistance Atherosclerosis Study.* Diabetes, Vol. 51, April 2002.

Handelsman, DJ, Crawford, BA. *Androgens Regulate Circulating Levels of Insulin-Like Growth Factor (IGF)-I and IGF Binding Protien-3 During Puberty in Male Baboons.* Journal of Clinical Metabolism, January, Vol. 81, No. 1, 1996.

Hansten, Philip. *Drug Interactions* 4*th* ed. London: Henry Kimpton Publishers, 1979.

Harper, Harold A., Ph.D. *Review of Physiological Chemistry* 7*th* ed. Los Altos: Lange Medical Publications, 1959.

Harris, J.R., ed. *Blood Cell Biochemistry, Erythroid Cells.* New York: Plenum Press, 1990.

Harrington, James and Carter-Su, Christin. *Signaling Pathways Activated By the Growth Hormone Receptor.* Trends in Endocrinology, August, Vol. 12, No. 6, 2001.

Harrison, George R. *How Things Work.* New York: William Morrow and Co., 1941.

Hayes, Francis J. A*romatase Inhibition in the Human Male Reveals a Hypothalamic Site of Estrogen Feedback.* Journal of Clinical Endocrinology and Metabolism, Vol. 85, No. 9, pgs 3027-3035, 2000.

Heitzer, Thomas. *Tetrahydrobiopterin Improves Endothelium-Dependent Vasodialtion in Chronic Smokers.* Circulation Research, Vol. 86, edition 36, 2000.

Heller, Richard F., M.S., Ph.D., et al. *The Carbohydrate Addict's Healthy Heart Program.* New York: Ballentine Publishing Group, 1999.

Hendrickson, James E., M.D. *The Molecules of Nature.* New York: W.A. Benjamin, 1965.

Hiramatsu, R, and Nisula, BC. *Erythrocyte-associated Cortisol: Measurement, Kinetics of Dissociation and Potential Physiological Significance.* Journal of Clinical Endocrinology and Metabolism, June, Vol. 64, No. 6, pgs 1224-32, 1987.

Hiramatsu, Ryoh and Nisula, Bruce C. *Uptake of Erythrocyte-Associated Component of Blood Testosterone and Corticosterone to Rat Brain.* Journal of steroid biochemistry, pgs 383-87.

Hiramatsu, R. *Uptake of Erythrocytes-Associated Component of Blood Testosterone and Corticosterone to Rat Brain.* J of Steroid Biochemistry Mol Biol, March, Vol. 383, No. 7, 1991.

Hiramatsu, Ryoji, et al. *Erythrocyte-Associated Cortisol: Measurement, Kinetics of Dissociation, and Potential Physiological Significance.* Journal of Clinical Endocrinology and Metabolism, 1987.

Hoffman, David. *The Complete Illustrated Holistic Herbal.* New York: Barnes&Noble, Inc, 1996.

Hunt, Valerie V. *Infinite Mind: The Science of Human Vibrations of Consciousness.* Malibu, CA: Malibu Publishing Co, 1996.

Isaacson, Robert L., et al. *Toxin-Induced Blood Vessel Inclusions Caused by the Chronic Administration of Aluminum and Sodium Fluoride and Their Implications for Dementia.* Annals New York Academy of Sciences.

Jacob, Stanley, M.D., et al. *The Miracle of MSM The Natural Solution for Pain.* New York: G.P. Putnam's Sons, 1999.

Jacobson, GM. *17 Beta-Estradiol Transport and Metabolism in Human Red blood cells.* J Clin Endocrinology and Metab., February, Vol. 40, Issue 2, 1975.

Jawetz, Ernest, M.D., Ph.D, et al. *Review of Medical Microbiology 15th ed.* Los Altos: Lange Medical Publications, 1982.

Jin, Weijun, et al. *Lipases and HDL Metabolism.* Trends in Endocrinology, Vol. 13, No. 4, May 2002.

Jones, T.W.H. *Dictionary of the Bach Flower Remedies.* Essex, England: C.W. Daniel Company Limited, 1995.

Junqueira, Luis C., M.D., et al. *Basic Histology 3rd ed.* Los Altos: Lange Medical Publications, 1980.

Kamat, Amrita, et. al. *Mechanisms in Tissue-Specific Regulation of Estrogen Biosynthesis in Humans.* Trends in Endocrinology and Metabolism, Vol. 13, April, pgs 122-128, 2002.

Kellner, Michael, et al. *Atrial Natriuretic Factor Inhibits the CRH-Stimulated Secretion of ACTH and Cortisol in Man.* Life Sciences, Vol. 60, 1992.

Kemper, Donald, ed. *Healthwise Handbook.* Idaho: Healthwise, Inc. 1976.

Keough, Carol, ed. *Future Youth.* Emmaus, PA: Rodale Press, Inc, 1987.

Khalsa, Dharma Singh, M.D., et al. *Brain Longevity*. New York: Time Warner Company, 1997.

Kirpichnikov, Dmitri, and James Sowers. *Diabetes Mellitus and Diabetes-Associated Vascular Disease*. Trends in Endocrinology and Metabolism, July, Vol. 12, No. 5, 2001.

Kishi, Yutaka, et al. *Alph-Lipoic Acid: Effects on Glucose Uptake, Sorbitol Pathway, and Energy Metabolism in Experimental Diabetic Neuropathy*. Diabetes, Vol. 48, October 1999.

Klaassen, Curtis D., Ph.D. *Casarett & Doull's Toxicology 6th ed*. McGraw-Hill Medical Publishing Division, 2001.

Klatz, Ronald, et al. *Grow Young with HGH*. New York: Harper Perennial, 1997.

Kotelchuck, David, ed. *Prognosis Negative*. New York: Vintage Books, 1976.

Kraemer, W.J., et al. *Effects of Heavy-Resistance Training On Hormonal Response Patterns In Younger VS. Older Men*. Journal of Applied Physiology, September, Vol. 87, No.3, 1999.

Krupka, R.M. and Deves, R. *Asymmetric Binding of Steroids to Internal and External Sites in the Glucose Carrier of Erythrocytes*. Biochem biophys Acta, Vol. 598, Issue 1, 1980.

Lacayo, Richard. *Testosterone*. TIME Magazine, April, pg 58, 2000.

Laughlin, Gail and Barret-Conner, Elizibeth. *Sexual Dimorphism in the Influence of Advanced Aging on the Adrenal Hormone levels: The Rancho Bernardo Study*. The Journal of Clinical Endocrinology and Metabolism, pgs 3561-3568, 2000.

Lasley, Bill L., et al. *The Relationship of Circultating Dehydroepiandrosterone, Testosterone, and Estradiol to Stages of the Menopausal Transition and Ethnicity*. The Journal of Clinical Endocrinology and Metabolism, Vol. 87, No. 8, 2002.

Leavelle, Dennis E., M.D., ed. *Mayo Medical Laboratories Interpretive Handbook*. Rochester, MN: Mayo Medical Laboratories, 1997.

Lee, John R., M.D., et al. *What Your Doctor May Not Tell You About Premenopause.* New York: Warner Books, Inc, 1999.

Lee, John R., M.D. *Natural Progesterone: the Multiple Roles of a Remarkable Hormone.* Sebastopol, CA: BLL Publishing, 1993.

Lehninger, Albert L. *Biochemistry.* New York: Worth Publishers, Inc, 1975.

LeShan, Lawrence, Ph.D. *Psychological States as Factors in the Development of Malignant Disease: A Critical Review.* New York Journal of Medicine, August 24, 1958.

Levitt, B.B. *Electromagnetic Fields.* New York: Harcourt Brace and Company, 1995.

Lewis, John G., et al. *Caution On The Use of Saliva Measurements to Monitor Absorption of Progesterone From Transdermal Creams in Postmenopausal Women.* Maturitas, Vol. 4, 2002.

Ley, Beth. *DHEA: Unlocking the Secrets to the Fountain of Youth.* California: BL Publications, 1996.

Lovern, J.A., *The Chemistry of Lipids of Biochemistry Significance.* London: Methuen & Co. LTD, 1955.

Lowe, John C., et al. *The Metabolic Treatment of Fibromyalgia.* Boulder, CO: McDowell Publishing Company, 2000.

Lowenthal, Albert A., M.D. *Endocrine Glands and Sexual Problems.* Chicago 1928.

Lorand, Arnold, M.D. *Old Age Deferred.* Philadelphia: F.A. Davis Publishers, 1911.

Maciocia, Giovanni. *Tongue Diagnosis in Chinese Medicine.* Seattle: Eastland Press, Inc, 1987.

Martin, Janet L., et al. *Insulin-Like Growth Factor Binding Protein-3 Is Regulated by Dihydrotestosterone and Stimulates Deoxyribonucleic Acid Synthesis and Cell Proliferation in LNCaP Prostate Carcinoma Cells.* Endocrinology, Vol. 141, No. 7, 2000.

Mauras, Nelly, et. al. *Estrogen Suppression in Males: Metabolic Effects*. The Journal of Clinical Endocrinology and Metabolism. Vol. 85, No. 7, pgs 2370-2377, 2000.

Mawatari, S. and Murakami, K. *Effects of Ascorbic Acid on Peroxidation of Human Erythrocyte Membranes by Lipoxygenase*. Nutrition Science Vitaminology, (Tokyo), December, Vol. 45, No. 6, pg 687, 1999.

McCann, Una D. *Brain Serotonin Neurotoxicity and Primary Pulmonry Hypertension From Fenfluramine and Dexfenfluramine*. JAMA, August, Vol. 278, No. 8, 1997.

McCarty, MF. *Androgenic Progestins Amplify the Breast Cancer Risk Associated with Hormone Replacement Therapy by Boosting IGF-I Activity*. Med Hypotheses, February, Vol. 56, No. 2, 2001.

McCarty, MF. *Modulation of Adipocyte Lipoprotein Lipase Expression as a Strategy for Preventing or Treating Visceral Obesity*. Med Hypotheses, August, Vol. 57, No. 2, 2001.

McEvoy, Gerald K., Pharm.D, ed. *AHFS Drug Information, 2001*. Bethesda, MD: American Society of Health-System Pharmacists, Inc, 2001.

McEvoy, Gerald K., Pharm.D, ed. *AHFS Drug Information, 1986*. Bethesda , MD: American Society of Health-System Pharmacists, Inc, 1986.

Mchedlishvili, G. *New Evidence for Involvement of Blood Rheological Disorders in Rise of Peripheral Resistance in Essential Hyperttension*. Clinical Hemorheology Microcirculation, Vol. 17, Issue 1.

McIntosh, M., et al. *Opposing Actions of Dehydroepiandrosterone and Corticosterone in Rats*. Proc Soc Exp Biol Med, July, Vol. 221, No. 3, 1999.

McLaughlin, T., et al. *Carbohydrate Induced Hypertriglyceridemia: An Insight into the Link between Plasma Insulin and Triglyceride Concentrations*. The Journal of Clinical Endocrinology and Metabolism. Vol .85, No. 9, pgs 3085-3088, 2000.

Mellon, Cynthia H. and Griffin, Lisa D. *Neurosteroids: biochemistry and clinical significance.* Trends in Endocrinology and Metabolism, Vol.13, pgs 35-43, 2002.

Mendelsohn, Robert S., M.D. *Confessions of a Medical Heretic.* New York: Warner Books Inc., 1979.

Michalak, Patricia S. *Rodale's Successful Organic Gardening, Herbs.* Emmaus, PA: Rodale Press, 1993.

Mindell, Earl L., R.Ph.D, Ph.D., et al. *Dr. Earl Mindell's Secrets of Natural Health.* Illinois: Keats Publishing, 2000.

Minear, Ralph E. M.D. *The Joy of Living Salt Free.* McMillian Publishing, 1984.

Mokken FC, et. al. *The Clinical Importance of Erythrocyte Deformability, a Hemorheologically Parameter.* Annals of Hematology, Vol. 64, Issue 3, 1992.

Morales, AJ. et al. *The Effects of Six Months Treatment with a 100 mg Daily Dose of Dehyroepiamdrosterone (DHEA) on Circulating Sex Steroids, Body Composition and Muscle Strength in Age-Advanced Men and Women.* Clinical Endocrinology (Oxf), October, Vol. 49, No. 4, 1998.

Morin, Laurie C., *Endocrine and Metabolic Effects of Metaformin vs. Ethinyl-Cyproterone acetate in Obese Women with Polycystic Ovary Syndrome: A Randomized Study.* The Journal of Clinical Endocrinology and Metabolism. Vol. 85, No. 9, pgs 3161-3168, 2000.

Morley J.E., et al. *Potentially Predictive and Manipulable Blood Serum Correlatives of Aging in the Healthy Human Male: Progressive Decreases in Bioavailable Testosterone, Dehydroepiamdrosterone Sulfate, and the Ratio of Insulin-Like Growth Factor 1 to Growth Hormone.* Pro Natl Acad Sci USA, July, Vol. 94, No.14, 1997.

Moss, Ralph W. *The Cancer Industry.* New York: Paragon House, 1989.

Monte, Tom, et al. *World Medicine.* New York: F.P. Putnam's Sons, 1993.

Munzer, T., et al. *Effects of GF and/or Sex Steroid Administration on Abdominal Subcutaneous and Visceral Fat in Healthy Aged Women and Men.* J Clin Endocirinol Metab, August, Vol. 86, No. 8, 2001.

Muramoto, Naboru. *Healing Ourselves.* New York: Avon Books, 1973.

Mullenix, Phyllis J., *Neurotoxicity of Sodium Fluoride in Rats.* Neurotoxicology and Teratology, Vol. 17, No. 2, 1995.

Murray, Michael, N.D., et al. *Encyclopedia of Natural Medicine.* California: Prima Health, 1998.

Myss, Caroline, PhD, et al. *Creation of Health.* New York: Three Rivers Press, 1993.

Nam, S.Y., et al. *Low-Dose Growth Hormone Treatment Combined with Diet Restriction Decreases Insulin Resistance by Reducing Visceral Fat and Increasing Muscle Mass in Obese Type 2 Diabetic Patients.* Int J Obes Relat Metab Disord, August, Vol. 25, No. 8, 2001.

Nelson, David L., et al. *Lehninger Principles of Biochemistry.* 3rd ed. New York: Worth Publishers, 2000.

Netzer, Corinne T. *Encyclopedia of Food Values.* New York: Dell Publishing, 1992.

Nicklas, B.J., et al. *Testosterone, Growth Hormone and IGF-I Response to Acute and Chronic Resistive Exercise in Men Aged 55-70 Years.* Int. Journal of Sports Medicine, October, Vol. 16, No. 7, 1995.

Nitenberg A. Acetylcholine induced coronary vasoconstriction in young, heavy smokers with normal coronary arteriographic findings. Service d'Explorations Fonctionnelles, Unite 251, France.

Ody, Penelope. *The Complete Medicinal Herbal.* New York: Dorling Kindersley Inc, 1993.

Okada, Hidetaka, et. al. *Progesterone Enhances Interleukin-15 Production in Human Endometrial Stromal Cells in Vitro.* Journal of Clinical Endocrinology and Metabolism. Vol. 85, No. 12, pgs 4765-4770, 2000.

Ornstein, Robert, et al. *The Amazing Brain.* Boston: Houghton Mifflin Company, 1984.

O'Rourke, P.J. *Parliament of Whores.* New York: The Atlantic Monthly Press, 1991.

Pascal, Alana. *DHEA the Fountain of Youth Discovered?* California: Ben-Wal Printing, 1996.

Paolisso G., et al. *Insulin Resistance and Advancing Age: What Role For Dehydroepiandrosterone Sulfate?* Metabolism, November, Vol.46, No.11, 1997.

Peeke, Pamela, MD, MPH. *Fight Fat After Forty.* New York: Penguin Group, 2000.

Persson, SU. *Correlations Between Fatty Acid Composition of the Erythrocyte Membrane and Blood Rheology Data.* Scandinavian Journal of Clinical Laboratory Investigation, April, Vol. 56, Issue 2, 1996.

Pert, Candace B., Ph.D. *The Molecules of Emotion.* New York: Simon and Schuster, Inc, 1997.

Petersdorf, Robert G., M.D., et al. *Harrison's Principles of Internal Medicine tenth edition.* McGraw-Hill Book Company, 1983.

Pinchera, Aldo, M.D., ed. *Endocrinology and Metabolism.* London: McGraw-Hill International (UK) Ltd., 2001.

Pino, Ana M. et. al. *Dietary Isoflavones Affect Sex Hormone Globulin levels in Postmenopausal Women.* The Journal of Clinical Endocrinology and Metabolism, Vol. 85, No.8, pgs 2797-2800, 2000.

Porkert, Manfred, M.D., et al. *Chinese Medicine.* New York: Henry Holt and Company, 1982.

Pries, Axel R., et al. *Structural Autoregulation of Terminal Vascular Beds.* Hypertension, 1999.

Quillin, Patrick, PhD, RD, CNS, et al. *Beating Cancer with Nutrition. Rev Ed.* Tulsa, OK: Nutrition Times Press, Inc, 2001.

Rath, Matthias, M.D. *Eradicating Heart Disease.* San Francisco: Health Now, 1993.

Ravaglia, G., et al. *Regular Moderate Intensity Physical Activity and Blood Concentrations of Endogenous Anabolic Hormones and Thyroid Hormones in Aging Men.* Mech Aging Dev, February, Vol. 122, No. 2, 2001.

Ravel, Richard, M.D. *Clinical Laboratory Medicine. 6th ed.* St Louis: Mosby-Year Book, Inc, 1995.

Raynaud-Simon, A., et al. *Plasma Insulin-Like Growth Factor I Levels in the Elderly: Relation to Plasma Dehydroepiandrosterone Sulfate Levels, Nutritional Status, Health and Mortality.* J Gerontology, July-August, Vol, 47, No. 4, 2001.

Reaven, Gerald, M.D., et al. *Syndrome X.* New York: Simon & Schuster, 2000.

Reid, Daniel. *The Complete Book of Chinese Health & Healing.* Massachusetts: Shambhala Publications, Inc. 1994.

Reiss, Uzzi, M.D., et al. *Natural Hormone Balance for Woman.* New York: Pocket Books, 2001.

Remington, Dennis, M.D., et al. *Back to Health.* Utah: Publishers Press, 1986.

Rifkind, Richard, et al. *Fundamentals of Hematology. 2nd ed.* Illinois: Year Book Medical Publishers, Inc. 1980.

Robbins, John. *Reclaiming Our Health: Exploding the Myth and Embracing the Source of True Healing.* Tiburon, CA: HJ Kramer Inc, 1998.

Robbins, Stanley L., M.D., et al. *Pathologic Basis of Disease. 2nd ed.* Philadelphia: W.B. Saunders Company, 1979.

Rodale, J.I., et al. *The Health Seeker.* Emmaus, PA: Rodale Books, Inc. 1972.

Rodale, J.I., ed. *Health Builder.* Emmaus, PA: Rodale Press, Inc., 1971.

Roggenkamp, HG. *Erythrocyte Rigidity in Healthy Patients and Patients with Cardiovascular Disease Risk Factors.* KWH, Oct, Vol. 64, pgs 1091-6, 1986.

Rojo, Ruth N.D. *Why is it harder to lose weight as we age?* Journal of Longevity Vol. 7, No. 9, 2001.

Rosedale, Ron. *Presentation at the Health Institute's boulder-Fest.* August 1999 seminar.

Rosenfeld, Isadore, M.D. *The Complete Medical Exam.* New York: Simon & Schuster, 1978.

Rosmond, R, and Bjortorp, P. *The Interactions Between Hypothalamic-Pituitary-Adrenal Axis Activity, Testosterone, Insulin-Like Growth Factor I and Abdominal Obesity with Metabolism and Blood Pressure in Men.* Int Journal Obes Relat Metab Disord, December, Vol. 22, No. 12, 1998.

Rosmond, Roland, et al. *Stress-Related Cortisol Secretion in Men: Relationships with Abdominal Obesity and Endocrine, Metabolic and Hemodynamic Abnormalities.* Journal of Clinical Endocrinology and Metabolism, February, Vol. 83, No. 6, 1998.

Ross, A.C., and Gordon, M.B., Chb, MFHom. *Homeopathy An Introductory Guide.* Northamptonshire: Thorsons Publishers Limited: 1976.

Rowen, Robert L., M.D. *How to Control High Blood Pressure Without Drugs.* Charles Scribner and Sons, 1986.

Rubin, Philip, ed. *Clinical Oncology sixth edition.* American Cancer Society, 1983.

Ruiz, Gomez F. *Treatments with progesterone analogues decreases macrophage Fcgamma receptors expression.* Clinical Immunopathology, December, Vol. 89,No. 3, pgs 231-9, 1998.

Russell, A.L. *Glycoaminoglycan (GAG) Deficiency in Protective Barrier as an Underlying, Primary Cause of Ulcerative Colitis, Crohn's Disease, Interstitial Cystitis and Possibly Reiter's Syndrome.* Medical Hypotheses, Vol. 52, No. 4, 1999.

Ryan, Graeme B., M.B., B.S., Ph.D., et al. *Inflamation*. Kalamazoo, MI: The Upjohn Company, 1977.

Sapolsky, Robert M. *Stress, the Aging Brain, and the Mechanisms of Neuron Death*. Cambridge, MA: The MIT Press, 1992.

Sapolsky, Robert M. *The Trouble with Testosterone*. New York: Simon and Shuster, Inc, 1997.

Sarno, John E., M.D. *The Mindbody Prescription*. New York: Warner Books, Inc, 1998.

Schofield, Janice F. *Discovering Wild Plants*. Bothell, WA: Alaska Northwest Books, 1989.

Simpson, Leslie O. *Red Cell and Hemorheological Changes in Multiple Sclerosis*. Pathology, Vol. 19, pgs 51-55, 1987.

Secomb, T. W. *A Model For Red Cell Motion in Glycocalyx-lined Capillaries*. American Journal of Physiology, Vol. 274, H1016-H1022, 1998.

Sahelian, Ray, M.D. *DHEA Youth in a Bottle?* Lets Live, October, 1996.

Scala, James, Dr., Ph.D. *High Blood Pressure Relief Diet*. NAL Books, 1988.

Schechter, Michael, M.D., et. al. *Oral Magnesium Therapy Improves Endothelial Function in Patients with Coronary Artery Disease*. Circulation, Nov. 7, 2000, pgs 2353-2358, 2000.

Scholl, B.F., PhG, M.D., ed. *Library of Health*. Philadelphia: Historical Publishing, Inc, 1932.

Schwarzbein, Diana, M.D., et al. *The Schwarzbein Principle*. Deerfield Beach, FL: Health Communications, Inc, 1999.

Sears, Barry, Ph.D., et al. *Enter the Zone*. New York: HarperCollins Publishers, Inc, 1995.

Sheally, C.N., M.D., Ph.D., ed. *The Complete Family Guide to Alternative Medicine*. New York: Barnes & Noble, Inc., 1996.

Shippen, Eugene, M.D., et al. *The Testosterone Syndrome.* New York: M. Evans and Company, Inc, 1998.

Signorello, LB., et al. *Hormones and Hair Patterning In Men: A Role for Insulin-Like Growth Factor 1?* Journal of the American Academy of Dermatology, February, Vol. 40, No. 2, 1999.

Sobel, David S., M.D., et al. *The People's Book of Medical Tests.* New York: Simon and Schuster, 1985.

Solerte, Sebastiano Bruno, et al. *Dehydroepiandrosterone Sulfate Enhances Natural Killer Cell Cytotoxicity in Humans Via Locally Generated Immunoreactive Insulin-Like Growth Factor I.* The Journal of Clinical Endocrinology & Metabolism, Vol. 84, No. 9, 1999.

Song, Linda Z.Y.X., M.D., et al. *Heart-Focused Attention and Heart-Brain Synchronization:Energetic and Physiological Mechanisms.* Alternative Therapies, September, Vol. 4, No. 5, 1998.

Sorrentino, Sandy, M.D., Ph.D., et al. *Coping with High Blood Pressure.* Dembner Books, 1986.

Spector, Walter G. *An Introduction to General Pathology. 2nd ed.* Edinburgh, Scotland: Churchill Livingstone, 1980.

Stelfox, Henry Thomas, M.D., et al. *Conflict of Interest in the Debate Over Calcium-Channel Antagonists.* The New England Journal of Medicine, January 8, 1998.

Stewart, Paul M. and Tomlison, Jeremy W. *Cortisol, 11B-Hydroxysteroid Dehydrogenase Type 1 and Central Obesity.* Trends in Endocrinology and Metabolism, April 2002, pgs.94-96.

Stites, Daniel P., M.D., et al., eds. *Medical Immunology 9th ed.* Stamford, CT: Appleton & Lange, 1997.

Stuart, J. *Erythrocyte Rheology.* J Clinical Pathology, Vol. 38, Issue 9, 1985.

Study Links High Carbohydrates to Cancer. Associated Press (April 2002)

Takaya, Kazuhiko, et. al. *Ghrelin Strongly Stimulates Growth Hormone (GH) Release in Humans.* The Journal of Clinical Endocrinology and Metabolism. Vol. 85. No. 12 pages 4908-4911, 2000.

Theodosakis, Jason, M.D., M.S., M.P.H., et al. *The Arthritis Cure.* New York: Affinity Communications Corporation, 1998.

Thomas, Lewis. *The Lives of a Cell.* New York: Bantam Books, 1974.

Thrailkill, K.M. *Insulin-Like Growth Factor-I in Diabetes Mellitus: its Physiologic, Metabolic Effects, and Potential Clinical Utility.* Diabetes Technol Ther, Spring, Vol. 2, No. 1, 2000.

Tilford, Gregory L. *Edible and Medicinal Plants of the West.* Missoula: Mountain Press Publishing Company, 1997.

Tilford, Gregory L. *From Earth to Herbalist.* Missoula: Mountain Press Publishing Company, 1998.

Tiller, William A. *Cardiac Coherence: A New, Noninvasive Measure of Autonomic Nervous System Order.* Alternative Therapies, January, Vol. 2, No. 1, 1996.

Tintera, John, M.D. *The Hypoadrenocortical State and Its Management.* Yonkers, New York, Vol.55, No. 13, 1955.

Tissandier, O., et al. *Testosterone, Dehydroepiandrosterone, Insulin-Like Growth Factor 1, and Insulin in Sedentary and Physically Trained Aged Men.* Eur J Appl Physiol, July, Vol. 85, No. 1-2, 2001.

Tsuda, K. et al. *Electron Paramagnetic Resonance Investigation on Modulatory Effect of 17Beta-estradiol on Membrane Fluidity of Erythrocytes in Postmenopausal Women.* Arteriosclerosis Thromb Vasc Biol, August, Vol. 21, No. 8, pgs 1306-12, 2001.

Tsuji, K. *Specific Binding and Effects of Dehroepiandrosterone Sulfate (DHEA-S) on Skeletal Muscle Cells: Possible Implication for DHEA-S Replacement Therapy in Patients With Myotonic Dystrophy.* Life Science, Vol. 65, No.1, 1999.

Tyler, Varro E., Ph.D., Sc.D. *Herbs of Choice.* New York: Pharmaceutical Products Press, 1994.

VanHaaften, M., et al. *Identification of 16-alpha Hydroxyestrone as a Metabolite of Estriol.* Gynecol Endorinol, Vol. 2, 1988.

Veldhuis, Johannes D., et al. *Estrogen and Testosterone, But Not a Nonaromatizable Androgen, Direct Network Integration of the Hypothalamo-Somatotrope (Growth Hormone)-Insulin-Like Growth Factor I Axis in the Human: Evidence from Pubertal Pathophysioogy and Sex-Steroid Hormone Replacement.* Journal of Clinical Endocrinology and Metabolism, Vol. 82, No.10, 1997.

Vendola, K., et al. *Androgens Promote Insulin-Like Growth Factor-I and Insulin-Like Growth Factor-I Receptor Gene Expression in the Primate Ovary.* Hum Reprod, September, Vol. 1, No. 9, 1999.

Viveiros, M.M., Liptrap, R.M. *ACTH Treatment Disrupts Ovarian IGF-I and Steroid Hormone Production.* Journal of Endocrinology, Vol.164, 2000.

Volek J.S., et al. *Body Composition and Hormonal Responses to a Carbohydrate Restricted Diet.* Metabolism, July, Vol. 51, No. 7, 2002.

Vondra, K., et al. *Role of the Steroids, SHBG, IGF-I, IGF BP-3 and Growth Hormone in Glucose Metabolism Disorders During Long-Term Treatment with Low Doses of Glucocorticoids.* Cas Lek Cesk, February, Vol. 141, No. 3, 2002.

Wallach, Jacques, M.D. *Interpretation of Diagnostic Tests 6th ed.* New York: Little, Brown and Company, 1996.

Warrier, Gopi. *The Complete Illustrated Guide to Ayurveda.* New York: Barnes & Noble, 1997.

Watkins, Alan D., et al. *The Impact of a New Emotional Self-Management Program on Stress, Emotions, Heart Rate Variability, DHEA and Cortisol.* Integrative Physiological and Behavioral Science, April-June, Vol. 33, No. 2, 1998.

Weast, Robert C., Ph.D. *Handbook of Chemistry and Physics 56th ed.* Cleveland, OH: CRC Press, Inc, 1975.

Weil, Andrew, M.D. *Natural Health, Natural Medicine.* Boston: Houghton Mifflin Company, 1990.

Weil, Andrew, M.D. *Health and Healing.* New York: Houghton Mifflin Company, 1995.

Weil, Andrew, M.D. *Spontaneous Healing.* New York: Alfred A. Knopf, Inc., 1995.

Weil, Andrew, M.D. *Eating Well for Optimum Health.* New York: Alfred A. Knopf, Inc., 2000.

Wheelwright, Edith G. *Medicinal Plants and their History.* New York: Dover Publications, Inc., 1974.

Whitaker, Julian M.D. *Dr. Whitaker's Guide to Natural Healing.* Rocklin, CA: Prima Publishing, 1995.

Whitaker, Julian, M.D. *DHEA helps regulate the immune system.* Health and Healing, September, Vol. 8, No. 9, 1998.

Wild, Russell, ed. *The Complete Book of Natural and Medicinal Cures.* Emmaus, PA: Rodale Press, 1994.

Wilson, Helen E., and White, Ann. *Prohormone: Their Clinical Relevance.* Trends in Endocrinology and Metabolism, Vol. 9, pgs. 396-402, 1998.

Golden, G.A. et al. *Rapid and Opposite Effects of Cortisol and Estradiol on Human Erythrocyte Na+, K+-ATPase Activity: Relationship to Steroid Intercalation Into The Cell Membrane.* Life Science, Vol. 65, No.12, pgs. 1247-55, 1999.

Wood, D. & J. *The Incredible Healing Needles.* New York: Samuel Weiser Inc., 1974.

Wood, Ian. *Pro-Inflammatory Mechanisms of a Nonsteroidal Anti-Inflammatory Drug.* Trends in Endocrinology, March, Vol. 13, No. 2, 2002.

Wood, Ian, et al. *Natural Hormone Replacement.* California: Smart Publications, 1997.

Wood, Ian, et al. *The Patient's Book of Natural Healing.* California: Prima Health, 1999.

Wright, Jonathan V., M.D., et al. *Natural Hormone Replacement for Women Over 45.* Petaluma, CA: Smart Publications, 1997.

Wright, Jonathan V., M.D. and Gaby, Alan, M.D. *Nutritional Therapy in Medical Practice.* Doubletree Seattle Airport Hotel, October 16-19.

Yen, SS, and Laughlin, GA. *Aging and the Adrenal Cortex.* Exp. Gerontol, Nov-Dec, Vol. 33, No. 7-8, 1998.

Youl, Kang H., et al. *Effects of Ginseng Ingestion on Growth Hormone, Testosterone, Cortisol, and Insulin-Like Growth Factor I Responses to Acute Resistance Exercise.* J Strength Cond Res, May, Vol. 16, No. 2, 2002.

Zachrisson, I., et al. *Determinants of Growth in Diabetic Pubertal Subjects.* Diabetes Care, August, Vol. 20, No. 8, 1997.

Zager, PG, et al. *Distribution of 18-hydroxycorticosterone between red blood cells and plasma.* J Clin Endocrinology Metab, January, Vol. 62, pgs 84-89, 1986.

Zborowski, Jeanne V., et. al. *Bone Mineral Density, Androgens, and the Polycystic Ovary: The Complex and Controversial Issue of Androgenic Influence in the Female Bone.* Vol. 85, No. 10, pgs 3496-3506, 2000.

INDEX

About the Author

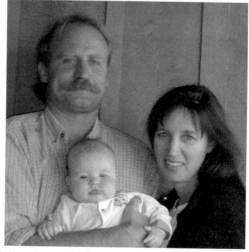

William B. Ferril, M.D. has a bachelor of science in biochemistry and received his doctorate in medicine at UC Davis, California. He completed his postgraduate education at Sacred Heart Medical Center in Spokane, Washington.

Most of the past seventeen years, he practiced in Montana on the Flathead Indian Reservation where he gained experience on the topics in this book. He works with chiropractors, naturopaths, acupuncturist, and homeopaths. Two of his special interests are herbal and organic farming.

His wife, Brenda, received her doctorate at Western States Chiropractic College in Portland, Oregon. They live with their son, Conner, in western Montana.

COMING SOON

Dancing on Tears by G. S. Wilcox

Has your father ever wished you dead?

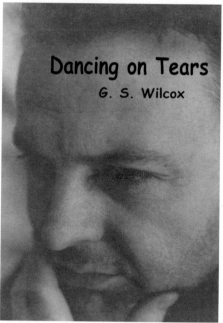

The nineteen-year old held the baby at arm's length - the child, his nemesis. He didn't want the child. He only wanted his wife, Hanna. Baby Katherine represents Lowell Marshall's worst fears--alienation from his wife, responsibility, and emotional commitment--poverty. He is forced through experiences of love and passion to evaluate why he is so fearful of the child. Why is he driven by the ghosts of his past?

Through years of agony and torture, Kate's fear, anger, and hatred of herself are directed toward him. She challenges his very soul at every turn. Strength and weakness impel them. He drives her away.

In his cleared vision, he sees he has created his own worst enemy, a child in his own image. He is shocked to see the extent of the damage he has done. Through the events that unfold, he realizes there are only two things one can share, passion and fear.

Age sixty-seven, Dr. Marshall is in a coma, Kate by his side. Together they transcend the boundaries of time and space and share the triumph of their relationship--transformation from anger and hate to love and passion for life.

Together father and daughter begin a communication of heart and spirit that is magical. Together they travel as one and share an intimate relationship of perception, revelation, and acceptance.

As Kate talks to her dad, there is a knowing for both of them that these inspired moments are the last they will ever share. With the acceptance comes immortality.

Dancing on Tears is a love story between a father and daughter, between parents and children of all ages. It is a story about life that touches the soul and heals the wounds of the heart.

From The Bridge Medical Publisher

Let your patients discover how *alternative medicine* provides affordable, effective, and healing treatment. This book also reveals how the business of mainstream medicine results in expensive, symptom control treatment.

Name   : _____.
Address: _____.
City: _____State: ____Zip: _____.
Phone :_____.

Quantity: _____ . X $50. US
per book =
Price   : _____.
Shipping: _____$7. 00 per book
Total   : _____.

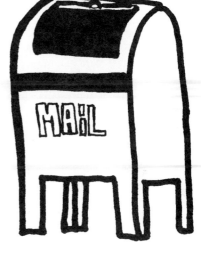

We accept credit cards, checks, or
money orders

The Bridge Medical Publisher,
200½ Wisconsin Ave.
Whitefish, MT 59937

(406) 863-9906 www.thebodyheals.com   **info@thebodyheals.com**